CURRENT REVIEW OF
ASTHMA

CURRENT REVIEW OF
ASTHMA

Edited by

MICHAEL A. KALINER, MD

Professor
Department of Medicine
George Washington University School of Medicine
Washington, DC
Medical Director
Institute for Asthma and Allergy
Wheaton, Maryland
Chevy Chase, Maryland

With 37 contributors

CM
CURRENT
MEDICINE

Current Medicine, Inc., Philadelphia

BS

Current Medicine, Inc.

400 Market Street
Suite 700
Philadelphia, PA 19106

Developmental Editor .... *Teresa M. Giuliana*
Commissioning Supervisor .... *Annmarie D'Ortona*
Illustrator .... *Wieslawa Langenfeld, Maureen Looney*
Cover Design.. *William C. Whitman, Jr.*
Design and Layout .... *Christine Keller-Quirk, Bill MacAdams*
Indexing .... *Prottsman Indexing Services, Inc.*
Production .... *Margaret La Mare*

Current review of asthma / edited by Michael A. Kaliner; with 25 contributors.
   p. ; cm.
  Includes bibliographical references and index.
  ISBN 1-57340-195-1 (hard cover : alk. paper)
   1. Asthma. I. Title: Asthma. II. Kaliner, Michael A.
  [DNLM: 1. Asthma. WF 553 C9758 2003]
  RC591 .C87 2003
  616.2′38--dc21

2002031071

ISBN 1-57340-195-1
ISSN 1542-1007

Printed in the United States by IPC.
5 4 3 2 1

8/27/04

Preface

To conceive of, engineer, and mold an idea into a book requires a huge amount of effort from authors, editors, and publishers. However, to finally sit down and read the book is an amazing feeling, especially when the final product is as good as this one. *Current Review of Asthma* is up-to-date, useful, complete, and worthwhile. It is an excellent resource for those who provide care for asthmatic patients and those interested in state-of-the-art information on asthma. The book joins *Current Review of Allergic Diseases* and *Current Review of Rhinitis*, a series characterized by its timeliness, clinical slant, and practical usefulness.

Asthma is such an important disease that a relevant work like this one will have a broad appeal. The chapters on epidemiology, pathology, airway remodeling, and pathophysiology are concise and provide in-depth information about the disease and how treatment might influence these processes. Discussions on concomitant diseases such as allergy, sinusitis, rhinitis, gastroesophageal reflux, and bronchitis are critical for the successful management of asthma. Each of these chapters is worth careful reading.

The core of the book is the focus on treatment. Each of the modalities available today is reviewed in detail. Corticosteroids, leukotriene modifiers, bronchodilators, anti-IgE, and other treatment choices are summarized in a useful fashion. Because much of the advance in asthma therapy has been based upon guidelines created by the National Heart, Lung, and Blood Institute, several chapters are devoted to the guidelines and their application to currently available treatment choices. These are insightful and important chapters. Finally, there is a chapter I have always wanted to write on pearls gleaned from 30 years of asthma treatment, which might be of interest to some readers.

Current Review of Asthma is the most timely book possible. The contributors, well-known scientists and clinicians, were asked to aim their chapters at practitioners who wanted to know everything clinically relevant about asthma. Sections of this book will prove invaluable both to the practitioner who cares for asthma as only a part of his practice as well as the asthma specialist.

An editor is never certain what can come from a book. Ideally, a book focused on asthma could influence asthma treatment and both save lives and make asthma management more effective. For the sake of the millions of asthmatic patients, it is my hope that the *Current Review of Asthma* will be successful in helping clinicians manage this important disease.

Michael A. Kaliner, MD
Chevy Chase, Maryland

Contributors

Peter J. Barnes, DM, DSc, FRCP

Professor and Head
Department of Thoracic Medicine
National Heart and Lung Institute
Imperial College
Royal Brompton Hospital
London, England

Thomas Bell, MD

Former Director of Montana
    Medical Research, LLC
Missoula, Montana
Former Assistant Director of the
    National Asthma Center
Denver, Colorado
Current Consultant in Informatics
    for Allergy and Asthma

Joseph T. Belleau, MD

Fellow
Department of Allergy and Immunology
University of Tennessee, Memphis
Memphis, Tennessee

Michael S. Blaiss, MD

Clinical Professor
Departments of Pediatrics and Medicine
University of Tennessee, Memphis
Memphis, Tennessee

Eugene R. Bleecker, MD

Professor
Department of Internal Medicine
Co-Director, Center for
    Human Genomics
Wake Forest University Health Sciences
Winston-Salem, North Carolina

Homer A. Boushey, MD

Professor
Department of Medicine
University of California, San Francisco
Staff Physician
Moffitt-Long Hospital
San Francisco, California

G. Daniel Brooks, MD

Clinical Fellow
Department of Medicine
Division of Allergy and Immunology
University of Wisconsin School
    of Medicine
Madison, Wisconsin

Robert K. Bush, MD

Professor
Department of Medicine
Division of Allergy and Immunology
University of Wisconsin School
    of Medicine
Chief, Allergy Division
William S. Middleton VA Hospital
Madison, Wisconsin

William J. Calhoun, MD

Associate Professor
Department of Pulmonary, Allergy, and
    Critical Care Medicine
University of Pittsburgh Medical Center
Director, Asthma, Allergy, and Airway
    Research Center
Comprehensive Lung Center
Pittsburgh, Pennsylvania

Thomas B. Casale, MD

Professor
Department of Internal Medicine
Center for Allergy, Asthma,
    and Immunology
Creighton University School of Medicine
Omaha, Nebraska

Lary Ciesemier, DO

Assistant Instructor
Department of Internal Medicine
Center for Allergy, Asthma,
    and Immunology
Creighton University School of Medicine
Omaha, Nebraska

Cori Copilevitz, MD

Fellow
Department of Allergy and Immunology
Saint Louis University School
    of Medicine
Saint Louis, Missouri

Kerry L. Drain, MD

Staff Physician
Spokane Allergy and Asthma Clinic
Spokane, Washington

Athena Economides, MD

Director of Pediatrics
Institute for Allergy and Asthma
Chevy Chase, Maryland

Elizabeth A. Erwin, MD

Fellow
Department of Allergy and Immunology
Asthma and Allergic Diseases Center
University of Virginia Health System
Charlottesville, Virginia

Peter J. Gergen, MD, MPH

Senior Medical Officer
Center for Primary Care and Research
Agency for Healthcare Research
    and Quality
Rockville, Maryland

Nicholas J. Gross, MD, PhD

Professor
Departments of Medicine and
    Molecular Biochemistry
Loyola University Stritch School
    of Medicine
Chicago, Illinois

Elliot Israel, MD

Associate Professor
Department of Pulmonary Medicine
Harvard Medical School
Director, Respiratory Therapy
Director, Clinical Research,
    Pulmonary Department
Harvard Medical School
Boston, Massachusetts

Michael A. Kaliner, MD

Professor
Department of Medicine
George Washington University School
    of Medicine
Washington, DC
Medical Director
Institute for Asthma and Allergy
Wheaton, Maryland
Chevy Chase, Maryland

Esther L. Langmack, MD

Assistant Professor
Department of Medicine
University of Colorado Health
    Sciences Center
National Jewish Medical and
    Research Center
Denver, Colorado

James T. C. Li, MD, PhD

Professor
Department of Medicine
Mayo Medical School
Rochester, Minnesota

Gailen D. Marshall, Jr., MD, PhD

Associate Professor
Department of Internal Medicine
Division of Allergy and Clinical
    Immunology
University of Texas Medical School
Chief, Allergy and Immunology Service
Memorial Hermann Hospital
Houston, Texas

Richard J. Martin, MD

Professor
Department of Medicine
University of Colorado Health
    Sciences Center
National Jewish Medical and
    Research Center
Denver, Colorado

Herman Mitchell, PhD

Adjunct Professor
Department of Biostatistics
University of North Carolina School
    of Public Health
Senior Research Scientist
Rho, Inc.
Chapel Hill, North Carolina

Harold S. Nelson, MD

Professor
Department of Medicine
University of Colorado Health
    Sciences Center
Denver, Colorado

Jennifer Altamura Namazy, MD

Fellow
Scripps Clinic
La Jolla, California

Jill Ohar, MD

Professor
Department of Medicine
Center for Human Genomics
Wake Forest University Health Sciences
Winston-Salem, North Carolina

Thomas A. E. Platts-Mills, MD, PhD

Professor
Department of Medicine
Head, Division of Allergy
    and Immunology
Director, Asthma and Allergic
    Diseases Center
University of Virginia Health System
Charlottesville, Virginia

Jonathan Sadeh, MD

Fellow
Department of Pulmonary and Critical
    Care Medicine
Harvard Medical School
Boston, Massachusetts

Michael Schatz, MD, MS

Clinical Professor
Department of Medicine
University of California San Diego
Chief, Department of Allergy
Kaiser Permanente Medical Center
San Diego, California

Ronald A. Simon, MD

Staff Physician
Scripps Clinic
La Jolla, California

Raymond G. Slavin, MD, MS

Professor
Department of Internal Medicine
Director, Division of Allergy
    and Immunology
Saint Louis University School
    of Medicine
Saint Louis, Missouri

Mark R. Stein, MD

Chief, Allergy Section
Good Samaritan Medical Center
West Palm Beach, Florida
Allergy Associates of the Palm Beaches
North Palm Beach, Florida

Stephen A. Tilles, MD

Clinical Assistant Professor
Department of Medicine
University of Washington School
    of Medicine
Executive Director
ASTHMA, Inc.
Seattle, Washington

Robert G. Townley, MD

Professor
Department of Medicine
Creighton University School of Medicine
Omaha, Nebraska

Rajeev Venkayya, MD

Assistant Professor
Department of Medicine
Division of Pulmonary &
    Critical Care Medicine
University of California, San Francisco
Chief, Severe Asthma Clinic
San Francisco General Hospital
San Francisco, California

Martha V. White, MD

Research Director
Institute for Allergy and Asthma
Wheaton, Maryland

Contents

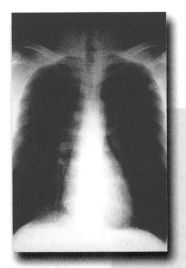

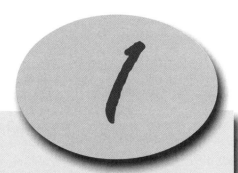

Epidemiology

Peter J. Gergen and Herman Mitchell

This chapter does not represent the policy of the Agency for Healthcare Research and Quality (AHRQ). The views expressed are those of the authors, and no official endorsement by AHRQ is intended or should be inferred.

DEFINITION OF ASTHMA

The epidemiology of asthma may appear confusing and contradictory to casual readers. What we call asthma is probably not a single disease; instead, it is a heterogeneous group of diseases with different etiologies and outcomes. A large part of early-onset wheezing has been found to be attributable to preexisting small airway size [1] or viral infections [2] and does not persist [3••]. Wheezing with onset after the first few years of life tends to be more often associated with atopy and persists to a greater degree than early-onset wheezing [3••]. At present, no reliable means exist to differentiate between these subgroups of asthmatic patients.

Epidemiologic studies have used a number of different definitions of asthma: a reported diagnosis with or without a doctor's confirmation, the report of certain symptoms, the presence of bronchoreactivity in response to a number of tests (*eg*, methacholine, exercise), or any combination of these definitions. In order to study active asthmatic patients, researchers have required that symptoms occur within a defined period of time (usually 12 months) or that the study participants are currently taking asthma medications.

Each of these approaches has its strengths and weaknesses. Using a diagnosis of asthma with or without a physician's confirmation presumes an individual has been correctly evaluated, assigned the diagnostic label, and reported the diagnosis when asked. Studies have shown that a large amount of active asthma is undiagnosed in both children and adults and that similar sets of symptoms may not be assigned the same diagnosis.

The use of symptoms avoids the problem of diagnostic labeling but introduces other problems. Wheeze is the most common symptom of asthma; however, not all asthmatic patients wheeze. A cough variant asthma has been reported among children in whom the predominant feature is cough that responds to bronchodilator therapy [4]. Bronchoreactivity as measured by response to exercise or histamine has been proposed as a gold standard for asthma. Population studies, however, have shown that this measure does not have a high degree of sensitivity and specificity. In one school-based study of 7- to 10-year-old children in New Zealand, 41% of the children with bronchoreactivity had no current asthma symptoms, and 42% of children with the diagnosis of asthma and current symptoms did not have bronchoreactivity [5].

BURDEN OF ASTHMA

With the recognition of its increasing prevalence, the monitoring of asthma in the United States population has received considerable attention over the past several decades. A number of nationally representative surveys and datasets offer the clearest picture of the changing burden of asthma among the United States population.

The prevalence of asthma in the United States is tracked using the National Health Interview Survey (NHIS). In 1996, there were estimated to be 14.6 million asthmatic patients in the United States, with 4.4 million younger than 18 years of age using a 12-month prevalence measure [6]. In 1997, the NHIS changed the asthma portion of the survey to identify a lifetime prevalence of asthma and a 12-month prevalence of asthma attacks. In 1997, the NHIS reported 26.7 million people with a lifetime prevalence of asthma and 11.1 million with asthma attacks in the past 12 months. The 1999, the NHIS found 10.5 million persons reporting an asthma attack in the preceding 12 months. No information on the lifetime prevalence of asthma from the 1999 survey has been released yet [7•].

Most childhood asthma begins before 5 years of age. A review of medical records of the Mayo Clinic found the highest incidence of asthma occurred in the first year of life, with incidence rates decreasing throughout childhood and reaching their lowest levels among adults [8]. During the life cycle, the incidence of asthma for men versus women changes. Before puberty, boys have a higher incidence of asthma than girls. The rates equalize during puberty, and women have a higher incidence rate of asthma after puberty [9•].

Asthma prevalence is found to vary with race or ethnicity and urbanity. In national surveys, blacks reported higher rates of asthma than whites [7•]. Hispanics reported wide discrepancies in prevalence; Mexican American children in the Southwest reported some of the lowest rates of asthma in the United States, but Puerto Rican children living on the East Coast of the United States reported some of the highest rates [10]. Other studies [11] suggest that the racial differences may reflect, at least in part, diagnostic acquisition rather than true differences in disease prevalence. A survey of 9- to 11-year-old children in Philadelphia found white and black children reported the same prevalence of persistent wheeze. But among the children with wheeze, the black children were more likely to have received the diagnosis of asthma [12].

Based on data from the NHIS, the self-reported prevalence of asthma increased 73.9% between 1980 and 1996. During the period of 1997 to 1999, the most recent data using the redesigned asthma questions, reported asthma attacks in the previous 12 months decreased for both whites (40.5 to 37.6 per 1000) and blacks (45.4 to 42.7 per 1000), which may reflect better asthma control but not necessarily a reduction in asthma prevalence [7•].

International prevalence comparisons are hard to make because of differences in definitions, data collection, and cultural understandings of asthma and wheeze. An international effort during the 1990s, the International Study of Asthma and Allergies in Childhood (ISAAC), developed a simple asthma questionnaire with which investigators around the world were encouraged to survey 6- to 7- and 13- to 14-year-old children at schools in their cities. The investigators were allowed to translate the questionnaire into their local language. The reported asthma and wheeze prevalences from 56 countries revealed a 15-fold range in the prevalence. Asthma and wheeze were highest in the developed world. Australia and New Zealand had the highest levels. North America was second followed by Western Europe and South America [13].

Asthma can have a significant impact on an individual's life. In 1994 to 1996, an estimated 14 million school days were lost as a result of asthma among children 5 to 17 years of age. Among this age group, 23.6% of the children with asthma reported some activity limitation as a result of their asthma. During this same time period among adults, 14.5 million workdays were lost as a result of asthma, and 14.6% of the adults with asthma reported some activity limitation as a result of their asthma [7•].

Data on asthma utilization patterns in the United States are available from two national surveys: the National Hospital Discharge Survey and the National Health Care Survey. In 1999, approximately 478,000 asthma hospitalizations were recorded. Rates were highest among children, with approximately 39% of all asthma hospitalizations occurring in patients younger than 15 years of age. However, there is a second lower peak of asthma hospitalizations in persons 65 years of age and older [14]. Hospitalization rates are elevated in urban areas with high levels of poverty or minority populations [15]. Readmissions can account for up to 20% of hospitalizations, and the readmission rate is higher in the younger age group [16].

Asthma hospitalization rates increased during the 1980s until they stabilized at a rate of approximately 19.5 per 10,000 population. The rate of asthma hospitalization remained around 19.5 per 10,000 population from 1985 through 1995, and then the rate began to decrease. In 1999, the asthma hospitalization rate had decreased to 17.6 per 10,000 population [7•]. The length of stay for an asthma hospitalization has also decreased in recent years.

In contrast to hospitalizations, the number of emergency room visits for asthma continue to increase. During 1999, there were approximately 2 million asthma-related emergency room visits. This represented a 26% increase since 1992 [17]. Emergency room visit rates are highest in minorities and young children [7•].

Visits to private doctors' offices for asthma show a somewhat different picture. During 1999, there were approximately 9.5 million visits for asthma [18]. This level has remained relatively constant since the early 1990s, when the reported increase in ambulatory care visits during the 1980s leveled off [19].

Asthma mortality is of great interest because deaths from the disorder are believed to be preventable. During 1999, 4657 deaths were attributed to asthma in the United States [20]. In contrast to hospitalizations, asthma mortality primarily affects adults, with approximately 78% occurring at or after 45 years of age. The ratio of black to white mortality has increased from 2 in 1979 to 2.6 in 1998 [20]. The United States asthma mortality rate of approximately two deaths per 100,000 population is low compared with rates up to seven to nine deaths per 100,000 population in other parts of the world; the highest rates are noted in New Zealand, West Germany, and Norway [21].

When deaths in the United States were classified under the International Classification of Disease (ICD)-9 coding system, asthma mortality between 1979 and 1998 increased from 2598 deaths (age-adjusted rate of 1.3 per 100,000 population) to 5438 (age-adjusted rate of 2.0 per 100,000 population) [20]. The United States reached an asthma mortality rate of two per 100,000 population in the period between 1987 and 1989. The rate has remained stable since then. Because of increasing population in the United States, the number of asthma deaths continued to increase until 1994, when the number stabilized at approximately 5500. In 1999, the United States adopted the ICD-10 to classify mortality, and asthma mortality decreased from 5438 in 1998 to 4657 in 1999. A large portion of this decrease can be attributed to coding changes in ICD-10, which result in fewer deaths being assigned an underlying cause of asthma.

Reviewing the previous sections on the burden of asthma, one might easily conclude that the severity of asthma has increased at least through the early to mid 1990s and has reached a plateau or even possibly begun to decrease. However, asthma mortality and health care use are as much a reflection of asthma control as is intrinsic severity. Asthma control reflects the access to appropriate health care, the use of medications, and environmental controls. Data from a number of sources imply that asthma severity has not increased despite the rising prevalence. Repeat surveys in 1991 and 1999 using the ISAAC questionnaire among 8- to 9-year-old students in Sheffield, England found an increase in the reported prevalence of current asthma 10.3% to 13.0%. When looking at the changes in reported wheezing frequency in the previous 12 months, the increase was confined to children who reported one to three attacks per year, but no increase was seen in the group reporting more than three attacks per year. Thus, the data suggest that the

increase in prevalence was confined to the milder group of asthmatic patients [22••]. Data from the United States, as reported in the NHIS, indicate that although the total school absences attributed to asthma increased from 6.6 million in 1980 to 1982 to 14 million in 1994 to 1996, the school absence days per child asthma year decreased from 4.9 to 3.7. Similar conclusions can be drawn when examining activity limitation caused by asthma; for children ages 5 to 17 years, the prevalence decreased from 27.2% to 23.6% during this same time period. For adults, the prevalence of limitation of activity remained stable during this time at approximately 14% [7•].

It appears that the burden of asthma in the United States is undergoing a change, with some data sources indicating a leveling off of the increase and others showing actual decreasing trends in some of the measures of asthma. Only in the coming years, with the availability of additional data, will it be come clearer whether or not the burden of asthma is actually decreasing in the United States.

NATURAL HISTORY

Wheeze is a common symptom among children in their early years. For some children, this symptom may indicate asthma that may well continue throughout their lives. However, many children (50% to 60%) who wheeze during their first few years of life will not continue to wheeze after 6 years of age [3••,23]. Children whose wheezing begins after the first few years of life tend to have a higher probability of developing other manifestations of atopy (*eg*, skin test reactivity) and have bronchial hyperresponsiveness than children whose wheezing starts in the first several years of life [24,25].

Despite the many variations in study design, changes in asthma definition, and the age of initial assessment, there is a surprising agreement regarding the general level of asthma remission. Even in studies with cohorts that began in the 1930s, it appears that approximately 50% of children with asthma are no longer symptomatic as adults [26,27]. A variety of factors have been associated with the persistence of asthma, including early onset, severity, coexisting atopy such as eczema, allergic rhinitis, family history of atopy, and lower pulmonary function test results [24,28,29].

However, this remission in asthma may not be permanent. Carefully designed prospective studies have shown that asthma symptoms frequently disappear during adolescence only to return in adulthood [30]. Even during adulthood, asthma can remit, although at a lower frequency than during childhood [31]. Adults with asthma have been found to have a faster decline in pulmonary functions such as FEV_1 (forced expiratory volume in 1 second) compared with patients without asthma [32]. Some patients who continue to show symptoms of asthma throughout their lives will have irreversible lung function impairment with airway remodeling [25]. There is speculation that early and appropriate treatment with inhaled steroids prevents this permanent airway remodeling. Further studies are needed to clarify this issue.

SEASONALITY

Asthma has been shown to have a strong seasonal component that appears to vary by the age group and outcome measured. Asthma symptoms, hospitalizations, and emergency room visits are highest in the autumn and winter and are lowest in the summer, especially in younger individuals [33,34]. In the United States, asthma mortality appears to be highest during the winter months for individuals older than 65 years of age; for individuals younger than 35 years of age, asthma mortality appears to be higher during the summer [35].

GENETICS VERSUS THE ENVIRONMENT

Genetics play an important role in asthma. For many years, it has been reported that individuals with asthma have a higher probability of having a parent or sibling with asthma than those without asthma. The risk of asthma in children increases as the number of parents with asthma increases, up to a sixfold increase if both parents have asthma. A parental history of asthma compared with other allergic diseases is more predictive of development of asthma in their children. Maternal factors seem more important than paternal, at least through 5 years of age [36].

The search for genes associated with asthma is underway, and a variety of candidate genes have been identified. To date, a number of interesting findings have come to light. Genetic polymorphism appears to play a role in response to treatment (*eg*, certain polymorphisms on the β_2-adrenergic receptor have been associated with poor responses to regular inhaled β-agonist treatment) [37••]. Different characteristics of the asthmatic state may have a different genetic basis, such as IgE (immunoglobulin E) and airway responsiveness [38].

Twin studies have long been used to determine the relative importance of environment and heredity on disease development. The reported heritability estimate of asthma has ranged from 35.6% [39] to 75% [40]. However, a preliminary report [41] indicates that the presence of asthma in the adoptive parents was a risk factor for asthma development among their adoptive children, implying that the home environment was an important factor in the development of asthma.

Other evidence for the role of the environment on the development of asthma comes from studying migrant populations, which allows comparisons of the development of asthma between two relatively homogenous groups of individuals living in different environments. For example, a study of children living on Tokelau, an island in the Pacific Ocean, and children of Tokelau ori-

gin living in New Zealand found that the Tokelaun children living in New Zealand had about double the prevalence of asthma as the Tokelaun children living in Tokelau [42]. This was true even when the children were new immigrants to New Zealand.

RISK FACTORS FOR ASTHMA
Allergy

In the 1940s, Rackemann [43] suggested there were at least two distinct subgroups: extrinsic asthmatic patients who tend to start earlier in life (before 30 years of age) and have other associated allergic manifestations, and intrinsic asthmatic patients who tend to have onset of their disease later in life (after 40 years of age) and do not have associated allergic manifestations. Burrows *et al.* [44] reported that asthma at all ages is related to IgE. Other forms of atopy, such as infantile eczema and hay fever, have also been associated with asthma.

Sensitivity to indoor allergens, such as dust mites, cats, cockroaches, and alternaria, consistently has been related to both the presence of asthma and asthma severity [45–48]. Outdoor allergens seem to play a more limited role [49].

The role that early exposure to allergen plays in the development of asthma is unclear. A longitudinal study [50] of English children up to 11 years of age found increased levels of house dust mites to be associated with the development of asthma. In another larger longitudinal study [51••], early exposure to indoor allergens was not associated with the development of asthma at 7 years of age. Other data regarding early exposure to high levels of cat allergen have reported the development of tolerance instead of sensitization [52••].

Environmental Factors

AIR POLLUTION
Air pollutants have been extensively studied with regard to asthma. Air pollutants such as SO_2, NO_2, particulates, ozone, and acid aerosols have been found to be associated with changes in asthma morbidity such as increases in doctor and emergency room visits, peak flow changes, and hospitalizations [53,54]. Exercising at times of high ozone levels is correlated with the development of asthma [55]. Changing traffic patterns have also been associated with changing asthma symptoms. A study that monitored acute asthma episodes among Medicaid recipients found a decrease in the rate of attacks during the Atlanta Summer Olympics, which the authors correlated with decreased commuter traffic and ozone levels associated with Olympics-related driving restrictions [56]. Although specific pollutants have been studied in isolation, air pollution usually is not caused by a single agent, and the interaction of these pollutants has been shown to be important in asthma.

A unique insight into the role of air pollution in asthma can be gained at looking at the comparison of East and West Germany before reunification. East Germany had higher levels of diesel exposure, SO_2, and particulate than West Germany, yet it had lower levels of asthma and allergen skin test reactivity [57]. More recent data from former East Germany found that as SO_2 and total suspended particles decreased, the reported rates of cough and irritation of the airways decreased but asthma and wheeze remained unchanged [58].

ENVIRONMENTAL TOBACCO SMOKE

Exposure to environmental tobacco smoke (ETS) is associated with an approximate doubling of the prevalence of asthma [59]. ETS exposure also plays a role in the severity of asthma. Reduced pulmonary function and more reported acute exacerbations were found to be related to ETS exposure among asthmatic patients attending an allergy clinic [60]. However, the data are less clear for the role of ETS as a trigger of asthma attacks. Studies that have looked at the changes in ETS exposure did not find corresponding changes in acute attacks of asthma [61].

With regard to the development of asthma, less consistent results have been found. In Arizona, ETS exposure was only associated with the development of asthma if mothers had less than 12 years of education but not among the children of more highly educated women [62]. In Canada, only children with atopic dermatitis exposed to ETS developed asthma, but others exposed to ETS did not [63]. Longitudinal studies conducted in New Zealand and Norway have not found ETS to be associated with the development of asthma [64,65]. Because childhood asthma is an allergic disease, one would expect that if ETS were responsible for the development of asthma, ETS should also increase the atopic status of individuals. In a cohort study from birth to age 6 years, exposure to maternal smoking increased the risk of asthma but not the risk of allergen skin test reactivity [66].

What role does ETS play in asthma? ETS appears to sensitize preexisting asthmatic patients to other triggers of asthma attacks rather than causing the development of new asthma [67]. Asthmatic patients "sensitized" by exposure to ETS experience more wheezing than nonsensitized asthmatic patients. This increase in wheezing would increase the chances that an undiagnosed asthmatic would be diagnosed and increase the perceived severity of all asthma.

Infections

Respiratory infections have been recognized as one of the most important triggers for asthma attacks in both children and adults [68,69]. Untreated infections of the respiratory tract such as sinusitis can make asthma more difficult to control. Recent studies, however, have shown that infections early in life may help focus the immune system and be protective for later asthma development. This protective effect of early infection is commonly referred to as the hygiene theory and is covered in a later section.

Birthweight

Low birthweight has been associated with the development of asthma early in life through the period of adolescence [70,71]. Low birthweight is not associated with an increase in allergen skin test reactivity later in life [70,71]. Although the association between low birthweight and asthma may be the consequence of residual abnormality in pulmonary structure or function in low birthweight infants, a 7-year longitudinal study found the development of asthma among children born at less than 1500 grams was independent of perinatal factors such as respiratory morbidity [72].

Obesity

Obesity has been related cross-sectionally to an increase in asthma prevalence, symptoms, medication use, and health care use [73–75]. Longitudinal studies have reported that the development of obesity is associate with an increased risk for developing asthma [76] and that weight loss improves pulmonary function and asthma symptoms [77].

Further evidence has clarified the role that obesity plays in asthma. Obesity has been found neither to be related to airway hyperreactivity [75] nor allergen skin test reactivity [73,74]. Thus, the mechanism through which obesity impacts on asthma appears to be mechanical rather than allergic. Further work has found that obesity, regardless of its mechanism of action, is not responsible for the recent trends in asthma [78].

Psychologic Factors

The early contributions of psychologists to our understanding of asthma focused on the notion of an "asthmatic personality" and the role of "emotions" as a precipitating factor in asthma exacerbations. Although this early research direction has proven to be of limited value, the relationship of psychologic adjustment to asthma morbidity has been shown to be quite important. Children with asthma are more likely to have psychologic problems and difficulties of social adjustment [79]. Similarly, measures of the psychologic status of parents have also been related to asthma symptoms of their children [80]. Depression among the parents of children with asthma has been shown to be associated with their child's asthma severity [81] and leads to more visits for emergency asthma treatment [82••]. Adherence failure is suggested as a major pathway by which these factors influence asthma morbidity [80] because increased psychologic difficulties may interfere with adherence to medical care plans and the consistency of filling prescriptions and keeping physician appointments. Although psychologic dysfunction may increase the severity of asthma, it is also likely that a child's asthma severity contributes to the caretaker's psychologic difficulties. In a longitudinal study design, Weil *et al.* [83••] have shown that psychologic adjustment influences subsequent asthma morbidity as well as being a result of the asthma severity itself.

More recently, the emerging area of psychoneuroimmunology has changed the focus of psychologic factors from their role as potential correlates, or causes, of asthma symptoms to their impact as mediators of the complex immune response to inflammation [84]. Especially relevant to asthma is the early work in this area that revealed an interesting impact of stress on viral disease [85], with college students having more respiratory infections during stressful examination periods. Given the clear relationship between asthma and viral infection [4,68], these studies are especially relevant to asthma. This link between stressors and asthma exacerbation has been supported and expanded by more recent work [86]. Stress, such as specific negative and stressful life events [87] as well as general measures of perceived stress [88], has now been clearly related to asthma exacerbation and severity. The complex nature of the interaction of stressors and immunology is an active area of recent research in both human and animal models [89–91].

Diet

Studies examining the effect of breastfeeding on the development of asthma have reported conflicting results, but a recent meta-analysis concluded that breastfeeding was generally protective against the development of asthma [92]. In addition, specific dietary components have been studied. Antioxidants (*eg*, vitamins C and E) in the diet have been inversely associated with bronchial reactivity, wheezing, and allergen skin test reactivity [93]. Other research has suggested that sodium in the diet contributes to bronchial reactivity [94].

Weather Conditions

Certain weather conditions such as low humidity and low temperature have been shown to be associated with increased use of emergency room visits and hospitalizations for asthma [95]. Asthma outbreaks have been associated with thunderstorms, possibly because of the increased levels of allergens put into the air by the weather disturbances [96].

TRENDS IN RISK FACTORS

The changing epidemiology of asthma provides the opportunity to compare the changes in the reported asthma risk factors to determine the role they are playing. Data are available on a number of the asthma risk factors during the period of the observed increase in asthma. Outdoor air pollution does not appear to play an important role in the increase in asthma in the United States because pollutant levels have been decreasing during the time of the increase. Between 1987 and 1996, the ambient concentrations of a number of pollutants decreased: nitrogen dioxide by 10%, ozone by 15%, and sulfur dioxide by 37%. Between 1988 and 1996, ambient particulate matter (PM10) decreased by 25% [97]. Similarly, cigarette smoking does not appear

to be driving the increase in asthma in the United States because cigarette smoking has been decreasing during the time of the well-documented asthma increase. Between 1965 and 1998, the percent of active smokers dropped from 41.9% to 24.0% among individuals 18 years of age and older [98]. There is little information regarding temporal trends in allergen levels. A longitudinal study [50] that reported that exposure to house dust mites was associated with the development of asthma found no change in the household levels of mites over the 10-year period of the study. Additionally, breastfeeding has remained stable in the United States since the early 1980s. In 1981 to 1983, the National Survey of Family Growth reported that 58.1% of babies in the United States were breastfed, although it fluctuated a few percentage points during the intervening years. From 1993 and 1994, the percent was still 58.1% [98]. Attendance at organized daycare, which is associated with an increased exposure to viral infections—an important trigger of asthma attacks—has increased for children of working mothers from 13% in 1977 to 29.4% in 1994 [99]. Changing family size has been discounted as an important contributor to the change in asthma [100].

POVERTY AND HEALTH CARE

Poverty and minority status are consistently reported to be related to increased asthma morbidity and mortality [7•]. There is no evidence that asthma is intrinsically a different disease among the various racial and ethnic groups in the United States. However, is asthma more prevalent in poor communities? Although asthma prevalence rates have been reported to be very high in poor urban areas, with a high percentage of minority residents [101], equally high rates have been reported in less urban areas with low levels of poverty and minority residents [102].

The observed variation in health care use related to asthma may more accurately reflect differences in the control of asthma rather than true differences in asthma prevalence. Access to and receipt of appropriate care can make a substantial difference in the type and amount of health care used by an individual with asthma. For example, variation in hospital rates for asthma among three cities in the United States was found to be related to the quality of primary care received [103], but almost 80% of visits for asthma to the emergency room were found to be potentially preventable with better self-management training [104].

The impact of appropriate treatment has been demonstrated in a number of studies. Use of inhaled steroids was associated with a decrease in hospitalizations [105], and treating coexisting allergic rhinitis in patients with asthma appears to be related to a decrease in asthma emergency room visits [106]. As expected, studies that compared specialty care with primary care have reported better outcomes for asthma patients treated by the specialists [107]. When examined in detail, the important difference between specialists and primary care physicians appears to be a greater emphasis on asthma education; the use of inhaled steroids; and the use of ancillary devices such as spacers and peak flow meters among the specialists. Because the majority of asthma care in the United States is provided by primary caregivers, more emphasis must be paid to train primary care doctors to properly treat patients with asthma.

Although the majority of poor and inner-city children have access to care through Medicaid and similar programs, more than 50% of these families have reported significant difficulty in actually getting medications, making appointments, and getting to their physician's office or clinic [108]. Even if a child has access to a private physician's office for asthma care, he or she may receive differing care based on income, race, or ethnicity [109]. The quality of asthma care received by poor and minority individuals is clearly inadequate, especially with regard to medication usage.

PREVENTION OF ASTHMA

Primary prevention is the prevention of disease development. A number of different strategies have been attempted to achieve primary prevention of asthma. One controlled trial [110] tested the effect of eliminating certain food allergens, and another [111] combined food allergen avoidance with dust mite reduction efforts. Neither study was successful in preventing the development of asthma in the first 4 to 7 years of life. More promising results have been found in clinical trials dealing with the treatment of patients with hay fever. Clinical trials looking at the treatment of hay fever with immunotherapy [112••] or cetirizine [113] have found that children who received the respective therapies developed asthma at a lower rate than children in the control group who did not receive treatment.

Secondary prevention deals with the amelioration of symptoms after a disease has developed. Secondary prevention has proved to be more doable than primary prevention in patients with asthma. Beneficial types of secondary prevention include providing specialty care [107], training clinic staff to follow asthma treatment guidelines [114], and providing nurse case managers [115] to empower patients to be better self-managers and advocates [116]. It is clear from these studies that there are many different points along the patient–provider continuum where one might successfully intervene. No one intervention is optimal for all situations. The choice of an intervention should be based on the population served, the existing medical system, and the availability of resources.

IS ASTHMA A DISEASE OF MODERN CIVILIZATION?

The observation that early exposure to infection may be protective of subsequent asthma development, the hygiene hypothesis, has received considerable recent attention. This hypothesis attempts to explain the recent asthma trends and international differences in asthma by a change in exposure to infectious agents. The hygiene hypothesis was first proposed by Strachan [117] to explain the decreased prevalence of hay fever in later-born children in large families. As first proposed, earlier exposure to infectious agents brought into the home by older siblings was thought to be protective against the development of asthma and other forms of atopy. Further studies of this phenomenon have examined other organisms thought to play a protective role in the development of asthma [118••]. Suspected agents have included measles, tuberculosis, and vaccinations such as diphtheria-tetanus-pertussis and bacillus Calmette-Guérin; however, all of these have been found by further studies to not play roles in the development of asthma [119–121].

More recent work has moved from respiratory infections to focus on the impact of gut floral and orofecal-type infections (*eg*, hepatitis A, toxoplasmosis) [122] influencing the development of asthma and allergy. Another developing avenue is the observation that growing up on a farm is protective against the development of asthma and atopy. Early exposure to endotoxins or infectious agents has been speculated to play a role in this phenomena [123].

Future asthma research must focus on identifying individuals who are susceptible to the development of asthma and environmental factors that convert this susceptibility to a reality. Questionnaire-based assessments of asthma may be of limited value in making this determination. Yet unmade discoveries in the genetics of asthma or atopy may give us this ability. Additionally, it is a major challenge for asthma research to disentangle true etiologic factors from the mere correlates of the disease. This will only be accomplished by a greater emphasis on longitudinal studies and controlled, randomized clinical trials rather than the more common cross-sectional approach that dominates the field. Only by using such methodologies that permit causal determinations will we be able to understand the importance of specific risk factors in the development and continuation of asthma.

REFERENCES AND RECOMMENDED READING

Papers of particular interest, published recently, have been highlighted as:
• 　*Of importance*
•• 　*Of major importance*

1.　Tager IB, Hanrahan JP, Tosteson TD, *et al.*: Lung function, pre- and post-natal smoke exposure, and wheezing in the first year of life. *Am Rev Respir Dis* 1993, 147:811–817.

2.　Duff AL, Pomeranz ES, Gelber LE, *et al.*: Risk factors for acute wheezing in infants and children: viruses, passive smoke, and IgE antibodies to inhalant allergens. *Pediatrics* 1993, 92:535–540.

3.•• Martinez FD, Wright AL, Taussig LM, *et al.*: Asthma and wheezing in the first six years of life: the Group Health Medical Associates. *N Engl J Med* 1995, 332:133–138.
A prospective study looking at wheezing in the first 6 years of life.

4. Johnson D, Osborn LM: Cough variant asthma: a review of the clinical literature. *J Asthma* 1991, 28:85–90.

5. Pattemore PK, Asher MI, Harrison AC, *et al.*: The interrelationship among bronchial hyperresponsiveness, the diagnosis of asthma, and asthma symptoms. *Am Rev Respir Dis* 1990, 142:549–554.

6. Adams PF, Hendershot GE, Marano MA: Current estimates for the National Health Interview Survey, 1996. National Center for Health Statistics. *Vital Health Stat* 1999, 10.

7.• Mannino D, Homa D, Akinbami LJ, *et al.*: Surveillance for asthma: United States, 1980–1999. *MMWR* 2002, 51:1–14.
The latest CDC asthma surveillance report indicating that the rise in asthma exacerbations may be leveling off or even decreasing, suggesting a positive impact of new asthma treatments and interventions.

8. Yunginger JW, Reed CE, O'Connell EJ, *et al.*: A community-based study of the epidemiology of asthma I. Incidence rates, 1964–84. *Am Rev Respir Dis* 1992, 146:888–894.

9.• de Marco R, Locatelli F, Sunyer J, Burney P: Differences in incidence of reported asthma related to age in men and women: a retrospective analysis of the data of the European Respiratory Health Survey. *Am J Respir Crit Care Med* 2000, 162:68–74.
Data indicating that the incidence of asthma was higher in males during childhood, during puberty the incidence in both sexes was similar, while after puberty the incidence was higher in women.

10. Carter-Pokras OD, Gergen PJ: Reported asthma among Puerto Rican, Mexican-American, and Cuban children, 1982 through 1984. *Am J Public Health* 1993, 83:580–582.

11. Roberts EM: Racial and ethnic disparities in childhood asthma diagnosis: the role of clinical findings. *J Natl Med Assoc* 2002, 94(4):215–223.

12. Cunningham J, Dockery DW, Speizer FE: Race, asthma, and persistent wheeze in Philadelphia schoolchildren. *Am J Public Health* 1996, 86:1406–1409.

13. Worldwide variations in the prevalence of asthma symptoms: the International Study of Asthma and Allergies in Childhood (ISAAC). *Eur Respir J* 1998, 12:315–335.

14. Popovic JR: 1999 National Hospital Discharge Survey: Annual Summary with detailed diagnosis and procedure data. National Center for Health Statistics. *Vital Health Stat* 2001, 12.

15. Gottlieb DJ, Beiser AS, O'Connor GT: Poverty, race, and medication use are correlates of asthma hospitalization rates: a small area analysis in Boston. *Chest* 1995, 108:28–35.

16. Goldring J, Hanrahan L, Anderson H, Remington P: Asthma hospitalizations and readmissions among children and young adults: Wisconsin, 1991–1995. *MMWR* 1997, 46:726–729.

17. Burt CW, McCaig LF: Trends in hospital emergency department utilization: United States, 1992–99. National Center for Health Statistics. *Vital Health Stat* 2001, 13.

18. Cherry DK, Burt CW, Woodwell DA: National Ambulatory Medical Care Survey: 1999 summary: advance data from vital and health statistics, no. 322. Hyattsville, MD: National Center for Health Statistics; 2001.

19. Schappert SM: National Ambulatory Medical Care Survey: 1991 and 1992 summary: advance data from vital and health statistics, nos. 230 and 253. Hyattsville, MD: National Center for Health Statistics; 1994.

20. U.S. Vital Statistics Mortality 1979 through 1999: http://wonder.cdc.gov. Accessed April 15, 2002.

21. Sears MR: Worldwide trends in asthma mortality. *Bull Int Union Tuberc Lung Dis* 1991, 66:79–83.

22.•• Ng Man Kwong G, Proctor A, Billings C, *et al.*: Increasing prevalence of asthma diagnosis and symptoms in children is confined to mild symptoms. *Thorax* 2001, 56:312–314.
A study tracking the trend in asthma prevalence among 8- and 9-year-old children in Sheffield, England between 1991 and 1999.

23. Brooke AM, Lambert PC, Burton PR, *et al.*: The natural history of respiratory symptoms in preschool children. *Am J Respir Crit Care Med* 1995, 152:1872–1878.

24. Rhodes HL, Thomas P, Sporik R, *et al.*: A birth cohort study of subjects at risk of atopy: twenty-two-year follow-up of wheeze and atopic status. *Am J Respir Crit Care Med* 2002, 165:176–180.

25. Reed CE: The natural history of asthma in adults: the problem of irreversibility. *J Allergy Clin Immunol* 1999, 103:539–547.

26. Park ES, Golding J, Carswell F, Stewart-Brown S: Preschool wheezing and prognosis at 10. *Arch Dis Child* 1986, 61:642–646.

27. Rackeman FM, Edwards MC: Asthma in children: a follow-up study of 688 patients after an interval of 20 years. *N Engl J Med* 1952, 246:815–823.

28. Gerritsen J, Koeter GH, de Monchy JG, Knol K: Allergy in subjects with asthma from childhood to adulthood. *J Allergy Clin Immunol* 1990, 85:116–125.

29. Strachan D, Gerritsen J: Long-term outcome of early childhood wheezing: population data. *Eur Respir J* 1996, 21(suppl):42–47.

30. Strachan DP, Butland BK, Anderson HR: Incidence and prognosis of asthma and wheezing illness from early childhood to age 33 in a national British cohort. *Br Med J* 1996, 312:1195–1199.

31. Panhuysen CI, Vonk JM, Koeter GH, *et al.*: Adult patients may outgrow their asthma: a 25-year follow-up study. *Am J Respir Crit Care Med* 1997, 155:1267–1272 (published erratum appears in *Am J Respir Crit Care Med* 1997, 156:674).

32. Lange P, Parner J, Vestbo J, *et al.*: A 15-year follow-up study of ventilatory function in adults with asthma. *N Engl J Med* 1998, 339:1194–1200.

33. Kljakovic M: The pattern of consultations for asthma in a general practice over 5 years. *NZ Med J* 1996, 109:48–50.

34. Gergen P, Mitchell H, Lynn H: Understanding the seasonal pattern of childhood asthma: results from the National Cooperative Inner City Asthma Study (NCICAS). *J Pediatr* 2002, in press.

35. Weiss KB: Seasonal trends in US asthma hospitalizations and mortality. *JAMA* 1990, 263:2323–2328.

36. Litonjua AA, Carey VJ, Burge HA, *et al.*: Parental history and the risk for childhood asthma: does mother confer more risk than father? *Am J Respir Crit Care Med* 1998, 158:176–181.

37.•• Israel E, Drazen JM, Liggett SB, *et al.*: The effect of polymorphisms of the β_2-adrenergic receptor on the response to regular use of albuterol in asthma. *Am J Respir Crit Care Med* 2000, 162:75–80.
A study indicating that certain polymorphisms were found to be associated with poor to harmful responses to β-agonist therapy. These findings may lead to the development of tests to individualize the therapy for asthma.

38. Palmer LJ, Burton PR, Faux JA, *et al.*: Independent inheritance of serum immunoglobulin E concentrations and airway responsiveness. *Am J Respir Crit Care Med* 2000, 161:1836–1843.

39. Nieminen MM, Kaprio J, Koskenvuo M: A population-based study of bronchial asthma in adult twin pairs. *Chest* 1991, 100:70–75.

40. Harris JR, Magnus P, Samuelsen SO, Tambs K: No evidence for effects of family environment on asthma: a retrospective study of Norwegian twins. *Am J Respir Crit Care Med* 1997, 156:43–49.

41. Smith JM, Cadoret RJ, Burns TL, Troughton EP: Asthma and allergic rhinitis in adoptees and their adoptive parents. *Ann Allergy Asthma Immunol* 1998, 81:135–139.

42. Waite DA, Eyles EF, Tonkin SL, O'Donnell TV: Asthma prevalence in Tokelauan children in two environments. *Clin Allergy* 1980, 10:71–75.

43. Rackemann FM: A working classification of asthma. *Am J Med* 1947, 3:601–606.

44. Burrows B, Martinez FD, Halonen M, *et al.*: Association of asthma with serum IgE levels and skin-test reactivity to allergens. *N Engl J Med* 1989, 320:271–277.

45. Perzanowski MS, Sporik R, Squillace SP, *et al.*: Association of sensitization to Alternaria allergens with asthma among school-age children. *J Allergy Clin Immunol* 1998, 101:626–632.

46. Chan-Yeung M, Manfreda J, Dimich-Ward H, *et al.*: Mite and cat allergen levels in homes and severity of asthma. *Am J Respir Crit Care Med* 1995, 152:1805–1811.

47. Almqvist C, Wickman M, Perfetti L, *et al.*: Worsening of asthma in children allergic to cats, after indirect exposure to cat at school. *Am J Respir Crit Care Med* 2001, 163:694–698.

48. Rosenstreich DL, Eggleston P, Kattan M, *et al.*: The role of cockroach allergy and exposure to cockroach allergen in causing morbidity among inner-city children with asthma. *N Engl J Med* 1997, 336:1356–1363.

49. Targonski PV, Persky VW, Ramekrishnan V: Effect of environmental molds on risk of death from asthma during the pollen season. *J Allergy Clin Immunol* 1995, 95:955–961.

50. Sporik R, Holgate ST, Platts-Mills TAE, Cogswell JJ: Exposure to house-dust mite allergen (Der p I) and the development of asthma in childhood. *N Engl J Med* 1990, 323:502–507.

51.•• Lau S, Illi S, Sommerfeld C, *et al.*: Early exposure to house-dust mite and cat allergens and development of childhood asthma: a cohort study: Multicentre Allergy Study Group. *Lancet* 2000, 356:1392–1397.
A study determining that no association was found between early exposure to allergens and the development of asthma or wheeze by age 7 years.

52.•• Platts-Mills T, Vaughan J, Squillace S, *et al.*: Sensitisation, asthma, and a modified Th2 response in children exposed to cat allergen: a population-based cross-sectional study. *Lancet* 2001, 357:752–756.
A 1997 study providing evidence that in certain situations, natural exposure to allergens can produce tolerance.

53. Hajat S, Haines A, Goubet SA, *et al.*: Association of air pollution with daily GP consultations for asthma and other lower respiratory conditions in London. *Thorax* 1999, 54:597–605.

54. Neas LM, Dockery DW, Koutrakis P, *et al.*: The association of ambient air pollution with twice daily peak expiratory flow rate measurements in children. *Am J Epidemiol* 1995, 141:111–122.

55. McConnell R, Berhane K, Gilliland F, *et al.*: Asthma in exercising children exposed to ozone: a cohort study. *Lancet* 2002, 359:386–391.

56. Friedman MS, Powell KE, Hutwagner L, *et al.*: Impact of changes in transportation and commuting behaviors during the 1996 Summer Olympic Games in Atlanta on air quality and childhood asthma. *JAMA* 2001, 285:897–905.

57. von Mutius E, Martinez FD, Fritzsch C, *et al.*: Prevalence of asthma and atopy in two areas of West and East Germany. *Am J Respir Crit Care Med* 1994, 149:358–364.

58. Kramer U, Behrendt H, Dolgner R, *et al.*: Airway diseases and allergies in East and West German children during the first 5 years after reunification: time trends and the impact of sulphur dioxide and total suspended particles. *Int J Epidemiol* 1999, 28:865–873.

59. Weitzman M, Gortmaker S, Walker DK, Sobol A: Maternal smoking and childhood asthma. *Pediatrics* 1990, 85:505–511.

60. Chilmonczyk BA, Salmun LM, Megathlin KN, *et al.*: Association between exposure to environmental tobacco smoke and exacerbations of asthma in children. *N Engl J Med* 1993, 328:1665–1669.

61. Ogborn CJ, Duggan AK, DeAngelis C: Urinary cotinine as a measure of passive smoke exposure in asthmatic children. *Clin Pediatr* 1994, 33:220–226.

62. Martinez FD, Cline M, Burrows B: Increased incidence of asthma in children of smoking mothers. *Pediatrics* 1992, 89:21–26.

63. Murray AB, Morrison BJ: It is children with atopic dermatitis who develop asthma more frequently if the mother smokes. *J Allergy Clin Immunol* 1990, 86:732–739.

64. Lilljeqvist A-C, Faleide AO, Watten RG: Low birthweight, environmental tobacco smoke, and air pollution: risk factors for childhood asthma? *Pediatr Asthma Allergy* 1997, 11:95–102.

65. Horwood LJ, Fergusson DM, Hons BA, Shannon FT: Social and familial factors in the development of early childhood asthma. *Pediatrics* 1985, 75:859–868.

66. Oddy W, Holt P, Sly P, *et al.*: Association between breast feeding and asthma in 6-year-old children: findings of a prospective birth cohort study. *Br Med J* 1999, 319:815–819.

67. Strachan DP, Cook DG: Health effects of passive smoking. 5. Parental smoking and allergic sensitisation in children *Thorax* 1998, 53:117–123 (published erratum appears in *Thorax* 1999, 54:366).

68. Nicholson KG, Kent J, Ireland DC: Respiratory viruses and exacerbation of asthma in adults. *Br Med J* 1993, 307:982–986.

69. Johnston SL, Pattemore PK, Sanderson G, *et al.*: Community study of role of viral infections in exacerbations of asthma in 9–11 year old children. *Br Med J* 1995, 310:1225–1229.

70. Frischer T, Kuehr J, Meinert R, *et al.*: Relationship between low birth weight and respiratory symptoms in a cohort of primary school children. *Acta Paediatr* 1992, 81:1040–1041.

71. von Mutius E, Nicolai T, Martinez FD: Prematurity as a risk factor for asthma in preadolescent children. *J Pediatr* 1993, 123:223–229.

72. Darlow BA, Horwood LJ, Mogridge N: Very low birthweight and asthma by age seven years in a national cohort. *Pediatr Pulmonol* 2000, 30:291–296.

73. von Mutius E, Schwartz J, Neas LM, *et al.*: Relation of body mass index to asthma and atopy in children: the National Health and Nutrition Examination Study III. *Thorax* 2001, 56:835–838.

74. Belamarich PF, Luder E, Kattan M, *et al.*: Do obese inner-city children with asthma have more symptoms than nonobese children with asthma? *Pediatrics* 2000, 106:1436–1441.

75. Schachter LM, Salome CM, Peat JK, Woolcock AJ: Obesity is a risk for asthma and wheeze but not airway hyperresponsiveness. *Thorax* 2001, 56:4–8.

76. Castro-Rodriguez JA, Holberg CJ, Morgan WJ, *et al.*: Increased incidence of asthmalike symptoms in girls who become overweight or obese during the school years. *Am J Respir Crit Care Med* 2001, 163:1344–1349.

77. Stenius-Aarniala B, Poussa T, Kvarnstrom J, *et al.*: Immediate and long term effects of weight reduction in obese people with asthma: randomised controlled study. *Br Med J* 2000, 320:827–832.

78. Chinn S, Rona RJ: Can the increase in body mass index explain the rising trend in asthma in children? *Thorax* 2001, 56:845–850.

79. MacLean WE Jr, Perrin JM, Gortmaker S, Pierre CB: Psychological adjustment of children with asthma: effects of illness severity and recent stressful life events. *J Pediatr Psychol* 1992, 17:159–171.

80. Wade S, Weil C, Holden G, *et al.*: Psychosocial characteristics of inner-city children with asthma: a description of the NCI-CAS psychosocial protocol: National Cooperative Inner-City Asthma Study. *Pediatr Pulmonol* 1997, 24:263–276.

81. Creer TL: Self-management in the treatment of childhood asthma. *J Allergy Clin Immunol* 1987, 80:500–505.

82.•• Bartlett SJ, Kolodner K, Butz AM, *et al.*: Maternal depressive symptoms and emergency department use among inner-city children with asthma. *Arch Pediatr Adolesc Med* 2001, 155:347–353.
Controlling for income and asthma symptoms, emergency room utilization was found to be 30% higher for children whose mothers manifest higher symptoms of depression.

83.•• Weil CM, Wade SL, Bauman LJ, *et al.*: The relationship between psychosocial factors and asthma morbidity in inner-city children with asthma. *Pediatrics* 1999, 104:1274–1280.
A study demonstrating that children with greater psychologic problems have more asthma symptoms and poorer functional status.

84. Busse WW, Kiecolt-Glaser JK, Coe C, *et al.*: NHLBI Workshop summary: stress and asthma. *Am J Respir Crit Care Med* 1995, 151:249–252.

85. Cohen S, Tyrrell DA, Smith AP: Psychological stress and susceptibility to the common cold. *N Engl J Med* 1991, 325:606–612.

86. Liu LY, Coe CL, Swenson CA, *et al.*: School examinations enhance airway inflammation to antigen challenge. *Am J Respir Crit Care Med* 2002, 165:1062–1067.

87. Kilpelainen M, Koskenvuo M, Helenius H, Terho EO: Stressful life events promote the manifestation of asthma and atopic diseases. *Clin Exp Allergy* 2002, 32:256–263.

88. Wright RJ, Cohen S, Carey V, *et al.*: Parental stress as a predictor of wheezing in infancy: a prospective birth-cohort study. *Am J Respir Crit Care Med* 2002, 165:358–365.

89. Rietveld S, Everaerd W, Creer TL: Stress-induced asthma: a review of research and potential mechanisms. *Clin Exp Allergy* 2000, 30:1058–1066.

90. Sternberg EM: Neuroendocrine regulation of autoimmune/inflammatory disease. *J Endocrinol* 2001, 169:429–435.

91. Bienenstock J: Stress and asthma: the plot thickens. *Am J Respir Crit Care Med* 2002, 165:1034–1035.

92. Gdalevich M, Mimouni D, Mimouni M: Breast-feeding and the risk of bronchial asthma in childhood: a systematic review with meta-analysis of prospective studies. *J Pediatr* 2001, 139:261–266.

93. Bodner C, Godden D, Brown K, *et al.*: Antioxidant intake and adult-onset wheeze: a case-control study: Aberdeen WHEASE Study Group. *Eur Respir J* 1999, 13:22–30.

94. Burney PG, Neild JE, Twort CH, *et al.*: Effect of changing dietary sodium on the airway response to histamine. *Thorax* 1989, 44:36–41.

95. Jamason PF, Kalkstein LS, Gergen PJ: A synoptic evaluation of asthma hospital admissions in New York City. *Am J Respir Crit Care Med* 1997, 156:1781–1788.

96. Davidson AC, Emberlin J, Cook AD, Venables KM: A major outbreak of asthma associated with a thunderstorm: experience of accident and emergency departments and patients' characteristics: Thames Regions Accident and Emergency Trainees Association. *Br Med J* 1996, 312:601–604.

97. National air quality and emissions trends report, 1996. Office of Air Quality Planning and Standards. Research Triangle Park, NC 27711: U.S. Environmental Protection Agency; 1998.

98. National Center for Health Statistics. Health, United States, 2000 with Adolescent Health Chartbook. Hyattsville, MD; 2000.

99. Primary child child care arrangements used for preschoolers by families with employed mothers: U.S. Bureau of the Census. Internet Release data: January 14, 1998.

100. Wickens K, Crane J, Pearce N, Beasley R: The magnitude of the effect of smaller family sizes on the increase in the prevalence of asthma and hay fever in the United Kingdom and New Zealand. *J Allergy Clin Immunol* 1999, 104:554–558.

101. Crain EF, Weiss KB, Bijur PE, *et al.*: An estimate of the prevalence of asthma and wheezing among inner-city children. *Pediatrics* 1994, 94:356–362.

102. Sporik R, Ingram JM, Price W, *et al.*: Association of asthma with serum IgE and skin test reactivity to allergens among children living at high altitude: tickling the dragon's breath. *Am J Respir Crit Care Med* 1995, 151:1388–1392.

103. Homer CJ, Szilagyi P, Rodewald L, *et al.*: Does quality of care affect rates of hospitalization for childhood asthma? *Pediatrics* 1996, 98:18–23.

104. Wasilewski Y, Clark NM, Evans D, *et al.*: Factors associated with emergency department visits by children with asthma: implications for health education. *Am J Public Health* 1996, 86:1410–1415.

105. Donahue JG, Weiss ST, Livingston JM, *et al.*: Inhaled steroids and the risk of hospitalization for asthma. *JAMA* 1997, 277:887–891.

106. Adams RJ, Fuhlbrigge AL, Finkelstein JA, Weiss ST: Intranasal steroids and the risk of emergency department visits for asthma. *J Allergy Clin Immunol* 2002, 109:636–642.

107. Wu AW, Young Y, Skinner EA, *et al.*: Quality of care and outcomes of adults with asthma treated by specialists and generalists in managed care. *Arch Intern Med* 2001, 161:2554–2560.

108. Crain EF, Kercsmar C, Weiss KB, *et al.*: Reported difficulties in access to quality care for children with asthma in the inner city. *Arch Pediatr Adolesc Med* 1998, 152:333–339.

109. Ortega AN, Gergen PJ, Paltiel AD, *et al.*: Impact of site of care, race, and Hispanic ethnicity on medication use for childhood asthma. *Pediatrics* 2002, 109[1]:E1.

110. Zeiger RS, Heller S: The development and prediction of atopy in high-risk children: follow-up at age seven years in a prospective randomized study of combined maternal and infant food allergen avoidance. *J Allergy Clin Immunol* 1995, 95:1179–1190.

111. Hide DW, Matthews S, Tariq S, Arshad SH: Allergen avoidance in infancy and allergy at 4 years of age. *Allergy* 1996, 51:89–93.

112.•• Moller C, Dreborg S, Ferdousi HA, *et al.*: Pollen immuno-therapy reduces the development of asthma in children with seasonal rhinoconjunctivitis (the PAT study). *J Allergy Clin Immunol* 2002, 109:251–256.
A study providing evidence that primary prevention of asthma may be possible.

113. Early Treatment of the Atopic Child study: Allergic factors associated with the development of asthma and the influence of cetirizine in a double-blind, randomised, placebo-controlled trial: first results of ETAC. *Pediatr Allergy Immunol* 1998, 9:116–124.

114. Evans D, Mellins R, Lobach K, *et al.*: Improving care for minority children with asthma: professional education in public health clinics. *Pediatrics* 1997, 99:157–164.

115. Wissow LS, Warshow M, Box J, Baker D: Case management and quality assurance to improve care of inner-city children with asthma. *Am J Dis Child* 1988, 142:748–752.

116. Evans R III, Gergen PJ, Mitchell H, *et al.*: A randomized clinical trial to reduce asthma morbidity among inner-city children: results of the National Cooperative Inner-City Asthma Study. *J Pediatr* 1999, 135:332–338.

117. Strachan DP: Hay fever, hygiene, and household size. *Br Med J* 1989, 299:1259–1260.

118.•• Strachan DP: Family size, infection and atopy: the first decade of the "hygiene hypothesis." *Thorax* 2000, 55:2–10.
A critical review of subsequent data in support of or refutation of the hygiene hypothesis.

119. von Mutius E, Pearce N, Beasley R, *et al.*: International patterns of tuberculosis and the prevalence of symptoms of asthma, rhinitis, and eczema. *Thorax* 2000, 55:449–453.

120. Paunio M, Heinonen O, Virtanen M, *et al.*: Measles history and atopic disease. *JAMA* 2000, 283:343–346.

121. Anderson HR, Poloniecki JD, Strachan DP, *et al.*: Immunization and symptoms of atopic disease in children: results from the International Study of Asthma and Allergies in Childhood. *Am J Public Health* 2001, 91:1126–1129.

122. Matricardi PM, Rosmini F, Riondino S, *et al.*: Exposure to foodborne and orofecal microbes versus airborne viruses in relation to atopy and allergic asthma: epidemiological study. *Br Med J* 2000, 320:412–417.

123. Riedler J, Braun-Fahrlander C, Eder W, *et al.*: Exposure to farming in early life and development of asthma and allergy: a cross-sectional survey. *Lancet* 2001, 358:1129–1133.

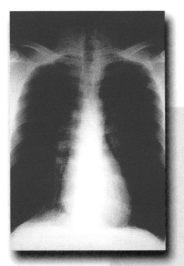

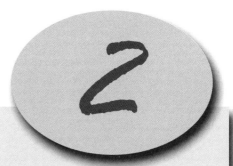

Costs of Asthma

Michael S. Blaiss and Joseph Belleau

Asthma is growing in incidence and severity throughout all regions of the United States and all the developed countries of the world. Health care costs are a major concern in this chronic disease because of the constant need for medications and the high use of emergency departments and hospitalizations for care. Another important aspect included in the total costs for asthma is indirect costs, which include missed work and school and early mortality associated with the disease. Understanding health care costs is paramount in developing strategies to ensure the best treatments at the optimal savings for society. This chapter begins with a general overview of the discipline of pharmacoeconomics and then reviews the cost aspects of asthma and discusses cost-effective approaches in its treatment.

OVERVIEW OF PHARMACOECONOMICS

As health care costs continue to escalate, the need to develop new ways to assess the worth of health care treatment has increased. This has led to the discipline of pharmacoeconomics. Pharmacoeconomics is the study of the comparative value of different pharmaceutical therapies in the management of a disease [1]. When evaluating the value of a medication, one needs to look beyond the purchase price and calculate the medication's total economic and health outcome on the patient populace [2]. This data can lead to informed decisions in managing patients and in developing policies for the public [3].

Health care costs can be divided into two major groups: direct and indirect [4]. Direct costs include all the monies spent on managing the disorder [5]. Along with the cost for medications, direct costs consist of all medical services, such as outpatient, hospital, and emergency department visits; physician fees; and laboratory procedures. Indirect costs take in all the non–health care expenditures linked with the illness. These are opportunity costs in that they are caused by a lack of monies received from missed "opportunities." Monies lost because of missing work and decreased productivity because of the illness are indirect costs. Also included in indirect costs are the economic value of missing school and unpaid caregivers' time to care for sick children.

Health care economists have developed several different methods to compare the total costs of different treatment modalities. The four most frequently used assessments are cost identification, cost benefit, cost effectiveness, and cost utility (Table 2-1).

The most commonly used approach in evaluating costs of treatment is cost-effectiveness analysis. This method compares the costs of different treatments in monetary units with the clinical results obtained with said treatment [6]. This analysis uses health outcomes, such as symptom-free days, use of short-acting β-agonists, and decreases in emergency department visits and hospitalizations, for assessing outcomes. This technique allows for the construction of a cost-effectiveness ratio, or the cost to achieve a particular outcome. For example, treatment A costs $1000 for 10 patients and increases symptom-free days by 50%; treatment B costs $2000 for 10 patients and increases symptom-free days by 90%. Treatment A has a cost-effectiveness ratio of 20 (1000/50) for each patient, and treatment B's cost-effectiveness ratio is 22.2 (2000/90). This approach can be used for other outcome measures in asthma to help determine the most cost-effective treatment for patients with asthma.

Table 2-1. ECONOMIC EVALUATIONS IN HEALTH CARE

Cost effectiveness
Costs are compared with clinical effects produced between different programs or treatments

Cost benefit
Costs are compared with benefits from a program or treatment as defined by society

Cost identification
Costs are compared between different programs or treatments

Cost utility
Costs are compared with quality-adjusted life years attained between different programs or treatments

PHARMACOECONOMICS OF ASTHMA

More than 15 million Americans are afflicted with asthma, with an incidence of around 3% to 4% of adults and 7% of children [7,8]. A recent Centers for Disease Control and Prevention (CDC) report of self-reported asthma suggested that the prevalence in the adult population might be as high in children as 7% in the United States [9]. Weiss *et al.* [7] estimated the total cost for asthma care in the United States to be $6.21 billion in 1990. They estimated $3.64 billion for direct costs of asthma care. These costs encompass physician costs, medication costs, laboratory procedures, imaging studies, hospitalizations, and emergency department care. Weiss *et al.* [7] computed indirect costs for asthma care at $2.57 billion. This figure represents loss of productivity caused by absence from school and work and premature death from asthma.

Weiss and Sullivan [10••] updated the calculations of the cost of asthma in the United States in 1994 and 1998, and the number grew to $12.7 billion in 1998. Table 2-2 shows the increase in costs caused by asthma in the United States from 1990 to 1998 from the Weiss studies [7,10••,11]. Although the total amount of money spent on asthma has increased significantly over the past decade, the cost per patient has actually decreased by 3.4% per individual patient on the basis of adjusted dollars. These expenses are a combination of direct and indirect cost of the illness.

A total of 56% of the total expenditures related to asthma, or $6.1 billion, was spent on direct medical costs. Direct costs are expenses generated in treating, preventing, and rehabilitating patients with asthma. Prescription drugs account for the greatest percentage of the total direct cost and have just recently exceeded hospitalizations as the most expensive direct expenditure [10••]. An estimated $2.5 billion is spent per year on medications. Despite the increased cost of medication, the reduction in total costs per patient is attributed to a

Table 2-2. COSTS OF ASTHMA IN THE UNITED STATES

Cost Item	Costs, *million $*		
Year	1990	1994	1998
Direct medical costs			
Hospital care	2044.9	2910.5	3323.5
Physician services	493.0	744.1	853.6
Prescriptions	1099.7	2452.0	3188.1
Total direct costs	3637.3	6107.6	7365.3
Indirect costs	2568.4	4640.6	7365.3
Total costs	6206.0	10748.3	12671.3

Adapted from *Weiss et al. [7]; Weiss and Sullivan [10••]; and Weiss et al. [11].*

decreased length of inpatient care. The decreased stay in the hospital combined with a fairly stable rate of hospital admissions, despite the increasing prevalence of the disease, reduces the overall per-patient charges.

Although the indirect costs of asthma account for only 43% of the total money spent, it is still estimated at $4.6 billion per year [10••]. The largest component of the indirect cost of asthma was loss of work, which is a combination of directly missed days of work that occur during an exacerbation and the loss of future potential earnings associated with both morbidity and mortality [12].

Although hospital charges can vary greatly, a study estimated a 3-day stay for status asthmaticus at $3000 [13]. Another report showed a 4-day charge of $6546 [14]. A study from New York State evaluated charges in teaching versus nonteaching hospitals in children with status asthmaticus [15]. In teaching hospitals, the costs were significantly but not meaningfully greater ($2459 vs $2271; $P = 0.001$).

Birnbaum *et al.* [16••] estimated the total costs of asthma to major employers in the United States by evaluating medical, pharmaceutical, and disability claims from 1996

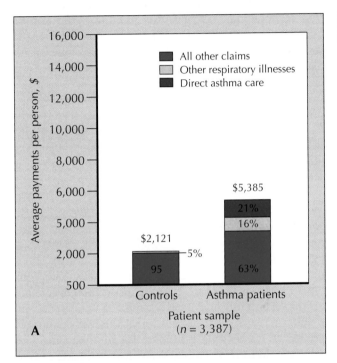

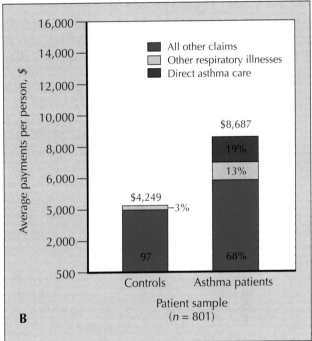

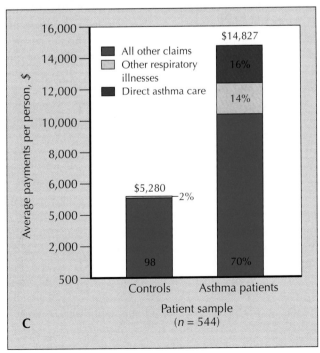

Figure 2-1.
Employer cost per asthma patient (including spouse, dependents, retirees less than age 65 years of age) for medical, pharmaceutical, and work-loss expenditures. (*Adapted from* Birnbaum *et al.* [16••].)

through 1998 (Fig. 2-1). They determined that $14,827 was the cost per asthmatic patient to the employer compared with $5280 spent on the control subjects. The study noted that asthmatic patients have approximately three times more medical claims, a higher average medication cost, and increased absenteeism. Additionally, more money was spent on disability than for average beneficiaries.

Individual annual costs vary for asthmatic patients. In 1997, Lenney [17] determined that in children with asthma, the yearly costs were greater than $1000. A yearly cost for each asthmatic child in an HMO in 1992 was $1060.32, compared with $563.81 for each nonasthmatic child [18]. As for individual costs of asthma, a small percentage of the total asthma population generates a majority of the costs. In one report, more than 70% of the total costs of asthma were generated by about 5% of patients [19]. Smith *et al.* [20] found that 80% of the resources for asthma were used by 20% of the asthma population. Unfortunately, even when high-cost patients with asthma are identified, these patients may not continue to be high-resource users over time. Nash *et al.* [21] found that in a pediatric Medicaid population, only 30% of asthmatic children who were high-cost patients continued to be the next year.

Leigh *et al.* [22] assessed direct and indirect costs associated with occupational asthma in the United States in 1996. They estimated that 15% of the asthma population was at risk for occupational asthma. The authors estimated that the burden of occupational asthma was $1.6 billion in total costs, with 74% related to direct costs and 26% to indirect costs. The authors stated that these numbers were conservative because they ignored costs associated with pain and suffering as well as the value of care rendered by family members.

Barnes *et al.* [23] reviewed cost studies of asthma from throughout the world. In 1990 US dollars, the cost per year for each asthmatic patient in Sweden is $1315; it is $1043 in the United Kingdom and $769 in Australia [24]. A study [25] estimated the total cost for asthma in Canada during 1990 to be between US$378 and US$486 million. Toelle *et al.* [26] evaluated the cost of asthma in children in Australia. The mean annual cost of asthma to the family was US$212.48 per asthmatic child, and 13.4 hours were spent obtaining treatment. A survey from Mexico from 1991 to 1996 demonstrated increasing costs for asthma care [27]. There was a significant increase in in-hospital care observed, ranging from US$14.5 million (1991) and US$19.8 million (1996) and a maximum of US$28.4 million (1994). A 1996 evaluation in Germany found total estimated costs were DM 5.81 billion related to asthma [28]. The major drivers of direct costs were outpatient-prescribed medicines followed by hospitalization. In the Netherlands, the cost for asthma care to the government was estimated to be more than US$100 million in 1993 [29].

Indirect costs of asthma ranged from 90% of total costs in a study from the United Kingdom to 30% in an Australian report [23]. The German study [28] suggested that 67% of total costs were indirect, but their calculations failed to consider outpatient physician costs.

Environmental Control in Asthma

The components of asthma management include environmental control, objective monitoring, patient education, pharmacologic therapy, and allergen immunotherapy. Environmental allergen avoidance procedures have been documented to play a role in cost-effective therapy in allergic asthmatic patients [30]. Studies have now shown that early exposure to possible allergens may increase the risk of developing allergic disorders [31]. Initiation of avoidance measures early in life may prevent or delay the development of allergic disorders [32]. Dust mite avoidance measures, such as removing carpeting and using encasing mattress covers, have been shown to improve pulmonary function and clinical symptomatology in patients with asthma sensitive to mites [33–35]. Cockroach infestation can lead to severe asthma problems, especially in the inner-city population. Vigorous abatement procedures to reduce cockroach levels in homes may prove valuable in cost-effective care [36].

Pharmaceutical Costs in Asthma

A mainstay of asthma management is appropriate pharmacologic therapy. With the publication of the National Heart, Lung, and Blood Institute's guidelines for long-term management of patients with asthma, clinicians have a stepwise approach to using medication depending on the severity of the patient's asthma [37]. Short-acting β-agonists, such as albuterol, are the most commonly prescribed medications for the treatment of patients with asthma. They are recommended for acute exacerbations and in the prevention of exercise-induced asthma. Patients who fall under any of the following categories are persistent patients with asthma and should be prescribed a long-term controller anti-inflammatory agent: 1) requiring short-acting β-agonists more than twice a week or going through more than two short-acting β-agonists canisters a year; 2) having nighttime symptoms more than twice a month; and 3) having a corticosteroid burst or unscheduled office visit for asthma twice a year or more. Anti-inflammatory medications include cromolyn, nedocromil, inhaled corticosteroids, and leukotriene receptor antagonists. Tables 2-3 and 2-4 show daily cost comparisons of these agents in the management of patients with mild persistent asthma [38]. It is important to note that these costs calculated from the average wholesale price might not actually be true indicators of a patient's cost.

Studies have shown that prescribing anti-inflammatory agents is an important cost-effective step in overall asthma management. Stempel *et al.* [39] analyzed drug use during the 12 months of 1993 in four health maintenance organizations with approximately 673,000 members. Health care costs were identified in asthmatic patients, ages 7 years and older, who used high doses of inhaled β-adrenergic agonists, defined as more than eight puffs per day. A total of 20,512 asthmatic patients was studied, with 5.3% receiving high doses of an inhaled bronchodilator. This group was then stratified by concurrent use of inhaled anti-inflammatory therapy. Members who used high doses of inhaled bronchodilators had annual charges for treatment related to their asthma that were three times higher than the average asthmatic patient ($1346.52 vs $447.42). The high β-agonist users had inpatient hospital and emergency department charges that grew proportionally as a percentage of total annual expenses. Konig and Shaffer [40] showed that for children with asthma, early treatment with anti-inflammatory medications with either cromolyn or inhaled corticosteroids, but not as-needed bronchodilators alone, improved the long-term prognosis of asthma and may reduce overall total costs. In another study [41], 310 adult patients with mild, moderate, or severe asthma were given nedocromil sodium for at least 1 year. After initiation of nedocromil sodium therapy, patients showed better asthma control as measured by improvements in pulmonary function scores and by reduced emergency department visits and hospital admissions.

Further data demonstrate that inhaled corticosteroid use has been shown to reduce hospitalizations and deaths in patients with asthma, demonstrating that inhaled corticosteroids are a cost-effective treatment [42•]. A Swedish study [43] documented inhaled corticosteroid use from 1978 to 1991 and showed that increased sales of inhaled corticosteroids were significantly correlated ($P < 0.01$) with a reduction in bed days caused by asthma. Rutten-van Molken *et al.* [44] determined the costs and effects of inhaled terbutaline plus placebo, inhaled terbutaline plus inhaled ipratropium, and inhaled terbutaline

plus inhaled beclomethasone in adults with moderate persistent asthma over a 2.5-year period. The treatment costs of the inhaled terbutaline plus inhaled beclomethasone therapy were higher, but total health care costs were lower in this group. Data document that inhaled corticosteroid use has been shown to reduce hospitalizations in patients with asthma, demonstrating that inhaled corticosteroids are a cost-effective treatment.

A study [45] evaluated Medicaid patients in Texas with asthma using continuously inhaled corticosteroids compared with asthma patients using other medications. The study was conducted from March 1996 through June 1998 and concluded that those treated with inhaled corticosteroids had an increase in prescription costs; however, this was offset by a decrease in all types of medical visits, especially acute care. Paltiel *et al.* [46] used a mathematical simulation mode to assess cost effectiveness of inhaled corticosteroids in patients with mild to moderate persistent asthma. Over a 10-year period, use of inhaled corticosteroids increased total health costs from approximately $5200 to $8400. The authors documented that costs for each symptom-free day gained by the patients was $7.50. They concluded that compared with treatment costs for other diseases, inhaled corticosteroids gave good value in adults with persistent asthma.

When new agents are approved for treatment of asthma, it is important that they be documented to be cost-effective. Suissa *et al.* [47] evaluated the clinical and economic effectiveness of the leukotriene receptor antagonist zafirlukast compared with placebo for mild to moderate asthma in 146 patients. The economic effectiveness outcomes were frequency and type of unscheduled health care contacts, use of β-agonist inhalers, consumption of nonasthma medications, and days of absence from work

Table 2-3. INHALED CORTICOSTEROIDS IN ASTHMA: COST PER DAY*

Agent	Cost per Day, $
Beclomethasone	2.84
Triamcinolone acetonide	2.54
Flunisolide	1.29
Fluticasone 44 µg	3.57
Budesonide	2.70
Fluticasone/salmeterol 100/50	2.86

*From 2002 Drug Topics Red Book [38] based on average wholesale price for treatment of mild persistent asthma in adults by the National Heart, Lung, and Blood Institute's guidelines (maximum dose). (Costs calculated from the average wholesale price may not be true indicators of the patient's true costs.)
(Adapted from 2002 Drug Topics Red Book [38].)

Table 2-4. OTHER CONTROLLER AGENTS IN ASTHMA*

Agent	Cost per Day, $
Zafirlukast	2.36
Montelukast	2.80
Nedocromil	3.28
Cromolyn	3.41
Theophylline 600 mg	1.45
Generic theophylline	0.44
Salmeterol	2.67

*Cost per day from 2002 Drug Topics Red Book [38] based on average wholesale price for treatment of mild persistent asthma in adults by the National Heart, Lung, and Blood Institute's guidelines (maximum dose). (Costs calculated from the average wholesale price may not be true indicators of the patient's true costs.)
(Adapted from 2002 Drug Topics Red Book [38].)

or school. The zafirlukast group had 55% fewer health care contacts and 55% fewer days of absence from work or school. They used 17% fewer canisters of inhaled β-agonists and 19% less nonasthma medication. Price *et al.* [48] assessed costs in the United Kingdom of adding montelukast, a leukotriene receptor antagonist, as chronic asthma therapy. Use of montelukast led to a significant reduction in use of short-acting β-agonist and antibiotics. Thus, montelukast was associated with a reduction of concomitant drug therapy costs. These data suggest that this medication group may have a cost-effective benefit in the treatment of asthma.

There have been several studies evaluating two of the most commonly used classes of anti-inflammatory medications in the treatment of asthma: inhaled corticosteroids and leukotriene receptor antagonists. When inhaled hydrofluoroalkane triamcinolone acetonide 450 µg/d was compared with oral montelukast 10 mg/d in a randomized, placebo-controlled, single-blinded, crossover study, it was concluded that both regimens improved morning and evening peak flows, nighttime β-2 agonist use, and symptoms compared with placebo [49].

Bukstein *et al.* [50] had similar results when they compared asthma-related expenditures between patients started on montelukast and fluticasone propionate. There was no significant difference in mean changes in total asthma-related health care costs, oral steroid prescriptions, hospitalizations, or emergency care between the two groups. However, the patients who took montelukast also demonstrated better adherence to their treatment and required fewer β-agonist prescriptions. When fluticasone propionate was compared with zafirlukast in patients with persistent asthma, Stempel *et al.* [51] showed that treatment with fluticasone propionate was more cost effective than treatment with zarfirlukast. The patients demonstrated a 70% reduced risk for hospitalization and 49% lower risk for emergency room visits. These results were reaffirmed in a second study [52] that compared the same two medications. The study showed that fluticasone propionate (88 µg twice a day) was more cost effective than zafirlukast (20 mg twice a day).

In patients with more moderate to severe persistent asthma, two or more controller agents may need to be prescribed for optimal asthma management. Stempel *et al.* [53] used a 24-month, pre- and postretrospective design in asthmatic patients continuously enrolled in 14 managed care plans to assess the costs associated with leukotriene modifier agents versus long-acting β-agonists added to inhaled corticosteroids for asthma control. Outcomes assessed were post-index pharmacy costs, rates of emergency department visits and hospitalizations, numbers of filled prescriptions for short-acting β-agonists, total asthma costs, and total health care costs. The total adjusted asthma costs were 63% higher for the patients who received leukotriene modifier agents than

for those who received long-acting β-agonists as add-on therapy with their inhaled corticosteroids. Wang *et al.* [54] compared the costs of several double controller therapies and found the least costly to be inhaled corticosteroids with mast cell stabilizing agents, such as cromolyn, followed by salmeterol, a long-acting β-agonist, and fluticasone, an inhaled corticosteroid.

Specific Allergen Immunotherapy in Asthma

Specific allergen immunotherapy as a treatment for asthma has been validated and data are accumulating to show it is a cost-effective treatment [55]. Calvo *et al.* [56] performed a study to attempt to further define the contribution of specific allergen immunotherapy in a pediatric asthmatic population. A total of 166 patients were treated with specific allergen immunotherapy, and 248 patients received no immunotherapy. The results were compared during 10 years of follow-up in both groups. There was a significant decrease in the number of acute crises in the treated group ($P < 0.05$). However, no differences were seen in the number of hospital admissions or in the quality of life between the treated and untreated groups. The treated group required significantly fewer drugs ($P < 0.05$). Thus, this study illustrates that specific allergen immunotherapy may be cost effective by reducing medication costs over time.

Abramson *et al.* [57] performed a meta-analysis of clinical trials of specific allergen immunotherapy to evaluate the effectiveness of this therapy in asthma. The results extracted included asthmatic symptoms, medication requirements, lung function, and bronchial hyperreactivity. Categorical outcomes were expressed as odds ratios. The combined odds of symptomatic improvement from immunotherapy with any allergen was 3.2. The odds for reduction in medication after mite immunotherapy was 4.2. The authors concluded that allergen immunotherapy is a treatment option in highly selected patients with allergic asthma. Creticos *et al.* [58] looked at 2-year use of ragweed immunotherapy in adult patients with asthma. There were reduced medication costs for asthma with immunotherapy, but the lower costs were counterbalanced by the costs of specific allergen immunotherapy.

Specific allergen immunotherapy may also represent an effective treatment that changes the natural course of allergic asthma in pediatric patients. Cantani *et al.* [59] performed a randomized, placebo-controlled trial with dust mite or pollen immunotherapy in 300 asthmatic children older than age 3 years. Children receiving specific allergen immunotherapy had significantly decreased drug usage, decreased asthma attacks, and improved quality of life. A European study [60] recently evaluated specific allergen immunotherapy in children with seasonal allergic rhinitis to determine if specific allergen immunotherapy can reduce the risk of development of asthma in that population. After 3 years of treatment, children in the specific allergen immunotherapy treatment group had statistically fewer asthma symptoms than the control group. This study is encouraging as a cost-effective way that specific allergen immunotherapy may prevent the development of asthma in the risk group of children with seasonal allergic rhinitis.

Bernstein [61•] evaluated the cost of specific allergen immunotherapy over a 5-year period compared with treatment with medication alone in three different medical centers in the United States. The average 5-year outlay to administer specific allergen immunotherapy was approximately $2000 compared with $6000 for medication alone. The combined total cost of specific allergen immunotherapy and medication compared with medication alone was less costly ($5000 vs $6000), assuming a minimal 50% efficacy for specific allergen immunotherapy and a 50% decrease medication usage. Unlike specific allergen immunotherapy, after 5 years of treatment, medication alone would have been effective only in controlling symptoms, with no effect on modifying the disease process. The lessening and possible disappearance of symptoms after long-term specific allergen immunotherapy should lead to significant cost savings [62]. A study [63] from Germany also documented the economic advantage of specific allergen immunotherapy. This evaluation showed that specific allergen immunotherapy administered for 3 years was cost effective in patients who were sensitive to pollen and house dust mites and whose symptoms were not adequately controlled with medication.

Asthma Intervention Programs in Cost-effective Management

Many studies have documented the role of asthma intervention programs in children and adults in producing cost-effective management [64]. There have been many different types of programs that show at least short-term efficacy in controlling asthma costs. Evaluating these interventions from an economic standpoint has shown that these programs can produce cost-effective results in all patients with asthma, but they are highly beneficial when aimed at high-risk patients or those with multiple hospitalizations [65].

Bolton *et al.* [66] analyzed the cost effectiveness of a self-management training program in adult patients with asthma. The educational sessions cost $85 per person, which was offset by the $628 per person reduction in emergency room charges. A protocol to assess therapeutic benefit and cost saving in the treatment of patients with acute asthma in the emergency department over 1 year was compared with costs before implementation of the protocol [67]. Following the protocol reduced the length of stays in the emergency department, rate of hospitalization, and frequency of return visits to the emergency department in 24 hours. This reduced charges to patients and third-party payers by a total of $395,000.

George *et al.* [68•] studied 18- to 45-year-old patients who were hospitalized with a diagnosis of asthma and evaluated the cost effectiveness of an asthma education program. Subjects were randomized to either routine outpatient follow-up or to an inpatient education program that consisted of education, spirometry, a phone call 24 hours after discharge, and follow-up in 1 week as an outpatient. The results showed a markedly higher follow-up rate with outpatient appointments in the education program, 60% compared with 27%. The teaching program also showed a significant cost saving by reducing the number of emergency room visits and hospitalizations for the 6 months after the educational intervention.

Asthma programs based outside of clinic and hospital settings can be beneficial in reducing asthma costs. Burton *et al.* [69] showed that a work-site program improved asthma care. After the program was ended, significantly more employees reported using controller medications, the desired outcome, rather than reliever medications.

A major emphasis has been placed on the development of intervention programs for the indigent population that primarily uses emergency departments for asthma care. An outreach program was developed for an inner-city pediatric asthma population [70]. Patients were scheduled for one-on-one orientation visits with an asthma outreach nurse, and an individualized step-care treatment program was outlined for each patient. The outreach nurse maintained personal or telephone contact with the families on a regular basis to ensure compliance. This program resulted in the reduction of emergency department admissions by 79% and hospital admissions by 86%, with estimated savings of approximately $87,000.

Kelso *et al.* [71] created a major long-term therapeutic and educational intervention program in the emergency department for indigent adult black patients with asthma. Outcome measures assessed were emergency department visits and hospitalizations for 1 year after the emergency department intervention. These outcomes were compared with a retrospective control group of 22 patients. Although there was a significant decrease in both emergency department visits and hospitalizations in the intervention group, there was no significant change in either category in the control group.

Additionally, a Virginia-based asthma program for the Medicaid population showed improved asthma outcomes [72]. This large-scale study revealed that the rate of emergency visit claims for patients of participating physicians who received feedback reports decreased an average of 41% from the same quarter one year earlier compared with only 18% for comparison community physicians. The authors performed a cost-effectiveness analysis and estimated direct savings to Medicaid of $3 to $4 for every incremental dollar spent providing asthma disease management support to physicians.

REFERENCES AND RECOMMENDED READING

Papers of particular interest, published recently, have been highlighted as:
- • Of importance
- •• Of major importance

1. Drummond MF, Stoddart GL, Torrance GW: *Methods for the Economic Evaluation of Health Care Programmes.* New York: Oxford University Press; 1987.

2. McIvor RA: Pharmacoeconomics in pediatric asthma. *Chest* 2001, 120:1762–1763.

3. Sullivan SD: Cost and cost-effectiveness in asthma. *Immunol Allergy Clin North Am* 1996, 16:819–839.

4. Blaiss M, et al.: *Improving Allergy and Asthma Care Through Outcomes Management. Managed Care Focus Series.* Edited by Davis M. American Academy of Allergy, Asthma, and Immunology; 1997.

5. Luce BR, et al.: Estimating costs in cost-effectiveness analysis. In *Cost-effectiveness in Health and Medicine.* Edited by Gold MR, et al. New York Oxford University Press; 1996:176–213.

6. Gibaldi M, Sullivan SD: A look at cost-effectiveness. *Pharmacotherapy* 1994, 14:399–414.

7. Weiss KB, Gergen PJ, Hodgson TA: An economic evaluation of asthma in the United States [see comments]. *N Engl J Med* 1992, 326:862–866.

8. Centers for Disease Control and Prevention: asthma mortality and hospitalization among children and young adults—United States, 1980–1993. *Morbid Mortal Wkly Rep* 1996, 45:350–353.

9. Self-reported asthma prevalence among adults—United States, 2000. *Morbid Mortal Wkly Rep* 2001, 50:682–686.

10. •• Weiss KB, Sullivan SD: The health economics of asthma and rhinitis. I. Assessing the economic impact. *J Allergy Clin Immunol* 2001, 107:3–8.
This review characterizes the economic burden associated with asthma. The authors show the upward spiral of direct and indirect costs caused by asthma in the past decade.

11. Weiss KB, Sullivan SD, Lyttle CS: Trends in the cost of illness for asthma in the united states, 1985–1994. *J Allergy Clin Immunol* 2000, 106:493–499.

12. Gergen PJ: Understanding the economic burden of asthma. *J Allergy Clin Immunol* 2001, 107:445–448.

13. Brillman J, Tandberg D: Observation unit impact on ED admission for asthma. *Am J Emerg Med* 1994, 12:11–14.

14. DeSilva R: A disease management case study on asthma. *Clin Ther* 1996, 18:1374–1382.

15. Huang ZJ, LaFleur BJ, Chamberlain JM, et al.: Inpatient childhood asthma treatment: relationship of hospital characteristics to length of stay and cost: analyses of New York State discharge data, 1995. *Arch Pediatr Adolesc Med* 2002, 156:67–72.

16. •• Birnbaum HG, Berger WE, Greenberg PE, et al.: Direct and indirect costs of asthma to an employer. *J Allergy Clin Immunol* 2002, 109:264–270.
This economic evaluation documented the high financial burden of asthma to employers. A key point from this study was that wage-related costs caused by disability and sporadic absenteeism accounted for almost as much as did medical care costs for employers.

17. Lenney W: The burden of pediatric asthma. *Pediatr Pulmonol* 1997, 15(suppl):13–16.

18. Lozano P, Fishman P, VonKorff M, Hecht J: Health care utilization and cost among children with asthma who were enrolled in a health maintenance organization. *Pediatrics* 1997, 99:757–764.

19. Todd W: New mindsets in asthma: interventions and disease management. *J Care Manage* 1995, 1:2–8.

20. Smith D, Malone D, Lawson K: A national estimate of the economic costs of asthma. *Am J Respir Crit Care Med* 1997, 156:787–793.

21. Nash DR, Childs GE, Kelleher KJ: A cohort study of resource use by medicaid children with asthma. *Pediatrics* 1999, 104(2 pt 1):310–312.

22. Leigh JP, Romano PS, Schenker MB, Kreiss K: Costs of occupational COPD and asthma. *Chest* 2002, 121:264–272.

23. Barnes PJ, Jonsson B, Klim JB: The costs of asthma. *Eur Respir J* 1996, 9:636–642.

24. National Heart, Lung, and Blood Institute, National Institutes of Health, Socioeconomics, in Global Strategy for Asthma Management and Prevention: A NHLBI/WHO Workshop Report, N.P.N. 94-3276. Bethesda, MD: US Department of Health and Human Services; 1994.

25. Krahn MD, Berka C, Langlois P, et al.: Direct and indirect costs of asthma in Canada. *Can Med Assoc J* 1996, 154:821–831.

26. Toelle BG, Peat JK, Mellis CM, Woolcock AJ: The cost of childhood asthma to Australian families. *Pediatr Pulmonol* 1995, 19: 330–335.

27. Rico-Mendez FG, Barquera S, Cabrera DA, et al.: Bronchial asthma health care costs in Mexico: analysis of trends from 1991–1996 with information from the Mexican Institute of Social Security. *J Investig Allergol Clin Immunol* 2000, 10:334–341.

28. Weissflog D, Matthys H, Virchow JC Jr: Epidemiology and costs of bronchial asthma and chronic bronchitis in Germany. *Deutsch Med Wochenschr* 2001, 126:803–808.

29. Rutten van-Molken MP, Feenstra TL: The burden of asthma and chronic obstructive pulmonary disease: data from The Netherlands. *Pharmacoeconomics* 2001, 19:1–6.

30. Kuster PA: Reducing risk of house dust mite and cockroach allergen exposure in inner-city children with asthma. *Pediatr Nurs* 1996, 22:297–303.

31. Kuehr J, Frischer T, Meinert R, et al.: Sensitization to mite allergens is a risk factor for early and late onset of asthma and for persistence of asthmatic signs in children. *J Allergy Clin Immunol* 1995, 95:655–662.

32. Hide DW, Matthews S, Matthews L, et al.: Effect of allergen avoidance in infancy on allergic manifestations at age two years. *J Allergy Clin Immunol* 1994, 93:842–846.

33. van der Heide S, Kauffman HF, Dubois AE, de Monchy JG: Allergen reduction measures in houses of allergic asthmatic patients: effects of air-cleaners and allergen-impermeable mattress covers [see comments]. *Eur Respir J* 1997, 10:1217–1223.

34. Piacentini GL, Martinati L, Mingoni S, Boner AL: Influence of allergen avoidance on the eosinophil phase of airway inflammation in children with allergic asthma. *J Allergy Clin Immunol* 1996, 97:1079–1084.

35. Peroni DG, Boner AL, Vallone G, et al.: Effective allergen avoidance at high altitude reduces allergen-induced bronchial hyperresponsiveness. *Am J Respir Crit Care Med* 1994, 149:1442–1446.

36. Arruda LK, Vailes LD, Ferriani VP, et al.: Cockroach allergens and asthma. *J Allergy Clin Immunol* 2001, 107:419–428.

37. National Heart, Lung, and Blood Institute, National Asthma Education and Prevention Program: *Expert Panel Report 2: Guidelines for the Diagnosis and Management of Asthma.* Bethesda, MD: National Institutes of Health; Pub. No. 97-4051; 1997.

38. *2002 Drug Topic Red Book.* Montvale, NJ: Medical Economics Company; 2002.

39. Stempel DA, Durcannin-Robbins JF, Hedblom EC, *et al.*: Drug utilization evaluation identifies costs associated with high use of beta-adrenergic agonists. *Ann Allergy Asthma Immunol* 1996, 76:153–158.

40. Konig P, Shaffer J: The effect of drug therapy on long-term outcome of childhood asthma: a possible preview of the international guidelines. *J Allergy Clin Immunol* 1996, 98:1103–1111.

41. Thomas P, Ross RN, Farrar JR: A retrospective assessment of cost avoidance associated with the use of nedocromil sodium metered-dose inhaler in the treatment of patients with asthma. *Clin Ther* 1996, 18:939–952.

42.• Suissa S, Ernst P: Inhaled corticosteroids: impact on asthma morbidity and mortality. *J Allergy Clin Immunol* 2001, 107:937–944.
Inhaled corticosteroids are the first-line therapy for most patients with persistent asthma. This review article documents the cost-effectiveness of inhaled corticosteroids in decreasing hospitalizations and death and emphasizes the importance of these agents for improved asthma outcomes.

43. Gerdtham UG, Hertzman P, Jonsson B, Boman G: Impact of inhaled corticosteroids on acute asthma hospitalization in Sweden 1978 to 1991. *Med Care* 1996, 34:1188–1198.

44. Rutten-van Molken MP, Van Doorslaer EK, Jansen MC, *et al.*: Costs and effects of inhaled corticosteroids and bronchodilators in asthma and chronic obstructive pulmonary disease. *Am J Respir Crit Care Med* 1995, 151:975–982.

45. Smith M, Rascati KL, Johnsrud MT: Cost and utilization patterns associated with presistent asthma. *J Managed Care Pharm* 2001, 7:452–459.

46. Paltiel AD, Fuhlbrigge AL, Kitch BT, *et al.*: Cost-effectiveness of inhaled corticosteroids in adults with mild-to-moderate asthma: results from the asthma policy model. *J Allergy Clin Immunol* 2001, 108:39–49.

47. Suissa S, Dennis R, Ernst P, *et al.*: Effectiveness of the leukotriene receptor antagonist zafirlukast for mild-to-moderate asthma: a randomized, double-blind, placebo-controlled trial. *Ann Intern Med* 1997, 126:177–183.

48. Price DB, Ben-Joseph RH, Zhang Q: Changes in asthma drug therapy costs for patients receiving chronic montelukast therapy in the U.K. *Respir Med* 2001, 95:83–89.

49. Dempsey OJ, Kennedy G, Lipworth BJ: Comparative efficacy and anti-inflammatory profile of once-daily therapy with leukotriene antagonist or low-dose inhaled corticosteroid in patients with mild persistent asthma. *J Allergy Clin Immunol* 2002, 109:68–74.

50. Bukstein DA, Henk HJ, Luskin AT: A comparison of asthma-related expenditures for patients started on montelukast versus fluticasone propionate as monotherapy. *Clin Ther* 2001, 23:1589–1600.

51. Stempel DA, Meyer JW, Stanford RH, *et al.*: One-year claims analysis comparing inhaled fluticasone propionate with zafirlukast for the treatment of asthma. *J Allergy Clin Immunol* 2001, 107:94–98.

52. Menendez R, Stanford RH, Edwards L, *et al.*: Cost-efficacy analysis of fluticasone propionate versus zafirlukast in patients with persistent asthma. *Pharmacoeconomics* 2001, 19:865–874.

53. Stempel DA, O'Donnell JC, Meyer JW: Inhaled corticosteroids plus salmeterol or montelukast: effects on resource utilization and costs. *J Allergy Clin Immunol* 2002, 109:433–439.

54. Wang SW, Liu X, Wiener DJ, *et al.*: Comparison of prevalence, cost, and outcomes of a combination of salmeterol and fluticasone therapy to common asthma treatments. *Am J Manag Care* 2001, 7:913–922.

55. Alvarez-Cuesta E, Gonzelez-Mancebo E: Immunotherapy in bronchial asthma. *Curr Opin Pulm Med* 2000, 6:50–54.

56. Calvo M, Marin F, Grob K, *et al.*: Ten-year follow-up in pediatric patients with allergic bronchial asthma: evaluation of specific immunotherapy. *J Investig Allergol Clin Immunol* 1994, 4:126–131.

57. Abramson MJ, Puy RM, Weiner JM: Is allergen immunotherapy effective in asthma? A meta-analysis of randomized controlled trials [see comments]. *Am J Respir Crit Care Med* 1995, 151:969–974.

58. Creticos PS, Reed CE, Norman PS, *et al.*: Ragweed immunotherapy in adult asthma [see comments]. *N Engl J Med* 1996, 334:501–506.

59. Cantani A, Arcese G, Lucenti P, *et al.*: A three-year prospective study of specific immunotherapy to inhalant allergens: evidence of safety and efficacy in 300 children with allergic asthma. *J Investig Allergol Clin Immunol* 1997, 7:90–97.

60. Moller C, Dreborg S, Ferdousi HA, *et al.*: Pollen immunotherapy reduces the development of asthma in children with seasonal rhinoconjunctivitis (the PAT-study). *J Allergy Clin Immunol* 2002, 109:251–256.

61.• Bernstein J: Cost-benefit analysis of allergen immunotherapy. *Immunol Allergy Clin North Am* 2000, 20:593–607.
This review article gives the most comprehensive data to date illustrating the cost-benefit of specific allergen immunotherapy.

62. Nieto A, Alvarez-Cuesta E, Boquete M, *et al.*: The cost of asthma treatment in Spain and rationalizing the expense. *J Investig Allergol Clin Immunol* 2001, 11:139–148.

63. Schadlich PK, Brecht JG: Economic evaluation of specific immunotherapy versus symptomatic treatment of allergic rhinitis in Germany. *Pharmacoeconomics* 2000, 17:37–52.

64. Liljas B, Lahdensuo A: Is asthma self-management cost-effective? *Patient Educ Couns* 1997, 32(suppl 1):97–104.

65. Sullivan SD, Weiss KB: Health economics of asthma and rhinitis. II. Assessing the value of interventions. *J Allergy Clin Immunol* 2001, 107:203–210.

66. Bolton MB, Tilley BC, Kuder J, *et al.*: The cost and effectiveness of an education program for adults who have asthma. *J Gen Intern Med* 1991, 6:401–407.

67. McFadden ER Jr, Elsanadi N, Dixon L, *et al.*: Protocol therapy for acute asthma: therapeutic benefits and cost savings. *Am J Med* 1995, 99:651–661.

68.• George MR, O'Dowd LC, Martin I, *et al.*: A comprehensive educational program improves clinical outcome measures in inner-city patients with asthma. *Arch Intern Med* 1999, 159:1710–1716.
Although asthma disease management programs are beneficial, are they cost effective? The inpatient intervention program of an inner-city indigent population showed cost savings, with fewer emergency department visits and a higher rate of compliance with routine office visits.

69. Burton WN, Connerty CM, Schultz AB, *et al.*: Bank One's worksite-based asthma disease management program. *J Occup Environ Med* 2001, 43:75–82.

70. Greineder DK, Loane KC, Parks P: Reduction in resource utilization by an asthma outreach program. *Arch Pediatr Adolesc Med* 1995, 149:415–420.

71. Kelso TM, Self TH, Rumbak MJ, *et al.*: Educational and long-term therapeutic intervention in the ED: effect on outcomes in adult indigent minority asthmatics. *Am J Emerg Med* 1995, 13:632–637.

72. Rossiter LF, Whitehurst-Cook MY, Small RE, *et al.*: The impact of disease management on outcomes and cost of care: a study of low-income asthma patients. *Inquiry* 2000, 37:188–202.

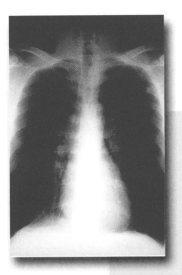

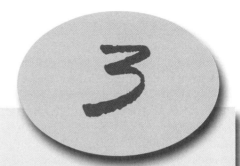

The Pathogenesis of Bronchial Asthma

Michael A. Kaliner

It is estimated that more than 15 million Americans currently have asthma. The incidence has increased by about 60% since the 1990s, not only in the United States but world-wide. Patients with asthma spent approximately $9.5 billion in 1997 on health care. Asthma is considered the greatest single cause of pediatric hospitalizations and the sixth most common cause for all hospitalizations, and is responsible for more than 5000 deaths per year (an increase of nearly 80% since the early 1990s) (Table 3-1).

The term *asthma* is derived from the Greek word for panting, or breathlessness, and thus might be considered a description of the primary symptom of this disease. Asthma can be defined clinically as recurrent airflow obstruction causing intermittent wheezing, breathlessness, chest tightness, and sometimes cough with sputum production. The National Asthma Education Panel, developed in conjunction with the National Heart, Lung, and Blood Institute, defined asthma in 1997 as having three components: airflow obstruction that is reversible (or nearly completely so), either spontaneously or in response to therapy; airway inflammation; and increased airway responsiveness to a variety of stimuli [1••].

CAUSES OF BRONCHIAL ASTHMA

Allergic Asthma

About 90% of asthmatic patients between 2 and 16 years of age are allergic, 70% of patients who are less than 30 years of age are allergic, and about 50% of those older than 30 years of age are concomitantly allergic [2]. Thus, coincidental allergies are by far the most common underlying condition leading to the development of asthma [3]. One should suspect allergy as a contributing factor when there is a family history of allergic diseases, when the clinical presentation includes seasonal exacerbations or exacerbations related to exposures to recognized allergens, when there is concomitant allergic rhinitis or other allergic disease, when a slight-to-moderate eosinophilia is present (300 to 1000/mm^3) or eosinophilia in the sputum is observed, or when the disease began at an early age or the patient is less than 40 years of age. Skin testing can be used to confirm IgE directed against incriminated allergens but does not establish a cause-and-effect relationship. Thus, patients may have a positive skin test but not have clinical symptoms of allergy or asthma when exposed to the incriminated allergen. Therefore, skin testing (or RAST [radioallergosorbent] testing) is only used to confirm the history and physical examination that suggest allergy. Levels of total IgE are of limited usefulness; only about 60% of allergic asthmatic patients have elevated IgE levels.

Because limiting exposure to allergens and allergy immunotherapy are both helpful in treating allergic asthmatic patients, a careful search for possible allergies is indicated in nearly all asthmatic patients. Current recommendations suggest that all asthmatic patients who wheeze more than 2 days per week should be evaluated by an allergist or other physician skilled in identifying allergic disease to institute prophylactic allergen avoidance measures.

It was once thought that allergic asthma was associated with a milder form of disease, but this contention has not been borne out. Allergic asthma is as severe as any other cause of asthma. Patients whose asthma began between the ages of 2 years and puberty generally have a good prognosis, while asthma appearing before 2 years of age may be of a more severe nature. Childhood asthma was once considered a disease that might be "outgrown." While some children with asthma do experience relief from asthma in their teens, asthma recurs in many patients between the ages of 20 and 40 years.

Table 3-1. ETIOLOGY OF BRONCHIAL ASTHMA

Causes of Bronchial Asthma

Allergic disease
  Allergic asthma
  Allergic bronchopulmonary aspergillosis
Infections
Bronchiolitis
  Upper respiratory tract infections
  Bronchitis
Industrial-occupational or environmental exposure
  Irritant exposures
  Allergen exposures
Chemical or drug ingestion
  Aspirin or other NSAIDs
  Sulfiting agents
  β-adrenergic antagonists
Vasculitis (Churg-Strauss allergic granulomatosis)
Idiopathic (intrinsic)

Conditions That May Worsen Asthma

Sinusitis
Gastroesophageal reflux disease
Pregnancy
Hyperthyroidism
Psychologic stress

Mast Cells and Asthma

The essential components of allergic reactions include allergens, IgE antibodies directed at antigenic determinants on the allergen, and activated mast cells that generate and release mediators and cytokines. Mast cell degranulation is followed by the late-phase reaction, involving activated lymphocytes and the infiltration of eosinophils [4,5•]. In order to initiate allergic responses, exposure to an appropriate antigen and a genetically determined capacity to respond with IgE production are required. Antigen presentation requires access of antigens to the mucous membrane, uptake by antigen-presenting cells, antigen processing, and stimulation of local antibody production. IgE production occurs in the same local environment as antigen presentation, probably in the draining lymph nodes. IgE production is regulated by locally produced helper factors thought to include cytokines produced by local Th2 helper cells. The IgE that is produced sensitizes mast cells in the same environment by binding to high-affinity receptors for IgE on the cell surface. Although no one is certain of the precise time involved, the production of sufficient IgE to render a subject allergic is thought to take several years or more [6,7].

Once sensitized, mast cells may degranulate upon subsequent allergen exposure. The bridging of IgE receptors by aggregation of IgE molecules bound to multivalent allergens initiates a biochemical reaction, which leads to the secretion of a range of chemical mediators from mast cells. These mediators then stimulate the surrounding tissues to elicit the allergic response [8•].

In man, the mast cell is found in the loose connective tissues of all organs, most notably around blood vessels, nerves, and lymphatics. Mast cells in the lung are found beneath the basement membranes of airways, near blood vessels in the submucosa, adjacent to submucous glands, scattered throughout the muscle bundles, in the intra-alveolar septa, and in the bronchial lumen. Mast cells appear in increased numbers in the epithelium after allergen exposure and are predominant in biopsies obtained during the allergy season. In the airways, there are about 20,000 mast cells/mm^3, and the mast cell represents 1% to 2% of alveolar cells [6,9].

Mediators of Anaphylaxis

There are four sources of mediators generated during the process of mast cell degranulation: preformed soluble molecules stored within the cytoplasmic granules, newly formed molecules quickly generated during the degranulation process, newly synthesized proteins transcribed over a period of hours after the initiation of degranulation, and macromolecular materials that derive from the granule matrix which may cause actions lasting for a prolonged period. The consequences of mediator release occur within minutes (immediate hypersensitivity) or may take hours to develop (late-phase allergic reactions) (Table 3-2).

The process of mast cell degranulation leads to transcription, synthesis, and secretion of potent cytokines over several hours, which likely contribute to the late-phase allergic response. Thus, mast cells synthesize and release interleukin (IL)-3, IL-4, IL-5, IL-6, IL-13, and IL-16 in addition to tumor necrosis factor and other inflammatory cytokines [8•,10]. Mast cells store IL-4 and secrete it as one of the granule mediators. Because IL-4 helps regulate IgE production, mast cell activation and release of IL-4 might assist IgE production [11,12].

Table 3-2. MAST CELL–DERIVED MEDIATORS

Preformed mediators rapidly released under
   physiologic conditions
  Histamine
  Eosinophil and neutrophil chemotactic factors
  Kininogenase
  Endothelin-1
  Arylsulfatase A
  Exoglycosidases
Mediators formed during the degranulation process
  Superoxide and other reactive oxygen species
  Leukotrienes C_4, D_4, E_4
  Prostaglandins$_2$, HETE$_5$, HHT
  Prostaglandin-generating factor of anaphylaxis
  Adenosine
  Bradykinin
  Platelet-activating factor
Mediators closely associated with the granule matrix
  Heparin, chondroitin sulfate E
  Tryptase
  Chymase
  Cathepsin G
  Carboxypeptidase
  Peroxidase
  Arylsulfatase B
  Inflammatory factors
  Superoxide dismutase
Cytokines transcribed after activation
  Interleukins-1, 2, 3, 4, 5, 6, 13, 16
  GM-CSF
  Macrophage inflammatory proteins 1α and 1β
  Monocyte chemotactic and activating factor
  TNF-α
  TCA-3
  Endothelin-1

*GM-CSF—granulocyte-macrophage colony-stimulating factor;
HETE—hydroxyeicosatetraenoic acid; HHT—hydroxyhepta-
decatrienoic acid; TNF—tumor necrosis factor.*

Once the allergic reaction is initiated, resident lymphocytes become activated, secreting their cytokines and chemokines. Eosinophils and some neutrophils are attracted to the area. They too release their granule contents, and the inflammatory process continues. The eosinophil infiltration is one of the specific hallmarks of asthma, and many investigators think that the eosinophils contribute to the pathogenesis of asthma [13,14••]. One of the clinical manifestations of this sequence of events is an increase in airway hyperreactivity [15]. There is data suggesting that increased airway reactivity after an allergen exposure is evident within a few hours and may last for weeks to months, suggesting prolonged inflammatory responses.

Allergens in Asthma

Inhalant allergens are most frequently involved in allergic respiratory diseases such as allergic rhinitis and asthma. These antigens, which directly impact on the respiratory mucosa, usually are derived from natural organic sources such as house dust, pollens, mold spores, and insect and animal emanations. Chemicals and irritants from the work place increasingly have been recognized as a cause of rhinitis, asthma, or both. These chemicals can act as allergens or irritants, or could influence the mucosal environment in such a manner as to predispose the individual towards developing an allergic response. Data suggest that diesel particulates can cause some patients to become allergic [16,17]. Inhalant allergic diseases may be episodic, seasonal (*ie*, hay fever), or perennial. The most important seasonal allergens are pollens. Despite popular belief, the heavy, sticky pollens of brightly colored flowers seldom cause allergy symptoms, as these pollen are spread by insects and not by wind currents. Exposure to nonseasonal allergens, mainly through inhalation but in some instances by ingestion, accounts for year-round allergies. Among the inhalants, dust mites, mold allergens, cockroaches, and animal emanations are responsible for most perennial allergic asthma.

Diagnosis of Allergy

Despite the development of in vitro methods of detecting IgE antibodies, skin testing (prick or intradermal) with appropriate allergens is the least time-consuming, most sensitive, most useful, and also the least expensive method to confirm the presence of allergen-specific IgE. Skin testing can be performed on infants as young as 1 to 4 months of age, although age dictates both the choice of allergens used and the clinical conditions for which they can be used. In infants under 1 year of age, food antigens are the likely offenders, causing eczema or asthma. Inhalant allergens are more likely to be involved after 2 to 4 years of exposure, although sensitization to indoor allergens can occur much more quickly. In exceptional cases, such as in patients with extensive eczema or marked dermatographism that negates use of skin tests, in vitro assays for serum IgE antibodies by radioallergosorbent, fluorescent-allergosorbent, multiple-thread allergosorbent, or enzyme-linked immunosorbent test techniques might be substituted for direct testing. With either in vitro testing or skin tests, however, it is essential that the relevance of the results be correlated to the patient's current clinical problems and their detailed history.

Allergic Bronchopulmonary Aspergillosis

Allergic bronchopulmonary aspergillosis (ABPA) was described in England as a progressive form of asthma leading eventually to pulmonary fibrosis. It was thought that the damp climate in England was responsible for the relatively frequent occurrence there and infrequent occurrence elsewhere. However, recent studies in the United States have revealed the presence of ABPA in the Midwest as well.

Compared to other forms of asthma, ABPA is seen infrequently and may be heralded by its specific clinical characteristics. There are five pulmonary disease patterns elicited by exposure to *Aspergillus* species: allergic asthma induced by exposure to mold spores in subjects with IgE antibodies directed at *Aspergillus* antigens; hypersensitivity pneumonitis in response to mold-spore inhalation in nonatopic patients who develop IgG-class antibodies and cellular immunity to *Aspergillus* antigens; a fungus ball or aspergilloma, a saprophytic colonization of a pre-existing cavity (as in old tuberculosis or sarcoidosis); invasive aspergillosis, an overwhelming diffuse pneumonia due to *Aspergillus* in an immunocompromised host; and ABPA, a subacute inflammatory reaction elicited by both IgE- and IgG-mediated immune responses directed at *Aspergillus* species growing in the respiratory tree. The precise incidence of ABPA in the United States is not known, but while

the disease is not rare, it is seen uncommonly. Diagnostic criteria for ABPA have been established and are summarized in Table 3-3 [18].

There are 5 stages of ABPA: stage 1 is the form of ABPA when the diagnostic criteria listed in Table 3-3 are met. The patient generally exhibits moderate to severe asthma, with purulent mucus production, eosinophilia, an abnormal chest radiograph, and high IgE levels. Skin testing to *Aspergillus* produces a positive immediate (and oftentimes late) reaction. The possible presence of bronchiectasis is analyzed by CT scans, and serologic testing for IgG antibodies directed at *Aspergillus* is performed. At this point, patients generally should be treated aggressively with corticosteroids, with a resultant remission (stage 2).

Once the patient has experienced a remission, corticosteroids are reduced to either every-other-day use or are removed entirely. At this stage, most experts continue patients on moderate doses of inhaled corticosteroids. Stage 3 occurs if an exacerbation eventuates, and may lead to the stage where chronic corticosteroids (either daily or every-other-day) are necessary (stage 4). Diffuse pulmonary fibrosis (stage 5) can develop or be the presenting stage at which ABPA is recognized. The importance of making the diagnosis of ABPA rests on the aggressive use of oral and inhaled corticosteroids to try to prevent the development of pulmonary fibrosis.

Infections

All patients with asthma may experience a worsening of their symptoms concurrent with upper respiratory tract infections, bronchitis, or influenza-type illnesses. Moreover, children may experience their initial asthma as a consequence of viral bronchiolitis, which commonly

---

Table 3-3. DIAGNOSTIC CRITERIA FOR ALLERGIC BRONCHOPULMONARY ASPERGILLOSIS

Primary criteria
  Asthma
  Eosinophilia (> 1000/mm^3)
  Positive immediate skin test reactions to *Aspergillus* antigen
  IgG antibodies to *Aspergillus* antigens
  Marked increase in IgE level
  Pulmonary infiltrates, often transitory
  Central, saccular bronchiectasis
  Elevated serum IgE and IgG to *Aspergillus fumigatus* compared
    to control groups
Secondary criteria
  Aspergillus in sputum
  History of expectorated brown plugs or specks
  Late-phase (or Arthus) skin test results to *Aspergillus* antigen

develops into chronic asthma. Finally, some patients have no clinical asthma except during concurrent respiratory infections. Some adult asthmatic patients trace their chronic asthma to a viral respiratory infection that led directly to chronic and oftentimes severe, nonallergic asthma [19].

Bronchiolitis

Bronchiolitis is an acute viral infection of the bronchioles, generally seen only in children less than 2 years of age. It is usually accompanied by upper respiratory tract symptoms, which may precede the lower respiratory tract involvement by 2 to 3 days. Patients experience cough (sometimes croup), dyspnea, rapid respirations, fever, and sometimes prostration. Physical examination reveals retractions, rapid respiration, occasional rales, and wheezing. Respiratory syncytial virus is the most frequent etiologic agent, but adenoviruses, rhinovirus, parainfluenza virus, and others may also cause the disease. It is thought that infections worsen asthma by reflexes triggered from the upper airway and sinuses, from direct effects of the virus on the airway epithelium, and possibly from IgE antibodies directed at the infectious agent. The common events are increased airway inflammation and increased airway hyperreactivity.

Occupational Asthma

The air we breathe may contain allergens of natural origin or allergens generated as a consequence of industrial or environmental processes. In addition, chemicals in the air may irritate the airways and lower the threshold for airway responsiveness. These same irritants may also be allergens for susceptible individuals. Besides industry-related exposure, modern life generates pollutants that linger in the air, generally in or around cities, which may damage the lungs. Thus, everyone is at risk of breathing potentially harmful substances, while asthmatic patients are at much greater risk of reacting adversely to them. Certain pollutants such as ozone increase airway reactivity even in normal subjects, and asthma may be exacerbated during pollution with either industrial or photochemical smog [20]. Approximately 2% to 15% of all cases of adult-onset asthma in men are of occupational origin (depending on the level of airway irritants and allergens in any working area).

Suspicion of occupational lung disease should be raised by the history of cough or chest tightness in relationship to the work place. In asthmatic patients, worsening of symptoms every week, especially early in the week, may be noted. Such suspicions can be strengthened by evidence of wheezing or abnormal pulmonary function after occupational exposure. Only a few appropriate occupation-related antigens are available for skin testing, so provocation with the suspected airborne chemical or particulate may be the only confirmatory test available. Some of the common occupational exposures leading to asthma are listed in Table 3-4.

The prevalence of occupational asthma varies with the exposure and the provocative agent. While only about 5% of workers regularly exposed to toluene diisocyanate develop asthma, 10% to 45% of workers exposed to relatively high concentrations of proteolytic enzymes in laundry detergent in the past were affected. The pattern of response may be immediate, late, or both. The underlying mechanism involves direct irritation and/or the induction of immunologic processes, including IgE- or IgG-type responses. Removal of the worker from the work place may reduce or reverse the airways disease, although there are many exceptions.

Chemical or Drug Exposure

ASPIRIN AND NSAIDs

It is estimated that 3% to 5% of asthmatic patients reliably will worsen after the ingestion of aspirin or other NSAIDs [21]. Ingestion of aspirin or other NSAIDs may provoke either of two responses: respiratory responses, including bronchorrhea, rhinorrhea, bronchospasm, conjunctivitis, lacrimation, and flushing, or urticaria and angioedema. Rarely, combinations of the two patterns are seen. Aspirin-sensitive patients may be recognized by the presence of nasal polyps, nonallergic rhinitis, persistent sinusitis, and asthma associated with moderate

Table 3-4. CAUSATIVE AGENTS IN OCCUPATIONAL ASTHMA

Category	Active Substance
Metal salts	Salts of platinum, nickel, chrome
Wood dusts	Oak, western red cedar (plicatic acid), redwood, mahogany
Vegetable dusts	Grain (mite, weevil), flour, castor bean, green coffee, gums, cottonseed, cotton dust
Industrial chemicals	Toluene diisocyanate, polyvinyl chloride, phthalic and trimellitic anhydrides, ethylene diamine
Pharmaceutical agents	Penicillins, phenylglycine acid chloride, ethylene diamine
Biologic enzymes	Bacillus subtilis, pancreatic enzymes
Animal and insect	Rodent urine protein, canine saliva or materials, feline saliva or secretions

eosinophilia (> 1000/mm^3). The frequency of NSAID sensitivity increases with age, although children and families have been described with clear-cut reactivity. There may be a wide range of associated allergies, but many subjects (about 50%) are not allergic.

The mechanism responsible for NSAID sensitivity appears to involve eicosanoid production (increased production of leukotrienes C and D) plus exaggerated responses to leukotrienes. NSAIDs inhibit the cyclo-oxygenase enzyme system responsible for prostaglandin formation, thereby reducing prostaglandin production and leading to increased production of lipoxygenase products. It has been suggested that NSAIDs cause asthma by reducing the formation of prostaglandins such as PGE that help maintain normal airway function while increasing the formation of asthma-provoking eicosanoids, including leukotrienes C and D. Recent work in humans has confirmed this suspicion, demonstrating that sensitive patients exposed to NSAIDs secrete excessive quantities of leukotrienes in their respiratory tract and develop both rhinitis and asthma.

Aspirin sensitivity should be suspected in any asthmatic patient with nasal polyposis, chronic sinusitis, and eosinophilia. The polyposis and sinusitis may precede the onset of recognized NSAID sensitivity by years. Under some circumstances, selected patients with this syndrome can be "desensitized" to NSAIDs by repeated oral challenges with aspirin, and may remain unresponsive to subsequent NSAID exposure if oral NSAIDs are given daily. Selective COX-2 inhibitors can be used safely in these subjects.

SULFITING AGENTS AND ASTHMA

Sulfiting agents include sulfur dioxide and any of its five sulfite salts, which are added to foods to prevent non-enzymatic browning, to inhibit growth of micro-organisms, to inhibit enzymatic activity, and to act as antioxidants and reducing agents, bleaching agents, processing aids, pH controls, and for stabilization. In 1986, in response to the recognition that sulfites could precipitate asthma, the Food and Drug Administration banned their use on fruits and vegetables served fresh. Other products, like beer and wine, are now labeled as containing sulfites. Sulfites are generally converted under acid conditions to sulfur dioxide, and are largely liberated during the processing and cooking of foods. It is thought that ingestion of sulfites leads to the liberation of sulfur dioxide in the mouth and stomach, which is then inspired. In very sensitive asthmatic patients, inhalation of sulfur dioxide, even in small amounts, provokes asthma attacks. It may be anticipated that only the most hyperresponsive asthmatic patients will react to ingested sulfites.

Sulfite sensitivity should be suspected in asthmatic patients who worsen in relationship to eating processed foods containing sulfites (*eg*, dried fruit, fruit juices, or processed potatoes) or wine and beer. Sulfite-sensitive asthmatic patients should be advised to wear an emblem identifying them as sulfite-sensitive and to carry a bronchodilator metered-dose inhaler and injectable epinephrine.

β-ADRENERGIC ANTAGONISTS

The β-adrenergic blocking agent, propranolol hydrochloride, was introduced in 1964, and it was immediately recognized that asthmatic patients were adversely affected by this drug. β-Adrenergic blocking agents are used to treat many diseases, such as glaucoma, migraine, hypertension, myocardial infarction, and tremor. The underlying mechanism by which β blockade induces asthma is thought to involve prevention of the normal β-adrenergic inhibitory influences on the parasympathetic ganglia in the airways. The reduction in β-adrenergic inhibitory influences at this level thereby allows relatively unimpaired cholinergic constrictor influences to develop. In the opinion of most specialists, asthmatic patients should not take β-adrenergic blocking agents. Of note, worsening of the status of a previously stable asthmatic patient should provoke inquiries as to other medications given by practitioners, in search of possible β-adrenergic blocking agent administration. There is an ever-widening use of β-blockers, and some β-blockers are now "hidden" in combination tablets, along with diuretics.

Vasculitis

In 1951, Churg and Strauss described a vasculitic process that had pathologic findings and clinical features warranting the designation of a separate disease entity, allergic angiitis and granulomatosis. Churg-Strauss syndrome is characterized pathologically by necrotizing vasculitis, tissue infiltration by eosinophils, and extravascular granulomas [22]. The disease has three phases, beginning with a prodrome of allergic asthma and allergic rhinitis that may exist for many years; the second phase includes eosinophilia along with the development of pulmonary eosinophilic infiltrates resembling Löffler's syndrome, eosinophilic pneumonia, or eosinophilic gastroenteritis; and the third phase is the vasculitic phase involving pulmonary vessels (96%), skin (67%), peripheral nerves (63%), gastrointestinal tract (42%), heart (38%), and kidney (38%).

Churg-Strauss syndrome affects males and females equally. The onset of the first stage, involving allergic rhinitis and asthma, occurs in young adults, while the vasculitis becomes apparent by age 35 to 50 years, and is suggested by the development of eosinophilia above 1500/mm^3, infiltrates in chest roentgenogram, sinusitis and otitis, hypertension, abdominal pain, purpura, urticaria, subcutaneous nodules, mononeuritis multiplex, general malaise, persistent low-grade fever, and weight loss. Many patients have an increased IgE level and the presence of rheumatoid factor. The prognosis in untreated patients is poor. Treatment generally consists of corticosteroids alone or combined with cytotoxic therapy.

Although Churg-Strauss syndrome is rare (occurring in approximately 1 of every 30,000 to 50,000 asthmatic patients), the recent introduction of leukotriene antagonists has led to an increased recognition of this disease. Thus, asthmatic patients who are weaned off oral corticosteroids and develop a flu-like syndrome with eosinophilia should be suspected of having Churg-Strauss syndrome [23]. In that circumstance, a chest radiograph is indicated to search for pulmonary infiltrates.

Idiopathic or Intrinsic Asthma

Up to 30% of asthmatic patients, particularly those over 30 years of age, have no apparent cause for their asthma. Their disease often begins with a severe upper or lower respiratory tract infection or sinusitis, and progresses to asthma in short order. Such patients often have coexistent sinusitis and nasal polyposis, as well as vasomotor rhinitis. It has been thought that such patients have a worse prognosis than other types of asthmatic patients, but this is certainly not predictable. In such patients, it is necessary to search for factors that might worsen asthma. Many patients with idiopathic asthma regularly produce mucus and have a history of tobacco smoking; such patients may have an asthmatic form of bronchitis.

CONDITIONS ASSOCIATED WITH EXACERBATIONS OF ASTHMA

Several clinical conditions are closely associated with and may worsen asthma by diverse mechanisms.

Sinusitis

An association between asthma and concomitant sinus disease has been recognized since the early part of the 20th century and has been reconfirmed repeatedly both in children and adults [24]. It is estimated that 60% to 75% of patients with severe asthma have concomitant sinusitis, and that 20% to 30% of sinusitis patients have asthma. Slavin [25] treated 33 adults with asthma and concomitant sinusitis medically or surgically. After therapy, 28 of 33 patients believed their asthma was improved, and 15 of 18 patients reduced their steroid requirement by 85%. Anecdotal observations suggest that the difficulty of treating asthmatic patients with sinusitis is proportional to the degree of sinusitis present. Physicians treating asthmatic patients should be alert to the possibilities that sinusitis frequently coexists in their patients, and that the severity of the sinusitis may influence the course of the bronchial asthma [25]. Although the precise mechanism by which sinusitis worsens asthma is not known with certainty, there is substantial evidence that a naso-sino-bronchial reflex exists that increases airway irritability and airflow obstruction.

In both children and adults, symptoms from acute sinusitis include purulent nasal discharge, persistent coughing (especially at night), and the presence of purulent mucus in the nasal vault and pharynx. Facial pain, headache, and fever occur less frequently. Most acute episodes of sinusitis follow upper respiratory infections, while some then develop into chronic or recurrent problems. Chronic sinusitis is associated with persistent or recurrent purulent nasal discharge, cough, headache or facial pressure, hyposmia, fetor oris, occasional fever, and worsening of asthma.

The physician should consider diagnostic studies for sinusitis whenever symptoms of upper respiratory infection or rhinitis are more protracted than expected, the patient has dull to intense throbbing pain over the involved sinus area, the patient's asthma is not responding appropriately to medications, or the patient has prolonged or persistent bronchitis that has failed to respond to appropriate therapy. On physical examination, edema and discoloration below the eyes may occasionally be observed. The nasal mucosa is inflamed, and a purulent discharge frequently is seen on the floor of the nose, beneath the middle turbinate, or draining down the throat.

Generally, radiographs with the findings of opacification, noticeable membrane thickening, or air-fluid levels within one or more sinuses confirm the suspicion of sinusitis. CT scans are much more sensitive than radiographs, provide better images, and are the diagnostic procedure of choice.

Gastroesophageal Reflux

The presence of gastroesophageal reflux (GERD) is suggested by heartburn, especially postprandial, that is increased on bending over, lying down, or straining. Confirmatory tests include radiographic demonstration of reflux, finding acid in the esophagus after instilling hydrochloric acid into the stomach, 24-hour monitoring of intraesophageal pH, or Bernstein's test, in which hydrochloric acid is dripped onto the lower esophagus and symptoms are elicited.

As many as 45% to 65% of adults and children with asthma have GERD [26]. The mechanism by which GERD produces asthma appears to involve triggering intraesophageal reflexes by acid stimulation, resulting in cholinergic reflexes into the airways and resultant bronchial constriction. While GERD may be asymptomatic in asthmatic patients, the strongest association is with nighttime asthma symptoms, especially night cough and nocturnal wheezing. GERD should be suspected in patients (especially children) with nocturnal exacerbations (especially cough) and recurrent heartburn. Effective management of GERD concomitantly may reduce asthma in some, but not all patients.

Pregnancy

Asthma complicates 4% of pregnancies, and is the most common chronic disease to do so [27]. About one third of pregnant asthmatic patients will improve during pregnancy, one third will be unchanged, and one third will worsen. Pregnancy is associated with an increase in tidal volume and a 20% to 50% increase in minute ventilation. This change has been attributed to a response to increased circulating progesterone, which acts as a respiratory stimulant. Arterial blood gases reflect a compensated respiratory alkalosis due to overventilation. Characteristic blood gases have a pH of 7.40 to 7.47, a partial arterial carbon dioxide pressure of 25 to 32 mm Hg, and a partial arterial oxygen pressure of 100 to 106 mm Hg.

Earlier studies suggested that the likelihood of prematurity and low-birth-weight infants and both perinatal and maternal death rates were increased in asthmatic women, but current studies do not confirm these problems in properly treated patients. The clinical course of asthma during pregnancy may be predicted by the behavior in the first trimester, and most patients have the same pattern of response with repeated pregnancies. When a pregnant asthmatic patient worsens, pulmonary emboli should always be considered as a possible cause.

The management of asthma in pregnancy involves the extensive use of inhaled medications and careful avoidance of any medication which might adversely affect the fetus. Because the uterus compromises the thoracic space late in pregnancy, it is very important to maintain excellent control of pregnant asthmatic patients throughout the pregnancy in order to avoid exacerbations during the last trimester.

PATHOPHYSIOLOGY

Pathologically, the airflow obstruction of asthma is due to combinations of bronchial smooth-muscle contraction, mucosal edema and inflammation, and viscid mucus secretion. The disease involves inflammation of large and small airways but not alveoli [28]. Pathologic examination of asthmatic lungs reveals that small bronchi and bronchioles are principally involved, there is extensive airway denudation due to loss or thinning of the epithelium, and the goblet cells are often markedly hyperplastic. The basement membrane is thickened due to the deposition of sub-

basement membrane collagen, and the lamina propria is infiltrated with CD4+ lymphocytes, mast cells, eosinophils, and neutrophils. The smooth muscle is hyperplastic and contracted. The submucous glands are hyperplastic and are actively secreting mucus. The airway lumen is often filled with secretions containing mucus, edema fluid, eosinophils, inspissated mucus plugs, Charcot-Leyden crystals, and Curschmann's spirals (Table 3-5).

The pathophysiologic event causing asthma is a reduction in small airway diameter. This abnormality leads to an increase in airway resistance, which makes it difficult for inspired air to escape the lungs, leading to a reduction in forced expiratory volumes and flow rates and hyperinflation of the lung with air trapping. The increase in the work of breathing creates a sense of breathlessness and generates inequities of alveolar ventilation and perfusion, which causes hypoxemia. Initially, blood gases exhibit reduced carbon dioxide levels, reflecting overventilation in an attempt to maintain oxygen levels. If airflow obstruction worsens or persists, hypoxemia develops. The last and most dangerous change in blood gases is hypercarbia, a sign of impending respiratory failure.

Associated with the dynamics of air trapping are ECG changes reflecting P pulmonale, and with hypoxemia, increases in pulmonary arterial pressures. These changes may lead to pulsus paradoxus. The presence of pulsus paradoxus, and the need to use the accessory muscles of respiration, reflect the severity of the airflow obstruction and may be useful clinical signs.

Because airway obstruction occurs within minutes of an inciting event and can reverse itself within minutes of treatment with β-adrenergic agonists, it is likely that airway smooth muscle constriction contributes significantly to airflow obstruction. Of the recognized factors capable of causing bronchial smooth muscle contraction, mast cell mediators and several neurohormones are probably the most important.

Edema of airway mucosa is due to increased venular and capillary permeability with leakage of serum proteins into interstitial areas. In the earliest careful descriptions of asthmatic lungs, the presence of edema was the most striking abnormality. More recently, mucosal edema has been directly observed by bronchoscopy after airway antigen challenge, and plasma protein exudation after antigen challenge has been documented. These observations combine to support the growing appreciation of the importance of airway mucosal edema in asthma [29]. Vascular permeability occurs within several minutes of allergen challenge and persists for 30 to 60 minutes. The late-phase allergic reaction is thought to be due to a combination of edema of the airways and the presence of increased inflammatory cells.

The mucosa of patients who have died in status asthmaticus contains mixed cellular infiltrates consisting of eosinophils, neutrophils, macrophages, lymphocytes, mast cells, and plasma cells. In the airway lumen, admixed in the

Table 3-5. PATHOLOGY OF ASTHMA

Denudation of airway epithelium
Sub-basement membrane fibrosis and collagen deposition
Airway wall edema
Mast cell activation
Inflammatory cell infiltration
  Neutrophils
  Eosinophils
  Lymphocytes (Th2 cells)
Mucus hypersecretion
  Goblet cell hyperplasia
Mucus gland hyperactivity

abundant secretions are eosinophils and eosinophil-derived Charcot-Leyden crystals, neutrophils, and desquamated clumps of epithelial cells (Creola bodies). The same pathologic changes are found in the lungs of allergic or nonallergic asthmatic patients, suggesting that there is a commonality in the pathophysiologic events.

Recent biopsy studies of the airways of asthmatic patients after allergen challenge have shown that within minutes of allergen exposure, mast cells degranulate and release mediators detectable in the bronchoalveolar lavage fluid, the superficial vessels swell and become permeable, and edema is formed. Biopsies done several hours later reveal edema, the increased expression of adhesion molecules on blood vessels, and increased cells in the mucosa expressing molecules which can bind to the adhesion molecules. The mucosa initially becomes infiltrated with neutrophils, and, after 12 to 24 hours, with eosinophils. The eosinophil releases some of its granule contents, as reflected in the presence of major basic protein in airway biopsies or pathologic specimens. Eosinophil-derived proteins can cause epithelial denudation, mucus secretion, and irritability of the airway. Of all the infiltrating cells, the eosinophil is the most specific, being seen rather exclusively in asthma and not with other inflammatory diseases of the airway.

Biopsies have also indicated that the lymphocytes in the asthmatic mucosa are primarily CD4+, express genes for the production of IL-4 and IL-5 (suggesting that they are of the Th2 phenotype associated with increased inflammation, prolonged eosinophil survival, and increased IgE production), and become activated after allergen challenge. The cytokines produced by Th2 lymphocytes can not only enhance IgE production, but also support many of the pathologic events that occur in the airways of asthmatic patients. This population of lymphocytes appears to be specifically expanded in atopic subjects. Moreover, allergen exposure in allergic individuals is the stimulus for Th2 expansion during the late-phase allergic reaction and in airways of asthmatic patients. Thus, there is a growing body of evidence that allergy and asthma are associated with an expanded Th2 population of lymphocytes which act to support the events occurring in the asthmatic airway [30•,31•,32•].

Pathologic examinations of patients who have died in status asthmaticus almost always reveal diffuse collections of mucus, which appear to contribute significantly to obstruction of the airways. The precise mechanisms responsible for increased mucus production have only been partly defined.

One of the absolute features of asthma is an exaggerated nonspecific airway reactivity to a variety of irritating stimuli. Thus, asthmatic patients develop airway obstruction in response to natural exposures (cold air, exercise, irritating chemicals, laughing, and coughing) or to provocations in the laboratory (histamine, methacholine, cold air-hyperventilation). Airway hyperresponsiveness is found universally in asthmatic patients, in a portion of patients with chronic bronchitis, in some patients with allergic rhinitis, and in 3% to 8% of otherwise normal patients. There is a close correlation between the degree of increased responsiveness and disease severity; patients with the most reactive airways often require oral corticosteroids for control, while milder degrees of abnormality predict the requirement for fewer medications [15]. Hyperresponsiveness increases after allergen exposure, late-phase allergic reactions, viral infections (especially influenza-type infections), and ozone exposure. Conversely, airway hyperresponsiveness may return to normal after allergen avoidance, allergy immunotherapy, or treatment with cromolyn or inhaled or oral corticosteroids. In recent years, airway hyperresponsiveness and airway inflammation have become targets in asthma therapy, supporting the use of anti-inflammatory agents to reduce airway reactivity.

Denudation of airway epithelial surfaces with the appearance of epithelial clumps in expectorated secretions accompanies severe asthma. The denuded epithelial surfaces may be replaced by goblet cells, resulting in goblet cell hyperplasia and increased mucus secretion. The mechanism for epithelial desquamation has not been systematically examined, although several mediators might participate. Edema of the airway results in movement of edema fluid between epithelial cells and into the airway lumen. This process may also contribute to weakening the epithelial bond. Lymphocyte-derived cytokines may also contribute to these phenomena.

FACTORS PREDISPOSING TO ASTHMA

Genetic Factors

When differentiating asthma from other obstructive airways disease, it is always relevant to ask if family members experience the same symptoms. If the asthmatic patient is atopic, familial concordance is likely to be present, while nonallergic asthmatic patients have fewer tendencies for genetic transmission. While the specific gene encoding asthma has not been identified with certainty, research is currently underway [33,34].

Autonomic Dysfunction

An imbalance of the autonomic nervous system with a blunted β-adrenergic response and hyperresponsiveness of the α-adrenergic and cholinergic systems have been documented in asthmatic patients, although this defect is not unique for asthma. These data suggest that asthmatic patients have an inherently reduced ability to sustain open airways, and a tendency for airflow obstruction based upon an inherent defect in their autonomic balance [35].

In summary, the events causing asthma involve a very complex interaction between inflammatory cells, the responding cells in the airway, and the development of airflow obstruction and possibly airway remodeling.

There are still many ambiguous areas, but most events seem to have certain elements in common: the infiltration of eosinophils, activation of mast cells and lymphocytes, and the generation of airflow obstruction and airway hyperactivity.

REFERENCES AND RECOMMENDED READING

Papers of particular interest, published recently, have been highlighted as:
* *Of importance*
** *Of major importance*

1.•• National Heart, Lung, and Blood Institute, National Asthma Education and Prevention Program: *Expert Panel Report 2: Guidelines for the Diagnosis and Management of Asthma.* Bethesda, MD: National Institutes of Health, Pub. No. 97-4051; 1997.
Essential reading for anyone involved in asthma care. These reports revolutionized the understanding and treatment of asthma.

2. Kaliner MA, Lemanske R: Rhinitis and asthma. *JAMA* 1992, 268:2807.

3. Burrows B, Martinez FD, Halonen M, *et al.*: Association of asthma with serum IgE levels and skin test reactivity to allergens. *N Engl J Med* 1989, 320:271–277.

4. Holgate S: The cellular and mediator basis of asthma in relationship to natural history. *Lancet* 1997, 350(suppl 2):5–9.

5.• Lemanske RF, Kaliner M: Late phase allergic reactions. In *Allergy Principles and Practice*, edn 4. Edited by Middleton E, Reed CE, Ellis EF, *et al.* St. Louis: Mosby; 1993:320–361.
The most comprehensive review of the late-phase reaction.

6. White MV, Kaliner MA: Mast cells and asthma. In *Asthma: Its Pathology and Treatment.* Edited by Kaliner MA, Persson C, Barnes P. New York: Marcel Dekker; 1990:409–440.

7. Scott T, Kaliner MA: Mast cells in asthma. In *The Mast Cell in Health and Disease.* Edited by Kaliner MA, Metcalfe DD. New York: Marcel Dekker; 1992:575–592.

8.• Schwartz LB: Mast cells and basophils. In *Inflammatory Mechanisms in Allergic Diseases.* Edited by Zweiman B, Schwartz LB. New York: Marcel Dekker; 2002:3–42.
An excellent, current review of mast cells and basophils, published in a very interesting book cited several times in this bibliography.

9. Kaliner MA: Pathogenesis of asthma. In *Clinical Immunology: Principles and Practice.* Edited by Rich RR. St Louis: Mosby; 1996:909–923.

10. Costa JJ, Metcalfe DD: Mast cell cytokines. In *The Mast Cell in Health and Disease.* Edited by Kaliner MA, Metcalfe DD. New York: Marcel Dekker; 1992.

11. Bradding P, Feather IH, Howarth PH, *et al.*: Interleukin 4 is localized to and released by human mast cells. *J Exp Med* 1992, 176:1381.

12. Gauchat JF, Henchoz S, Mazzei G, *et al.*: Induction of human IgE synthesis in B cells by mast cells and basophils. *Nature* 365:340, 1993.

13. Robinson DS, Wardlaw AJ, Kay AB. Eosinophils. In *Inflammatory Mechanisms in Allergic Diseases.* Edited by Zweiman B, Schwartz LB. New York: Marcel Dekker; 2002:43–76.

14.•• Eapen SS, Busse WW. Asthma. In *Inflammatory Mechanisms in Allergic Diseases.* Edited by Zweiman B, Schwartz LB. New York: Marcel Dekker; 2002:325–354.
An excellent review of the role of inflammatory cells in asthma pathophysiology. Highly recommended for a current update that goes far beyond this chapter.

15. Louis R, Lau LC, Bron AQ, *et al.*: The relationship between airways inflammation and asthma severity. *Am J Respir Crit Care Med* 2000, 161:9–16.

16. Diaz-Sanchez D, Penichet-Garcia M, Saxon A: Diesel exhaust particles directly induce activated mast cells to degranulate and increase histamine levels and symptom severity. *J Allergy Clin Immunol* 2000, 106:1140–1146.

17. Polosa R: The interaction between particulate air pollution and allergens in enhancing allergic and airway responses. *Curr Allergy Rep* 2001, 1:102–107.

18. Rosenberg M, Patterson R, Mintzer R, *et al.*: Clinical and immunologic criteria for the diagnosis of allergic bronchopulmonary aspergillosis. *Ann Int Med* 1997, 86:405–411.

19. Papadopoulos NG, Johnston SL: The role of viruses in the induction and progression of asthma. *Curr Allergy Rep* 2001, 1:144–152.

20. Burnett RT, Dales RE, Raizenne ME, *et al.*: Effects of low ambient levels of ozone and sulfates on the frequency of respiratory admissions to Ontario hospitals. *Environ Res* 1994, 65:172–194.

21. Stevenson D, Simon RA, Zuraw B: Sensitivity to aspirin and non-steroidal anti-inflammatory drugs. In *Allergy: Principles and Practice*, edn 7. Edited by Middleton E, Ellis EF, Yunginger JW. St. Louis: Mosby. In press.

22. Katz P, Fauci AS: Systemic vasculitis. In *Immunological Diseases*, edn 4. Edited by Samter M. Boston: Little Brown; 1988.

23. Weller PF, Plaut M, Taggert V, Trontell A: The relationship of asthma therapy and Churg-Strauss Syndrome: NIH workshop summary report. *J Allergy Clin Immunol* 2001, 108:175–183.

24. Bresiani M, Paradis L, Des Roches A, *et al.*: Rhinosinusitis in severe asthma. *J Allergy Clin Immunol* 2001, 107:73–80.

25. Slavin RG: Nasal polyps and sinusitis. In *Inflammatory Mechanisms in Allergic Diseases.* Edited by Zweiman B, Schwartz LB. New York: Marcel Dekker; 2002:295–310.

26. Field SK, Underwood M, Brant R, Cowie RL: Prevalence of gastro-esophageal reflux symptoms in asthma. *Chest* 1996, 109:316–322.

27. Schatz M: Interrelationships between asthma and pregnancy: a literature review. *J Allergy Clin Immunol* 1999, 103:S330–S336.

28. Hamid Q, Song Y, Kotsimbos TC, *et al.*: Inflammation of small airways in asthma. *J Allergy Clin Immunol* 1997, 100:44–51.

29. Kaliner MA: Allergic inflammation and asthma. In *Progress in Allergy and Clinical Immunology*, vol 3. Edited by Johansson SGO. Seattle: Hogrefe and Huber; 1995:301–305.

30.• Lee NA, Gelfand EW, Lee JL: Pulmonary T cells and eosinophils: coconspirators or independent triggers of allergic respiratory pathology? *J Allergy Clin Immunol* 2001, 107:945–957.
An interesting discussion of the roles of infiltrating cells in asthma.

31.• Cameron L, Hamid Q: Regulation of allergic airways inflammation by cytokines and glucocorticoids. *Curr Allergy Rep* 2001, 1:153–163.
Highly recommended for anyone interested in the latest list of cytokines and their possible roles in asthma.

32.• Romangnani S: Lymphocytes. In *Inflammatory Mechanisms in Allergic Diseases.* Edited by Zweiman B, Schwartz LB. New York: Marcel Dekker; 2002:97–124.
A very current review by the scientist responsible for opening up our understanding of Th1 and Th2 lymphocytes.

33. Wjst M, Fischer G, Immervoll T, *et al.*: A genome-wide search for linkage to asthma. *Genomics* 1999, 58:1–8.

34. Ober C: Susceptibility genes in asthma and allergy. *Curr Allergy Asthma Rep* 2001, 1:174–179.

35. Lemanske RF Jr, Kaliner MA: Autonomic nervous system abnormalities and asthma. *Am Rev Respir Dis* 1990, 141:S157–S161.

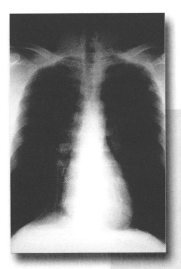

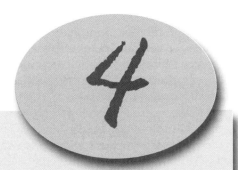

Airway Remodeling in Asthma

William J. Calhoun

In a general sense, the term *remodeling* means structural change to a tissue or organ that develops in response to physiologic or pathophysiologic processes. Thus, left ventricular hypertrophy can be considered a remodeling response to hypertension or aortic stenosis. In the airway, structural changes develop as a consequence of many chronic inflammatory diseases of the airway, including asthma. These structural, anatomic changes may or may not be associated with physiologic or functional alterations, which are discussed in this chapter. As applied to the airway in asthma, the term *remodeling* has taken on a misleadingly broader connotation to include irreversible airflow limitation, bronchial hyperresponsiveness, and a lack of physiologic improvement with otherwise effective asthma therapy. This chapter defines airway remodeling in the narrow sense of structural change of the airway as a consequence of asthma. Common changes of airway remodeling in asthma include thickening of the reticular basement membrane (RBM) (or lamina reticularis), goblet cell hyperplasia, altered matrix proteins, increased mass of airway smooth muscle, and increases in submucosal vasculature.

A relevant question is why airway remodeling is thought to be important; an important related question is what clinical significance is in airway remodeling. Patients with asthma virtually never complain of "remodeled airways." Rather, they have cough, breathlessness, shortness of breath, and wheezing. Patients may be concerned about the long-term effects of asthma or its treatment, but they often do not understand the underlying pathology. One answer lies in the possibility that structural changes of remodeling underlie key aspects of asthma pathophysiology, including airway hyperresponsiveness, mucus hypersecretion, and fixed airway obstruction. The data that link these critically important asthma outcomes with structural airway changes are not compelling, and they do not prove a linkage between remodeling and more traditional asthma outcomes. However, the data do raise important questions and may have substantial implications for understanding asthma and its consequences. Another answer involves the matter of therapeutics and the response of structural changes to asthma therapies. Current data are equivocal on this point but suggest that existing therapies may be able to alter at least some of the structural changes associated with remodeling.

Remodeling is exceedingly common in asthma [1••,2••]; it is present both in adults and children [3,4] and develops early in the disease process, perhaps even before the development of clinical symptoms [4]. In fact, thickening of the RBM is present in asthmatic patients in clinical remission free of symptoms or on asthma medications for at least 12 months [5] and in athletes with normal airway function [6], which suggests that the structural alterations in asthma are long standing. These same data, however, begin to raise the question of the relationship between remodeling and clinical disease activity in patients with asthma. If remodeling persisted, why was clinical quiescence seen? Collagen deposition is similar in patients with severe and mild asthma [7]. If structure dictates function, then the lack of correlation between remodeling and clinical asthma severity is puzzling. Finally, the relationship, if any, between inflammation and remodeling remains an enigma. This chapter highlights recent data that shed light on these questions.

PATHOLOGIC OBSERVATIONS IN AIRWAY REMODELING

Debate continues over the specific anatomic features that define the term *remodeling*. However, there is common agreement that remodeling includes, at least, many or all of the changes listed in Table 4-1 [2••,8,9] and shown in Figure 4-1. Remodeling occurs in both fatal and nonfatal asthma, but this chapter limits the discussion to changes observed in nonfatal asthma because these are of the most direct clinical relevance. Of these changes, the one receiving most attention, perhaps because it is relatively easy to measure using bronchoscopy and bronchial biopsies, is the thickness of the RBM. Histochemical measurements have shown that this structural change is not a thickened true basement membrane, which is composed of type IV collagen. Rather, the structural change in the lamina reticularis, or RBM, is a consequence of increases in types I, III, and V collagen, which are generally associated with healing and scar formation [3]. The implications of these findings are not entirely clear, but they suggest that attention should be paid to the mechanisms that regulate fibrosing and healing responses.

Changes in matrix proteins in the submucosal space, deep to the mucosa, are also well described. Deposition

of tenascin, one such structural protein, is increased in patients with asthma compared with control subjects and is further increased in allergic patients exposed to relevant allergens in season. Similarly, laminin appears to be increased in asthmatic versus control subjects [10]. Augmented collagen deposition may also be seen, but the finding is not as consistent as that observed in the lamina reticularis [7,11].

Descriptions of increases in smooth muscle mass date to as early as 1922 [12,13]. These increases are caused by both hypertrophy (*ie*, increased cell size) and hyperplasia (*ie*, increased cell number) [14]. The mechanisms by which these changes occur is the subject of active current research. Changes in smooth muscle mass have obvious implications for the regulation of airway tone and subsequent development of bronchial obstruction, but recent understanding of smooth muscle as an active participant in the inflammatory process [15–17] raises the possibility that the increased smooth muscle compartment may also play a role in enhancing or sustaining the inflammatory response in the airways of asthmatic individuals.

Finally, it is clear that increases in the volume of blood vessels occur in patients with asthma. This finding is the consequence of two processes: increased vessel number and vasodilation [18]. The presence of hypervascularity in patients with asthma is important for several reasons. First, vascular tone, vasodilation, and edema are susceptible to pharmacologic regulation on a short time frame. To the extent that these processes contribute to airway obstruction, they should be reversible within minutes to hours. Secondly, edema causes swelling, and such swelling may increase the apparent size of affected structures, such as the lamina reticularis or submucosal space, without a necessary increase in the matrix or structural proteins in that space. Hence, some of the described changes might be caused by edema, and conversely, some of the therapeutic effects could be caused by an effect on edema rather than an effect on protein content. Few studies of remodeling have considered this technical—but potentially important—concept.

POTENTIAL CLINICAL IMPLICATIONS OF AIRWAY REMODELING

As noted, "remodeled airways" is a very uncommon chief complaint of asthmatic patients. Patients have symptoms related to pathology and pathophysiology, which exist as consequences of their asthma. Thus, it is important to consider the consequences of a remodeled airway that are relevant to asthma symptoms. These potential concerns are summarized in Table 4-2. Perhaps the most common concern regarding the implications of airway remodeling is that of an irreversible decline in lung function. A seminal study by Peat *et al.* [19] demonstrated that some patients with asthma exhibited an exaggerated decline in lung function compared with

---

Table 4-1. PATHOLOGIC FEATURES ASSOCIATED WITH AIRWAY REMODELING

Thickened reticular basement membrane
   (*ie*, lamina reticularis)
Altered matrix proteins (*eg*, submucosal collagen,
   tenascin, elastin)
Increased smooth muscle mass
Increased vasculature
Increased mucous glands (*ie*, mucous metaplasia)
Altered expression of matrix proteoglycans

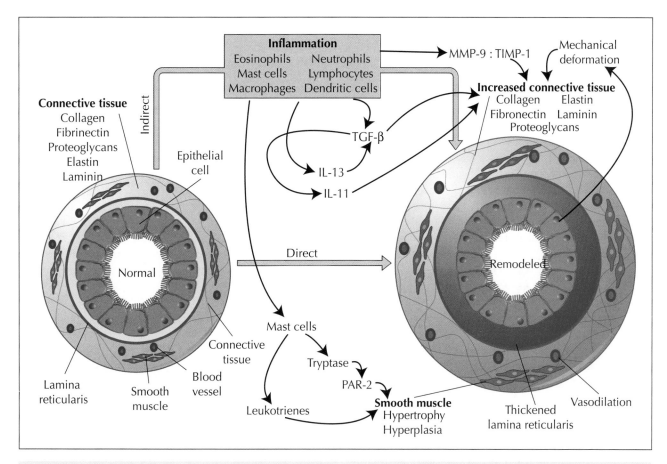

Figure 4-1.
A representation of a normal airway (*left*) and a remodeled airway (*right*). Components of the normal airway
relevant to the process of remodeling are labeled and
include the reticular basement membrane (RBM)
(or lamina reticularis), submucosal connective tissue and
proteoglycans, smooth muscle, and blood vessels.

Key processes in airway remodeling are highlighted by
ovals. Mechanisms implicated in remodeling are shown with
arrows. A key controversy is whether remodeling occurs indirectly as a consequence of inflammation and healing or as a
direct effect that is independent of inflammatory responses.

Note that the remodeled airway does not necessary have
a smaller diameter (fixed airflow obstruction), but increases in the thickness of the RBM, the amount of submucosal
connective tissue, smooth muscle volume, and size and
number of blood vessels are typical and nearly universal.

The recent demonstration that mechanical stress can
induce increased connective tissue is critically important
because the remodeled airway is predicted to subject
epithelium to increased mechanical stresses compared
with the normal airway. This pair of mechanisms may
serve as a positive feedback, or amplification, loop.

Table 4-2. POSSIBLE CLINICAL IMPLICATIONS OF AIRWAY REMODELING*

Fixed (irreversible) airway obstruction
Increased rate of decline of lung function
Increased bronchial hyperresponsiveness
Increased rate of exacerbation
Unresponsiveness to therapy
Abnormal mechanical properties of the airway

**None of the listed possibilities have been unambiguously
correlated with airway remodeling.*

appropriate control subjects. Several more recent studies
[20] have essentially confirmed these findings. Because of
the ubiquity of remodeling, these data have been
interpreted as linking abnormal lung function to the
structural changes of remodeling. However, other lines of
evidence argue against a clear relationship between structural changes and abnormal airway function. Most strik-
ingly, patients with severe, difficult to control asthma and
patients with mild asthma have comparable degrees of
collagen I and collagen III expression and similar degrees
of RBM thickening [7]. If remodeling were a principal
determinant of airway function or asthma severity, a difference between these two groups would be expected.
Only a single study [21] has found an association
between asthma severity and the degree of remodeling,
but that association was weak and the magnitude of

effect was small. Furthermore, the duration of asthma, another important clinical variable, was not related to the degree of remodeling. Thus, the nature of the relationship, if any, between remodeling and loss of lung function remains uncertain.

There are intriguing arguments to suggest that structural changes may be associated with the development of airway hyperresponsiveness [22]. Elegant mathematical modeling suggests that several features of the remodeled airway, such as increased wall stiffness, increased thickness of the wall internal to the smooth muscle layer, and decreased coupling of the airway to the retracting forces of the parenchyma may independently lead to hyperresponsiveness of the airway. However, the predictions of this modeling have not yet been researched in well-conducted clinical trials. This lack of association is perhaps not surprising because remodeling can be observed even in subjects with normal lung function and no airway hyperresponsiveness [6].

One report [23] does suggest that a specific aspect of remodeling is associated with airway hyperresponsiveness. Extracellular matrix consists of both structural proteins (*ie*, collagen, laminin, fibronectin, tenascin, and others) and proteoglycans (*ie*, lumican, biglycan, versican, hyaluronic acid, and others). Increases in proteoglycan deposition in the wall of asthmatic airways were seen in comparison to the airways of control subjects. Furthermore, there was a significant correlation in this study between airway hyperresponsiveness and the degree of deposition of various proteoglycans. These data argue in support of the Pare model in which structural changes do have functional implications; however, additional data are required.

Thus, despite appropriate and reasonable concern that the structural changes of remodeling may have important physiologic consequences, such as irreversible loss of lung function, accelerated decline in lung function, or increased bronchial hyperresponsiveness, a compelling body of data to prove the hypothesis is still lacking.

MECHANISMS AND CONCEPTS OF AIRWAY REMODELING

The mechanism (or mechanisms) by which the structural changes of remodeling occur are not known with certainty. What is clear is that they must be multiple because the process of remodeling involves many different cells and tissues that are regulated by different mechanisms. More fundamentally, controversy remains as to whether remodeling occurs as a response to inflammation or as a primary event initiated by a more proximal signal that could also initiate inflammation in parallel. This latter debate has an important clinical implication. If remodeling responses are a consequence of airway inflammation (*ie*, if inflammation is necessary for remodeling to occur), then of necessity, anti-inflammatory

therapy will have an antiremodeling effect. In contrast, if a more proximal signal initiates both inflammation and remodeling as parallel but separate processes, it is possible that anti-inflammatory therapy will have no effect on remodeling.

For conceptual simplicity, the identified mechanisms that have been linked to remodeling are grouped into four areas: growth factors, cytokines, mediators, and other factors. This review should not be considered exhaustive; instead, it is simply representative of the considerable existing and growing body of information on the process of remodeling.

Growth Factors in Airway Remodeling

Of the growth factors implicated in regulation of profibrotic responses and linked to airway remodeling, transforming growth factor-β (TGF-β) has been most closely associated with exaggerated fibroblast function and collagen synthesis. This product of macrophages and platelets attracts fibroblasts, enhances fibroblast proliferation, and induces brisk synthesis and release of matrix proteins. It is commonly identified at sites of fibrosis and wound healing. TGF-β is secreted in an inactive form but can be activated by a variety of processes, including proteolysis [24]. TGF-β mRNA expression is increased in asthmatic but not control subjects [25], and TGF-β protein expression is greater in asthmatic patients than in healthy patients and is further elevated by allergen challenge [26]. In addition, airway smooth muscle cells release biologically active TGF-β, which can function in an autocrine fashion to promote synthesis of collagen. In summary, TGF-β potently recruits fibroblasts, induces their proliferation, and augments their collagen production; moreover, it is produced by airway smooth muscle cells and macrophages and is present at increased levels in asthmatic compared with healthy patients. Thus, it is a plausible mediator of airway remodeling. However, proof of this concept requires agents that block TGF-β activity or signaling of its receptor in animal models of airway fibrosis and, ultimately, in human clinical trials.

Other structural proteins, such as fibronectin, can serve to promote fibroblast growth. After segmental allergen challenge, concentrations of fibronectin in bronchoalveolar lavage (BAL) fluid increase in relationship to histamine, a marker for the intensity of the allergic response. Furthermore, biochemical evidence suggests that the fibronectin is locally produced and is not a consequence of inflammation and vascular leak [27]. This information suggests that the initiation of allergic responses is associated with activation of pathways that enhance fibroblast function.

Cytokines in Airway Remodeling

An intriguing cytokine linked to airway remodeling is interleukin (IL)-11, a member of the IL-6 family. This pleotropic cytokine induces prominent thrombocytosis and has effects on bone and the liver. It is induced by a number of factors present in the asthmatic airway, including TGF-β, histamine, eosinophil major basic protein, and respiratory viruses [28]. Overexpression of IL-11 in mice produced a prominent increase in peribronchial fibrosis, suggesting that IL-11 could be involved in the pathogenesis of airway remodeling [29]. Moreover, these transgenic animals exhibited airway obstruction and hyperresponsiveness to methacholine. Collectively, these data support the participation of IL-11 in airway remodeling but do not prove unique causality.

Th2-like cytokines (*ie*, IL-4, IL-5, IL-13) have been linked to establishing and maintaining the eosinophil-rich inflammatory state that characterizes allergic and nonallergic asthma. Consequently, there has been interest in identifying mechanisms by which these same cytokines might foster remodeling. Of considerable interest, IL-13 appears to play a central role in fibrosis as well as inflammation. Using murine modeling, Wills-Karp *et al.* [30] have clearly shown that IL-13 is critically important to the process of fibrosis, at least in mice. Further evidence for the importance of IL-13 was developed using neutralizing antibodies. In a murine model of allergic airway inflammation and fibrosis, administration of anti–IL-13 antibodies was associated with significant diminution in airway collagen deposition and a possible physiologic correlate, airway hyperresponsiveness [31]. The mechanism by which IL-13 promotes fibrosis appears to involve epithelial cells, with specific induction and secretion of TGF-β by epithelium.

In a careful study of the effects of the epithelium on mesenchymal cells, including fibroblasts, Richter *et al.* [32] evaluated the effects of cytokines (including IL-4 and IL-13) and growth factors. They showed that IL-13 had little direct effect on fibroblast function, but IL-13 applied to epithelial cells induced brisk release of TGF-β, which then prominently augmented collagen release [32] (*see* Fig. 4-1). This evidence has strengthened support for the concept that epithelial injury and repair may be centrally important in the process of remodeling.

Recently, IL-17 has been shown to be increased in BAL cells from asthmatic patients compared with healthy patients. This memory T-cell–derived cytokine activates a wide variety of cells, including fibroblasts, for enhanced proinflammatory and profibrotic functions. Furthermore, IL-17 appears to be expressed by eosinophils [33]. These important observations suggest that eosinophilic inflammation may, in fact, be linked pathogenically to the process of airway fibrosis. The extent to which this association accounts for fibrosis in humans with asthma has yet to be established, but a biologically plausible mechanism has now been described.

Mediators in Airway Remodeling

Mast cells have been linked to asthma for decades, most prominently through the release of mediators, such as histamine and cysteinyl leukotrienes, when the cell is activated by cross linking of high-affinity IgE-receptors expressed on the surface. Mast cells are also a rich source of tryptases, proteases known to be released rapidly upon mast cell activation. However, the specific targets of these tryptases, particularly with respect to the pathogenesis of asthma, have remained elusive.

New information has recently become available that links activation of mast cells, tryptase release, and fibrogenesis in the airway. Tryptases exist predominantly in tetrameric form, which protects the molecule from degradation in tissue and enhances substrate specificity. Recent evidence suggests that tryptase may selectively destroy inhibitory neuropeptides (*eg*, vasoactive intestinal peptide and calcitonin gene–related peptide, which normally limit bronchoconstriction) and may thereby promote smooth muscle contraction [34•]. Of specific relevance to the question of remodeling, tryptase appears to cleave an extracellular piece of the protease-activated receptor type 2 (PAR-2), which exposes a new terminus that functions as a tethered ligand to stimulate PAR-2. This receptor has recently been shown to produce airway smooth muscle cell proliferation [35]. These data further suggest an important link between protease activity in general and the process of remodeling. Collectively, these data suggest an important contribution of tryptase to remodeling and imply that prevention of tryptase release or activity (or protease inhibition more generally) might be an effective anti-remodeling strategy. However, this suggestion has not yet been tested in a well-designed clinical trial.

Cysteinyl leukotrienes are extremely potent agonists for smooth muscle contraction and augment growth factor–induced smooth muscle proliferation. They also promote fibroblast proliferation and collagen synthesis. These data provide a biologically plausible link between activation of cysteinyl leukotrienes and the structural changes of remodeling. Cysteinyl leukotrienes are products of mast cells and eosinophils, both prominently implicated in the pathogenesis of asthma. Recent evidence also implicates this important class of mediators in remodeling responses in mice. Henderson *et al.* [36••] recently reported the effects of inhibition of cysteinyl leukotriene activity using the receptor antagonist montelukast in a murine model of allergic inflammation, airway hyperresponsiveness, and airway fibrosis. Not surprisingly, allergen alone produced significant increases in airway eosinophils, Th2-like lymphocytes and their cytokine products, mucus hypersecretion, and airway fibrosis. Montelukast treatment of these mice significantly reduced the allergen-driven changes and, for some outcome measures, essentially normalized the response to that of saline challenge alone. These data argue that cysteinyl leukotrienes have important effects in the airway beyond promoting smooth muscle contraction and mucus secretion, and raise the possibility that inhibiting cysteinyl leukotrienes could be an important component of an overall asthma therapeutic strategy, particularly with respect to structural changes. Of course, these data do not address the clinically important question of whether remodeling is reversible with leukotriene modifiers.

Taken together, the existing data strongly suggest an important role for mast cells and their secreted products in the process of airway wall remodeling in asthma. Interested readers are referred to an excellent review by Page *et al.* [37••].

Other Factors in Airway Remodeling

Repeated allergen exposure is one animal model of airway structural changes that has clear implications for human asthma. Clearly, human atopic asthmatic patients have repeated allergen exposures that can provoke repeated episodes of airway obstruction and inflammation. Two recent reports [36••,38] highlight the effects of prolonged and repeated exposure of the airway of sensitized animals to allergen. The Henderson model, referenced previously, used nine allergen challenges over the course of approximately 60 days in mice. The treated animals developed considerable evidence of airway fibrosis, which was ameliorated by montelukast [36••]. A different model with the same implicit hypothesis was reported by Palmans *et al.* [38]. Six allergen challenges in sensitized rats likewise generated expected eosinophilic inflammation and hyperresponsiveness to carbachol. In addition, peribronchial fibrosis was observed, as manifest as increased deposition of fibronectin and collagen [38].

Another important concept in airway remodeling is that of matrix-degrading enzymes (*ie*, matrix metalloproteinases [MMPs]) and their endogenous inhibitors (*eg*, tissue inhibitor of metalloproteinase-1 [TIMP-1]). Of the MMPs, MMP-9 has been most widely studied. It is increased in BAL fluids from patients with asthma compared with control subjects; furthermore, it is increased after segmental allergen challenges in patients with asthma. TIMP-1 is also increased by allergen challenges but not to the same degree as the degradative enzyme MMP-9 [39]. Of considerable interest, allergen challenge causes an increase in the ratio of MMP-9 to TIMP-1, suggesting that an important consequence of allergen challenge is the development of an environment in the airway that favors remodeling.

Further evidence of the potential importance of this mechanism is an older report by Vignola *et al.* [40] that showed a relationship between inflammatory airway disease severity, as measured by FEV_1 (forced expiratory volume in 1 second) and the ratio of MMP-9 to TIMP-1. Curiously, however, the ratio of MMP-9 to TIMP-1 was reduced in patients with disease states compared with healthy control subjects. These types of fundamental disparities in the published literature make the topic of remodeling confusing and controversial. It is not likely that one group of investigators is correct and another is incorrect; rather, it is likely that biologically important differences in patient populations and methods are currently unrecog-

nized. Clearly, putative biochemical markers of remodeling will require extensive validation to be useful to clinicians.

Finally, a factor as simple as mechanical stress appears to play an important role in inducing genes related to remodeling responses. Elegant experiments by Tschumperlin *et al.* [41] and Swartz *et al.* [42] have shown that mechanical stress of human airway epithelial cells in co-culture with fibroblasts at a level of stress that is comparable to that developed physiologically during bronchoconstriction causes increased release of fibronectin, MMPs, and collagen. The way that these mechanical signals are transduced to altered gene and protein expression has not been fully elucidated, but a role for divalent calcium and inositol 1,4,5-triphospate has been suggested [41,42].

EFFECTS OF THERAPY ON AIRWAY REMODELING AND MARKERS OF AIRWAY REMODELING

An important clinical question is whether currently available therapies reverse existing structural changes and whether they can prevent remodeling from occurring in the first place. In summary, there are no adequate, well-controlled clinical trials (in terms of size, duration of follow-up, and methodology) that confirm that any available asthma therapy changes or prevents structural changes of remodeling. There are, however, some thought-provoking data from clinical, animal, and biomarker studies that suggest that treatments may influence remodeling.

Corticosteroids

A number of studies have evaluated the question of whether inhaled corticosteroids (ICSs) alter the thickness of the lamina reticularis. Of these, only one has shown an effect, and that effect was of very modest degree [43]. In the study by Olivieri *et al.* [43], 250 μg of fluticasone twice daily for 6 weeks was compared with placebo in 17 patients. Reduction in inflammation was seen, and a significant change in the thickness of the RBM was also observed. However, the magnitude of the effect was only about 10%. Chu *et al.* [7] evaluated subjects with mild asthma who did not require ICSs and compared them with asthmatic patients who required modest doses of ICSs and with asthmatic patients with severe disease taking high-dose ICSs and oral steroids. No differences in submucosal collagen or its subtypes were seen. The older literature is more consistent with these findings by Chu *et al.* Thus, despite their considerable potency as anti-inflammatory agents of choice in asthma, the potential beneficial effects of ICSs on structural changes of remodeling have not yet been established.

Leukotriene Modifiers

There have been no controlled trials of the effect of leukotriene modifiers on remodeling in human asthma.

The data of Henderson *et al.* [36••], noted previously, suggest that administration of montelukast during the allergen challenge phase largely can prevent the development of airway remodeling that would otherwise occur. However, prevention of remodeling is a far different question—and probably an easier goal to reach—than treating patients with established peribronchial fibrosis. The animal data are provocative, but clinical data are lacking.

Long-acting β-Agonists

These agents are most important in asthma for their prominent bronchodilator effects and the control of symptoms that is thereby achieved. However, salmeterol also appears to have an effect on the vascularity of the airway wall, which is increased in patients with asthma. Three months of salmeterol, 50 μg twice daily, was evaluated using bronchial biopsies in 34 asthmatic patients. Treatment was associated with a significant reduction in the number of blood vessels in the airway wall in asthmatic patients; the treatment of 11 asthmatic patients with low-dose fluticasone had no effect on this parameter [44]. The clinical implications of this finding, if any, remain unclear. It is notable, however, that a potent inhaled steroid failed to alter airway wall vascularity. This finding suggests that multiple mechanisms leading to remodeling may be activated in patients with asthma, and that combination therapy may be a useful strategy, not just for control of airway function and symptoms but also for control of the process of remodeling.

CONTROVERSIES IN AIRWAY REMODELING

Important areas of the remodeling field remain highly controversial (Table 4-3). Most important among them is the question of whether the structural changes of remodeling have a clinically important outcome (*see* Table 4-2). If they do not, the question of remodeling may be "much ado about nothing." From a mechanistic standpoint, a critical question is whether remodeling represents a fibrogenic response to inflammation or if it develops independent of inflammation (*see* Fig. 4-1). There are critical clinical implications of this question: if remodeling is dependent on preexisting inflammation, then aggressive anti-inflammatory therapy, perhaps considerably more intense than currently in use, would be a logical and rational approach to controlling remodeling. In contrast, if remodeling can develop independent of the inflammatory response (perhaps having been triggered by an early injury such as mast cell activation or mechanical stress), then it will very likely be necessary to develop therapeutic strategies that deal specifically with fibrogenic mechanisms. Although much of the existing literature suggests that remodeling is most associated with inflammation, the provocative data from the Drazen group [40,41] suggesting that mechanical stress alone (which may be amplified by inflammation) can evoke gene expression changes plausibly linked to remodeling would argue that remodeling and inflammation may be separate processes.

REFERENCES AND RECOMMENDED READING

Papers of particular interest, published recently, have been highlighted as:
•   *Of importance*
•• *Of major importance*

1.•• Jeffery PK: Remodeling in asthma and chronic obstructive lung disease. *Am J Respir Crit Care Med* 2001, 164(suppl):28–38.
This paper represents the state of the art in airway remodeling. Although the focus is not exclusively asthma, the data presented and reviewed are of considerable interest. The author is a world authority on the histology of normal and diseased airways.

2.•• Busse W, Elias J, Sheppard D, Banks-Schlegel S: Airway remodeling and repair. *Am J Respir Crit Care Med* 1999, 160:1035–1042.
This review is more focused on the changes of the airway in asthma and has a somewhat broader view of the airway than the article by Jeffery [1].

3. Roche WR, Beasley R, Williams JH, Holgate ST: Subepithelial fibrosis in the bronchi of asthmatics. *Lancet* 1989, 1:520–523.

4. Pohunek P, Roche WR, Turzikova J, *et al.*: Eosinophilic inflammation in the bronchial mucosa of children with bronchial asthma. *Eur Respir J* 1997, 11(suppl):160.

5. van den Torrn WM, Overbeek SE, de Jongste JC, *et al.*: Airway inflammation is present during clinical remission of atopic asthma. *Am J Respir Crit Care Med* 2001, 164:2107–2113.

6. Karjalainen E-M, Laitinen A, Sue-Chu M, *et al.*: Evidence of airway inflammation and remodeling in ski athletes with and without bronchial hyperresponsiveness to methacholine. *Am J Respir Crit Care Med* 2000, 161:2086–2091.

7. Chu HW, Halliday JL, Martin RJ, *et al.*: Collagen deposition in large airways may not differentiate severe asthma from milder forms of the disease. *Am J Respir Crit Care Med* 1998, 158:1936–1944.

8. Elias JA: Airway remodeling in asthma: unanswered questions. *Am J Respir Crit Care Med* 2000, 161(suppl):168–171.

9. Vignola AM, Kips J, Bousquet J: Tissue remodeling as a feature of persistent asthma. *J Allergy Clin Immunol* 2000, 105:1041–1053.

Table 4-3. CONTROVERSIES AND FUTURE DIRECTIONS IN AIRWAY REMODELING

Is remodeling a physiologic response (*eg*, healing) or a pathologic event?

Is remodeling a consequence of inflammation or an independent process?

What are the clinically important consequences of airway remodeling in patients with asthma?

What are the effects of available asthma therapies on airway remodeling and its consequences?

10. Laitinen A, Altraja A, Kampe M, *et al.*: Tenascin is increased in airways basement membrane of asthmatics and is decreased by an inhaled steroid. *Am J Respir Crit Care Med* 1997, 156:951–958.

11. Carroll NG, Perry S, Karkhanis A: The airway longitudinal elastic fiber network and mucosal folding in patients with asthma. *Am J Respir Crit Care Med* 2000, 161:244–248.

12. Huber HL, Koessler KK: The pathology of bronchial asthma. *Ann Intern Med* 1922, 30:689–693.

13. Dunhill M: The pathology of asthma with special reference of changes in the bronchial mucosa. *J Clin Pathol* 1960, 13:27–33.

14. Ebina M, Takahashi T, Chiba T, Montomiya M: Cellular hypertrophy and hyperplasia of airway smooth muscles underlying bronchial asthma: a 3-D morphometric study. *Am Rev Respir Dis* 1993, 48:720–726.

15. Amrani Y, Moore PE, Hoffman R, *et al.*: Interferon-gamma modulates cysteinyl leukotriene receptor-1 expression and function in human airway myocytes. *Am J Respir Crit Care Med* 2001, 164:2098–2101.

16. Ammit AJ, Hastie AT, Edsall LC, *et al.*: Sphingosine-1-phosphate modulates human airway smooth muscle cell functions that promote inflammation and airway remodeling in asthma. *FASEB J* 2001, 15:1212–1214.

17. Ammit AJ, Hoffman RK, Amrani Y, *et al.*: Tumor necrosis factor alpha induced secretion of RANTES and IL-6 from human airway smooth muscle cells: modulation by cyclic adenosine monophosphate. *Am J Respir Cell Mol Biol* 2000, 23:794–802.

18. Li X, Wilson JW: Increased vascularity of the bronchial mucosa in mild asthma. *Am J Respir Crit Care Med* 1997, 156:229–233.

19. Peat JK, Woolcock AJ, Cullen K: Rate of decline in lung function in subjects with asthma. *Eur J Respir Dis* 1987, 20:171–179.

20. Lange P, Parner J, Vestbo J, *et al.*: A 15-year followup study of ventilatory function in adults with asthma. *N Engl J Med* 1998, 339:1194–1200.

21. Chetta A, Foresi A, Del-Donno M, *et al.*: Airway remodeling is a distinctive feature of asthma and is related to severity of disease. *Chest* 1997, 111:852–857.

22. Pare PD, Roberts DR, Bai TR, Wiggs BJ: The functional consequences of airway remodeling in asthma. *Monaldi Arch Chest Dis* 1997, 52:589–598.

23. Huang J, Olivenstein R, Taha R, *et al.*: Enhanced proteoglycan deposition in the airway wall of atopic asthmatics. *Am J Respir Crit Care Med* 1999, 160:725–729.

24. Munger JS, Harpel JG, Gleizes PE, *et al.*: Latent transforming growth factor-β: structural features and mechanisms of activation. *Kidney Int* 1997, 51:1376–1382.

25. Minshall EM, Leung DYM, Martin RJ, *et al.*: Eosinophil associated TGF-β1 mRNA expression and airways fibrosis in bronchial asthma. *Am J Respir Cell Mol Biol* 1997, 17:326–333.

26. Reddington AE, Madden J, Frew AJ, *et al.*: Transforming growth factor-β1 in asthma: measurement in bronchoalveolar lavage fluid. *Am J Respir Crit Care Med* 1997, 156:642–647.

27. Meerschaert J, Kelly EAB, Mosher DF, *et al.*: Segmental allergen challenge increases fibronectin in bronchoalveolar lavage fluid. *Am J Respir Crit Care Med* 1999, 159:619–625.

28. Zheng T, Zhu Z, Wang J, *et al.*: IL-11: insights in asthma from overexpression transgenic modeling. *J Allergy Clin Immunol* 2001, 108:489–496.

29. Tang W, Geba GP, Zheng T, *et al.*: Targeted expression of IL-11 in the murine airway causes lymphocytic inflammation, bronchial remodeling, and airways obstruction. *J Clin Invest* 1996, 98:2845–2853.

30. Wills-Karp M, Luyimbazi J, Xu X, *et al.*: IL-13: central mediator of allergic asthma. *Science* 1998, 282:2258–2261.

31. Blease K, Jakubzick C, Westwick J, *et al.*: Therapeutic effect of IL-13 immunoneutralization during chronic experimental fungal asthma. *J Immunol* 2001, 166:5219–5224.

32. Richter A, Puddicombe SM, Lordan JL, *et al.*: The contribution of IL-4 and IL-13 to the epithelial-mesenchymal trophic unit in asthma. *Am J Respir Cell Mol Biol* 2001, 25:385–391.

33. Molet S, Hamid Q, Davoine F, *et al.*: IL-17 is increased in asthmatic airways and induces human bronchial fibroblasts to produce cytokines. *J Allergy Clin Immunol* 2001, 108:430–438.

34.• Sommerhoff CP: Mast cell tryptases and airway remodeling. *Am J Respir Crit Care Med* 2001, 164(suppl):52–58.
This review of mast cell tryptases is full of important insights and three-dimensional molecular modeling. Readers interested in specifics of these important molecules are encouraged to read this article.

35. Berger P, Perng D-W, Thabrew H, *et al.*: Tryptase and agonists of PAR-2 induce the proliferation of human airway smooth muscle cells. *J Appl Physiol* 2001, 91:1371–1379.

36.•• Henderson WR Jr, Tang L-O, Chu S-J, *et al.*: A role for cysteinyl leukotrienes in airway remodeling in a mouse asthma model. *Am J Respir Crit Care Med* 2002, 165:108–116.
This is arguably the most important paper in the past year in the field of leukotriene biology. In a relevant animal model, the authors demonstrate important effects of antileukotriene therapy on inflammation and particularly on structural changes (ie, remodeling) of the airway.

37.•• Page S, Ammit AJ, Black JL, Armour CL: Human mast cells and airway smooth muscle interactions: implications for asthma. *Am J Physiol Lung Cell Molec Physiol* 2001, 281:1313–1323.
This lengthy review of mast cells and smooth muscle cells and their interactions is highly recommended for its readability, content, and insights.

38. Palmans E, Kips JC, Pauwels RA: Prolonged allergen exposure induces structural airway changes in sensitized rats. *Am J Respir Crit Care Med* 2000, 161:627–635.

39. Kelly EAB, Busse WW, Jarjour NN: Increased matrix metalloproteinase-9 in the airway after allergen challenge. *Am J Respir Crit Care Med* 2000, 162:1157–1161.

40. Vignola AM, Riccobono L, Miarbella A, *et al.*: Sputum metalloproteinase-9/tissue inhibitor of metalloproteinase-1 ratio correlates with airflow obstruction in asthma and chronic bronchitis. *Am J Respir Crit Care Med* 1998, 158:1945–1950.

41. Tschumperlin DJ, Drazen JM: Mechanical stimuli to airway remodeling. *Am J Respir Crit Care Med* 2001, 164(suppl):90–94.

42. Swartz MA, Tschumperlin DJ, Drazen JM: Mechanical stress is communicated between different cell types to elicit matrix remodeling. *Proc Nat Acad Sci U S A* 2001, 98:6180–6185.

43. Olivieri D, Chetta A, Del Donno M, *et al.*: Effect of short-term treatment with low-dose inhaled fluticasone propionate on airway inflammation and remodeling in mild asthma: a placebo-controlled study. *Am J Respir Crit Care Med* 1997, 155:1864–1871.

44. Orsida BE, Ward C, Li X, *et al.*: Effect of a long-acting beta agonist over three months on airway wall vascular remodeling in asthma. *Am J Respir Crit Care Med* 2001, 164:117–121.

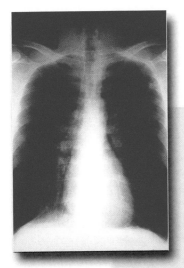

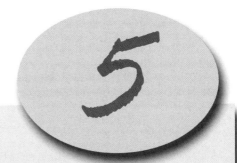

Asthma Diagnosis and Differential Diagnosis

Stephen A. Tilles and Harold S. Nelson

When a patient reports having dyspnea, cough, or wheezing, most clinicians appropriately consider asthma as a possible diagnosis. However, despite awareness in recent years of the increased prevalence of asthma, there is considerable epidemiologic evidence that asthma is underdiagnosed, particularly in children [1], adolescents [2], and elderly individuals [3,4]. Conversely, there are a variety of "masqueraders" that are often incorrectly diagnosed and inappropriately treated as asthma. In other patients, asthma symptoms fail to respond to treatment because of the presence of one or more additional diagnoses that complicate their asthma. When symptoms fail to respond to the usual asthma therapies, patients are often treated with increasing doses of systemic corticosteroids, resulting in unnecessary and sometimes permanent side effects. The potential magnitude of this problem is illustrated by the vocal cord dysfunction (VCD) experience at the National Jewish Medical and Research Center in Denver. Of all patients referred with "refractory asthma," nearly 10% were instead found to have a syndrome called VCD [5]. The largest published VCD case series from the same institution reported inappropriate prior treatment of such patients with prednisone averaging nearly 30 mg/d for more than 4 years [6••].

This chapter outlines how to establish an accurate diagnosis of asthma, including a review of clinical hallmarks and objective testing. The differential diagnosis of adult asthma is then discussed, with emphasis on the more common asthma masqueraders. Finally, the chapter addresses conditions that commonly complicate moderate to severe asthma.

ESTABLISHING THE DIAGNOSIS OF ASTHMA

Asthma is a heterogeneous disease with a variety of clinical presentations. Many patients develop atopic asthma and allergic rhinitis as children or young adults, often after a history of eczema during early childhood. Others present as children or adults without allergies, including some with coexisting chronic sinus disease, nasal polyposis, or acute bronchospastic reactions to aspirin and other NSAIDs. Still others present in middle or late adulthood after severe respiratory infections. Although each of these asthma phenotypes may present differently, they share fundamental clinical hallmarks. Familiarity with these asthma hallmarks enables clinicians to confidently establish the diagnosis and stage its severity. Table 5-1 outlines key indicators for considering the diagnosis of asthma and lists markers of undertreated asthma.

According to the National Heart, Lung, and Blood Institute's *Guidelines for the Diagnosis and Management of Asthma* [7•], a diagnosis of asthma requires a history of symptoms suggestive of airflow obstruction, and the symptoms and airflow obstruction should be at least partially reversible. Symptoms must include some combination of expiratory wheezing, cough, dyspnea, and chest tightness. Chronic symptoms often also include sputum production. The clinical pattern may be variable, but symptoms tend to occur or worsen in response to one or more of the following: exercise, cold air, irritants, viral respiratory infections, allergen exposure (*eg*, animal dander, dust mites, mold, or pollen), weather changes, and emotional stress. Symptoms, airflow obstruction, and asthmatic lung inflammation are all typically worse at night and may awaken patients in the early morning hours.

The physical examination findings in patients with asthma vary depending on the severity and chronicity of the disease. The findings may include hyperexpansion of the chest, expiratory wheeze, and a prolonged expiratory phase of breathing. However, a significant proportion of

patients with mild and moderate asthma has no abnormal physical findings on chest examination. Other physical findings that are not directly related to asthma but are common in asthma patients include nasal turbinate edema, nasal polyps, and eczematous dermatitis.

The principal objective methods for documenting airflow obstruction in symptomatic asthma are spirometry and peak expiratory flow (PEF) monitoring. A reduction in the FEV_1 (forced expiratory volume in 1 second) is the most accurate measurement of airflow obstruction by spirometry. Demonstrating improvement in FEV_1 in response to bronchodilator treatment is perhaps the most specific objective way to confirm the diagnosis of asthma. According to the American Thoracic Society's established criteria for the diagnosis of asthma [8], a significant bronchodilator response is defined as an improvement in FEV_1 by 12% of baseline and 200 mL. However, the upper 95% confidence interval for reversibility is 10% of predicted in nonasthmatic patients [9]. In a study that compared asthma with chronic bronchitis, a 15% increase in the percent of predicted FEV_1 in response to an inhaled bronchodilator had a specificity of 1.0 for asthma [10]. Therefore, expressing bronchodilator response as the increase in FEV_1 as percent of the predicted FEV_1 is a more specific method for confirming the diagnosis of asthma.

The forced vital capacity (FVC) is typically influenced much less by airflow obstruction than FEV_1; therefore, the ratio of FEV_1 to FVC is often decreased in patients with asthma. Examination of the flow volume loop verifies these spirometric changes. Airflow obstruction caused by asthma (and other intrathoracic obstructive processes) results in an increased concavity of the expiratory portion of the flow volume loop (Fig. 5-1). However, because asthma is often worse at night and in the early morning hours, many symptomatic patients feel well and have normal lung function during the day when they are not stressed with exercise or other triggering factors. Therefore, despite the value of spirometry in documenting airflow obstruction, normal values do not exclude the diagnosis of asthma.

A decrease in the PEF is also seen with intrathoracic airflow obstruction. Because a peak flow meter is inexpensive and designed for home use, it offers the advantage of unlimited measurements to aid in both diagnosis and treatment decisions. Although the accuracy of individual PEF measurements is limited by their dependence on technique and patient effort, properly performed PEF monitoring can be very useful. For example, in a study that compared 27 symptomatic asthmatic patients, five asymptomatic asthmatic patients, and five nonasthmatic patients [12], the degree of bronchial hyperreactivity (BHR) correlated with the magnitude of the morning reduction in PEF, the PEF response to bronchodilator, and diurnal PEF variation. This correlation between bronchial responsiveness and PEF was

Table 5-1. HALLMARKS OF ASTHMA

Symptoms
  Wheezing
  Dyspnea
  Cough
  Chest tightness
Factors that make asthma worse
  Exercise
  Cold air
  Viral upper respiratory infection
  Allergens
    Seasonal (*eg*, pollens, molds)
    Perennial (*eg*, dust mites, furry pets)
  Irritants
    Tobacco smoke
    Air pollution
    Airborne chemicals
Lung function
  Reversible airflow limitation and diurnal variation
    as measured by spirometry or peak flow meter
Markers of poor control
  Ongoing nocturnal awakening caused by
    asthma symptoms
  History of intubation or intensive care unit admission
  History of multiple emergency room visits or
    hospitalizations

also present among asymptomatic asthmatic patients. When the clinical history and spirometry fail to confirm the diagnosis, a reasonable approach is to instruct the patient to measure and record his or her PEF before taking bronchodilator medication in the morning and after bronchodilator medication in the afternoon or early evening for 1 to 2 weeks. A 12% or more average diurnal PEF variation is suggestive of asthma [12].

Assessing the response to empiric asthma therapy is a useful way to help confirm the diagnosis of asthma. For example, if exercise-induced asthma is suspected after the initial evaluation, the diagnosis is confirmed when a short-acting inhaled bronchodilator (*eg*, two puffs of albuterol 15 minutes before exercise) reliably prevents symptoms. Similarly, if the initial evaluation reveals a history compatible with moderate to severe asthma and

spirometry reveals chronic airflow obstruction without significant response to bronchodilator, it is appropriate to assess the response to a potent anti-inflammatory medication over time. Either a systemic corticosteroid (*eg*, prednisone 20 mg twice daily for 1 to 2 weeks) [13] or high-dose inhaled corticosteroid (*eg*, two to four puffs twice daily of either fluticasone propionate 220 µg/puff or budesonide turbuhaler for 3 to 4 weeks) would be expected to improve symptoms, FEV_1, and morning PEF if the patient has asthma. After the diagnosis is confirmed, a lower maintenance dose of anti-inflammatory medication would generally be appropriate.

Additional diagnostic testing may be appropriate, especially when the diagnosis is not clear. A chest radiograph in patients with asthma may be normal or show lung hyperinflation. High-resolution CT of the chest may

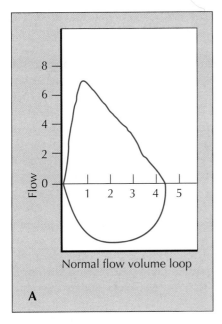

A Normal flow volume loop

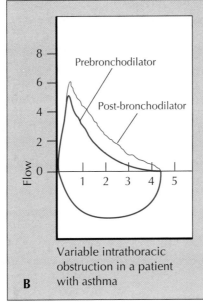

B Variable intrathoracic obstruction in a patient with asthma

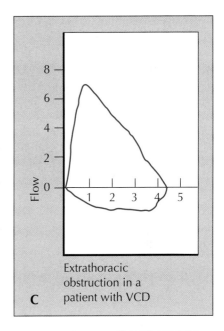

C Extrathoracic obstruction in a patient with VCD

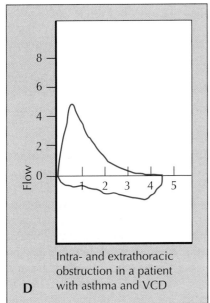

D Intra- and extrathoracic obstruction in a patient with asthma and VCD

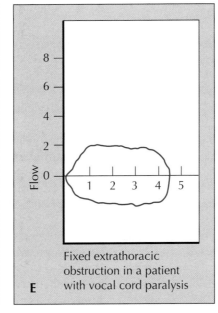

E Fixed extrathoracic obstruction in a patient with vocal cord paralysis

Figure 5-1.
Flow volume loops and airflow obstruction. *A*, Normal flow volume loop. *B*, Variable intrathoracic obstruction in a patient with severe asthma. *C*, Variable extrathoracic obstruction in a patient with vocal cord dysfunction (VCD). *D*, Variable intra- and extrathoracic obstruction in a patient with asthma and VCD. *E*, Fixed extrathoracic obstruction in a patient with vocal cord paresis. *Solid line* indicates baseline; *dashed line* indicates predicted. (*Adapted from* Tilles and Nelson [11].)

identify hyperinflation or more subtle findings such as bronchial wall thickening, air trapping, or even mild bronchiectasis. Formal pulmonary function study findings suggestive of asthma include airflow obstruction, increased lung volumes, and a normal or increased diffusion capacity for carbon monoxide (DLCO). Because of their expense, neither high-resolution CT of the chest nor formal pulmonary function studies are indicated in the initial work-up of patients who have typical asthma symptoms and reversible airflow obstruction.

Another important diagnostic tool is measurement of nonspecific BHR. BHR is a cardinal feature of symptomatic asthma regardless of severity. The diagnostic sensitivity of standardized bronchoprovocation protocols using inhaled methacholine or histamine approaches 100%; the degree of BHR correlates with asthma severity; and in individual patients, the improvement in the degree of BHR in response to asthma treatment may be the most accurate predictor of clinical outcome [14•]. Protocols also exist for provocation with exercise or inhaled allergen. However, BHR measurements have a variety of limitations that confine their appropriate use to a minority of patients suspected of having asthma. These include a poor specificity for asthma, relatively high cost (because of a requirement for an appropriate facility and personnel), and an exclusion of patients with severely compromised lung function because of safety concerns. Therefore, in practical terms, measurements of BHR are most helpful in patients without severe airflow obstruction in whom the history, physical examination, and other objective tests fail to establish the diagnosis. Figure 5-2 outlines an algorithm for establishing the diagnosis of asthma.

DIFFERENTIAL DIAGNOSIS

The differential diagnosis of asthma is quite long, and many asthma specialists carefully evaluate patients for an entire career without encountering some of the least common asthma masqueraders. On the other hand, in everyday practice, patients are frequently misdiagnosed as having asthma, resulting in both escalating doses of expensive and potentially harmful asthma medications and a failure to initiate appropriate therapy. Therefore, familiarity with a practical approach to differential diagnosis is essential. Tables 5-2 to 5-7 list asthma masqueraders and emphasize the more common diagnoses that are likely to be encountered. This chapter focuses on the differential diagnosis of adult asthma, but a pediatric list is included for reference.

Chronic obstructive pulmonary disease (COPD) is perhaps the disease most commonly confused with asthma in adults, and both emphysema and chronic bronchitis may be misdiagnosed as asthma. Because both COPD and asthma are common, there are many patients who suffer from both diseases. Although the symptoms and medical treatments of COPD and asthma overlap, there are important differences in long-term management and prognosis. Therefore, it is important to clarify the relative contribution of COPD and asthma to symptoms in individual patients.

The clinical similarities between COPD and asthma include symptoms (*ie*, dyspnea, wheezing, and cough), a susceptibility to worsening of symptoms with respiratory infections and exercise, and the presence of airflow obstruction on spirometry. However, the typical clinical patterns of the diseases differ significantly (*see* Table 5-2). COPD is a gradually progressive disease of elderly adults with a history of tobacco use whose baseline symptoms tend to be consistent day to day. Dyspnea in COPD typically occurs only with exertion. Asthma onset occurs more commonly during either childhood or young adulthood, and asthma symptoms are usually episodic, depend on a wider range of triggering factors, and may occur spontaneously while the individual is at rest. The nature of the exercise response in COPD and asthma also differs. In exercise-induced asthma, the symptoms usually worsen upon cessation of exercise, reflecting acute bronchospasm. For example, a patient with asthma may report the onset of an "attack" during or just after running. In contrast, a 60-year-old patient who reports a daily routine involving a 3-minute rest every two blocks while walking to work is much more likely to have COPD, cardiac disease, or another disease whose symptoms are proportional to oxygen demand.

Objective testing helps stage COPD and distinguish between COPD and asthma. Pulmonary function testing abnormalities common in patients with COPD but not asthma include a decreased baseline DLCO (corrected for alveolar volume) and a decreased FEV_1 that does not reverse significantly with either bronchodilator or corticosteroid treatment. Exercise challenge studies are often associated with a decrease in blood oxygen saturation rather than a significant decrease in FEV_1. Methacholine challenge can be useful to discriminate asthma from COPD when the baseline FEV_1 is normal or mildly reduced, but it loses its specificity when the FEV_1 is moderately reduced. In one study [15], 19 of 27 smokers with chronic bronchitis and a reduced FEV_1 had significant bronchial hyperreactivity to inhaled methacholine. Finally, the presence of significant sputum eosinophilia (*eg*, > 50% of total inflammatory cells) is expected in patients with asthma but is rarely seen in those with COPD.

As mentioned earlier, another important asthma masquerader is a syndrome called VCD. VCD is a nonorganic laryngeal disorder that involves paradoxical adduction of the vocal cords while a patient attempts to breathe. This results in some combination of dyspnea, cough, wheezing, throat tightness, and chest tightness. These symptoms are not life threatening, but they may be dramatic, resulting in multiple emergency room visits and even intubation in some patients. The incidence of VCD is unknown but often accounts for respiratory symptoms that fail to respond to asthma treatment in women and adolescent girls. VCD is a less common asthma masquerader in men and boys. The flow volume loop often reveals inspiratory truncation, suggesting extrathoracic airflow obstruction (*see* Fig. 5-2). Confirmation of the diagnosis requires direct visualization of paradoxical vocal cord motion. Because the laryngeal examination and flow volume loop in patients with VCD is often normal in the absence of symptoms, provocation of symptoms with methacholine, histamine, or exercise challenge is often required when the diagnosis is in question. Controlled VCD treatment trials have not been performed, although VCD management involves speech therapy focused on laryngeal relaxation. Many patients also benefit from psychotherapy.

There are distinct patient profiles for VCD. Newman *et al.* [6••] reported the largest and most thoroughly described series of laryngoscopically confirmed VCD patients in 1995. All of the patients had been referred to the National Jewish Medical and Research Center in Denver for refractory asthma, many having traveled from other parts of the United States after failing treatment despite the efforts of local asthma specialists. These 95 patients ranged in age from 22 to 55 years, and 84% of them were women. Of interest, just over 50% of them also had asthma (*see* "Conditions That Complicate Moderate to Severe Asthma"). Only one of the 42 VCD patients without asthma were men, and there was a strong association with prior psychologic trauma and ongoing psychiatric illness.

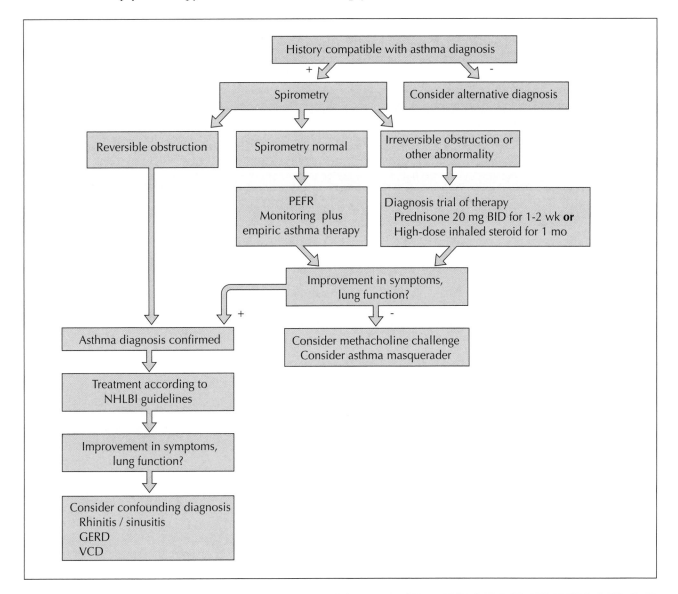

Figure 5-2.
Algorithm for establishing the diagnosis of asthma.
BID—twice a day; GERD—gastroesophageal reflux disease;

NHBLI—National Heart, Lung, and Blood Institute; PEFR—peak expiratory flow rate; VCD—vocal chord dysfunction.

Vocal cord dysfunction is also commonly mistaken for asthma in younger patients, particularly in response to exercise. In another case series from the National Jewish Medical and Research Center, Landwehr *et al.* [16] described seven adolescent athletes (six of them were girls) who had been referred for refractory exercise-induced asthma and were found to have VCD. Only one of the seven had significant bronchial hyperresponsiveness. All of them were outstanding students academically and, as with the adult series, there was a strong association with psychiatric illness.

Vocal cord dysfunction has also been shown to be common in less selected patient populations. In a report from a military pulmonary clinic, VCD was laryngoscopically confirmed in 15% of military recruits referred for exertional dyspnea during basic training [17]. Thirty percent of the patients were men. A large European study [18] used airway hyperresponsiveness to histamine to assess airflow obstruction using spirometric criteria in 441 subjects (54% of them were men) with cough, wheeze, or dyspnea without diagnosed asthma. Extrathoracic airflow obstruction was provoked in the majority of subjects and was more likely in patients with postnasal drip and pharyngitis. Other studies have described a very prominent association between VCD and otherwise occult gastroesophageal reflux disease [19,20]. Therefore, VCD occurs in a primary form, as a confounder of asthma, and in association with other disease processes that result in laryngeal irritation such as gastroesophageal reflux disease and rhinitis. Each of these forms of VCD results in symptoms that may be mistaken for asthma.

Distinguishing VCD symptoms from those caused by asthma is often difficult (*see* Table 5-2). Localization of symptoms to the throat, difficulty with inspiration rather than expiration, a lack of sputum production, and the absence of nocturnal worsening may help raise the suspicion for VCD. However, most patients with VCD primarily describe dyspnea and chest symptoms [6••] without relating an inspiratory versus expiratory component. Nocturnal episodes of VCD have also been reported [21]. Therefore, VCD should be considered as a possibility in any symptomatic patient who fails to respond to asthma treatment, especially if the patient is either an adolescent with exercise as the primary trigger

Table 5-2. COMPARISON OF ASTHMA, COPD, AND VCD*

	Asthma	COPD	VCD
History			
Age of onset	Any age	Elderly smokers	Adolescents and young adults
Classic symptoms	Wheezing, dyspnea, cough, worse at night	Dyspnea on exertion	Dyspnea, chest tightness, stridor
Relation of symptoms to the respiratory cycle	Exhalation > inhalation	Expiration > inhalation	Inhalation > exhalation
Localization of symptoms	Deep in chest	Deep in chest	Upper chest, throat
Physical examination findings during symptoms	Expiratory wheezing (posterior chest)	Expiratory wheezing (posterior chest)	Inspiratory wheezing or stridor (upper chest or throat)
Diagnostic test results			
Chest radiograph	Hyperinflation, bronchial thickening	Hyperinflation, hyperlucency	Normal
Pulmonary function testing	Increased lung volumes	Increased lung volumes	Normal lung volumes
	Reversible airflow obstruction	Irreversible airflow obstruction	Inspiratory airflow obstruction
	Increased DLCO	Decreased DLCO, neutrophils	Normal DLCO
Sputum examination	Eosinophils		Normal
Response to treatment			
Corticosteroids	Good	Poor	Poor
Bronchodilators	Good	Modest	Poor

Significant overlap in clinical presentation is possible. This table is a guide intended to represent the most common presentations of isolated disease. COPD—chronic obstructive pulmonary disease; DLCO—diffusion capacity for carbon monoxide; VCD—vocal cord dysfunction. Adapted from Tilles and Nelson [11].

or a woman with a history of anxiety or other psychologic problems.

Less common asthma masqueraders include relatively common diseases that occasionally present with symptoms suggestive of asthma (*eg*, coronary artery disease, congestive heart failure, recurrent pulmonary embolism) and uncommon diseases whose primary presentation overlaps significantly with asthma (*eg*, mechanical obstruction of the central airway, cystic fibrosis, bronchiolitis obliterans, bronchiectasis, hypersensitivity pneumonitis). Table 5-3 lists the typical presentations of less common asthma masqueraders and how they may be distinguished from asthma. Tables 5-4 and 5-5 list examples of diagnoses that obstruct airflow in large airways. Uncommon asthma masqueraders are listed in Table 5-6. Finally, a summary of the differential diagnosis of asthma in children is listed in Table 5-7.

CONDITIONS THAT COMPLICATE MODERATE TO SEVERE ASTHMA

The majority of patients with asthma have rhinitis, sinusitis, or both [22–24], and the evidence for a physiologic link between the upper and lower airway is plentiful. For example, nasal allergen provocation in patients with nonasthmatic allergic rhinitis results in

Table 5-3. LESS COMMON ASTHMA MASQUERADERS

Diagnosis	Presentation	Key to Differentiating from Asthma
CHF	Dyspnea on exertion, paroxysmal nocturnal dyspnea, occasionally wheezing, BHR	Examination findings: rales, edema, gallop rhythm
	Cardiac risk factors	Chest radiograph
		ECG
		Echocardiogram
Pulmonary embolism	Dyspnea, occasionally wheezing	Unilateral rales, leg edema, cord
	PE risk factors: oral contraceptive use, history of deep venous thrombosis, pregnancy, hypercoagulable state, immobility	V/Q scan
		Spiral CT scan
Cystic fibrosis	Dyspnea, cough, GI complaints	Sweat chloride test
	Airflow obstruction	DNA analysis
	Infertility	
	Poor growth	
Bronchiolitis obliterans	Cough, dyspnea	Bronchoscopy with BAL
	Irreversible airflow obstruction	Transbronchial biopsy
Bronchiectasis	Cough, dyspnea unresponsive to bronchodilator or corticosteroid	HRCT chest
	Recurrent pneumonia	
Hypersensitivity pneumonitis	Dyspnea after chronic exposure to organic antigen (*eg*, moldy hay, birds)	Resolution of symptoms upon removal from exposure
	Restriction on spirometry	Precipitating antibodies
Aspiration GERD	Recurrent pneumonia	Overnight esophageal pH probe
	Pulmonary fibrosis	Barium swallow
		HRCT chest
Central airway obstruction	Dyspnea, expiratory wheezing	Symptoms improve with heliox inhalation
	Symptoms not episodic	Bronchoscopy
	No diurnal variation	
Extrathoracic obstruction	Dyspnea, stridor, inspiratory wheezing	Laryngoscopy
	Truncation of the inspiratory portion of the flow volume loop	

BAL—bronchoalveolar lavage; BHR—bronchial hyperreactivity; CHF—congestive heart failure; GERD—gastroesophageal reflux disease; GI—gastrointestinal; HRCT—high-resolution computed tomography; PE—pulmonary embolism.

upregulation of bronchial adhesion molecules and an influx of eosinophils into the bronchial mucosa [25]. Conversely, allergen challenge directly into the lung in patients with allergic rhinitis results in an increase in nasal inflammation [26,27]. In patients with both allergic rhinitis and asthma, nasal corticosteroid treatment has been shown to prevent the increase in BHR associated with both experimental [28] and natural [29] allergen exposure. In a retrospective cohort study [30], nasal corticosteroid treatment was associated with a reduced risk of emergency department visits for asthma. These

observations suggest that there is "crosstalk" between the lung and nose and that using nasal corticosteroids to treat patients with rhinitis may improve asthma control.

The relationship between asthma and sinusitis is also quite strong, and the term *chronic hyperplastic eosinophilic sinusitis* (CHS) has emerged to describe the type of sinus disease that is often present in patients with severe asthma. In general, CHS is the result of neither infection nor allergen exposure, and it is often associated with nasal polyposis. In a recent study of 89 patients with severe asthma [31•], 84% had abnormal sinus CT scans, and the extent of sinus disease correlated with the level of eosinophils in both peripheral blood and sputum. Demonstrating long-term improvement in asthma control with CHS treatment has been difficult, but this may be caused by the inability to chronically deliver topical anti-inflammatory treatment (*eg,* corticosteroids) to the sinuses [32]. Although patients with CHS typically respond well to systemic corticosteroids, the disease usually recurs. Sinus surgery is often performed, although a rationale for surgery for this eosinophilic inflammation of the mucosa is lacking and a failure of surgery to achieve lasting improvement is common. A reasonable long-term approach to a patient with difficult-to-control asthma and chronic sinusitis is to treat with a combination of daily nasal saline irrigation and a topical nasal corticosteroid, reserving surgery for cases of severe obstructing nasal polyposis, osteomyelitis, bony erosion, or other expanding lesions. Subacute flares of bacterial sinusitis often result in asthma exacerbations and usually respond to treatment with a burst of systemic corticosteroid for 1 to 2 weeks plus an antibiotic for 2 to 4 weeks.

Another important confounding diagnosis to consider in asthma patients is gastroesophageal reflux disease (GERD). Approximately 75% of patients with asthma also have GERD [33••]. Possible explanations for this include autonomic dysregulation in asthma [34], a mechanical change in the relationship of the esophagus to

---

Table 5-4. CAUSES OF INTRATHORACIC CENTRAL AIRWAY OBSTRUCTION

Broncholithiasis
Endobronchial granulomatous disease
  Tuberculosis
  Sarcoidosis
Bronchomalacia
Foreign body
Web or stricture
Vascular ring
Tumor
Relapsing polychondritis
Extrinsic compression
  Tumor
  Vascular structure

Adapted from *Tilles and Nelson* [11].

Table 5-5. CAUSES OF EXTRATHORACIC AIRWAY OBSTRUCTION

Vocal cord dysfunction
Vocal cord paresis
Cricoarytenoid joint arthritis
Lymph node enlargement
Tumor
Tracheomalacia
Epiglottitis
Extrinsic compression
  Edema
  Hemorrhage
  Thyroid enlargement
  Tumor

Adapted from *Tilles and Nelson* [11].

Table 5-6. UNCOMMON ASTHMA MASQUERADERS

Pulmonary infiltration with eosinophilia
  Tropical eosinophilia
  Löffler's syndrome
  Chronic eosinophilic pneumonia
  Idiopathic hypereosinophilic syndrome
  Allergic bronchopulmonary aspergillosis
  Churg-Strauss syndrome
Metastatic carcinoid
Systemic mastocytosis
Lymphangioleiomyomatosis
Amyloidosis

the diaphragm caused by lung hyperinflation, or a reduction in lower esophageal sphincter tone by bronchodilator medicines. GERD also has the potential to trigger asthma symptoms and is a major reason for asthma symptoms that appear refractory to treatment. This is caused in part by a vagally mediated reflex bronchoconstriction [34] and also likely involves microaspiration and alterations in minute ventilation [35].

Treatment of patients with GERD has the potential for improving asthma control. In a literature review of studies evaluating the effects of GERD treatment on asthma outcomes, Field and Sutherland [36] pointed out that improvement of asthma symptoms was documented in 69% of treated subjects and asthma medication reduction was achieved by 62%. GERD treatment did not result in lung function improvements in any of the studies reviewed. Surgical treatment of GERD results in a similar degree of symptom improvement [37]. Therefore, treatment of GERD is warranted in patients with asthma. A 3-month trial of high-dose proton pump inhibitor therapy (*eg*, omeprazole 20 mg twice a day) is a reasonable approach to an asthma patient with GERD symptoms. A similar treatment trial is reasonable in patients with moderate to severe asthma without GERD symptoms. However, overnight esophageal pH monitoring is a more cost-effective way to document whether GERD is present. Referral to a gastroenterologist is appropriate when both symptoms and an abnormal overnight

esophageal pH persist despite 3 months of appropriate antireflux therapy [33••].

As mentioned previously, VCD often complicates difficult asthma. Compared with patients with refractory asthma alone, patients with asthma and VCD present with similar symptoms, medication histories, and spirometry, but are more likely to have been hospitalized [6••]. Laryngeal irritation caused by rhinitis or GERD is likely responsible for a significant proportion of VCD symptoms in these patients. Confirming the diagnosis of VCD requires laryngoscopic documentation of paradoxical vocal cord motion. However, terminal truncation of the inspiratory portion of the flow volume loop (*see* Fig. 5-2C) is suggestive of VCD and, with a typical history, sufficient to refer the patient for a trial of speech therapy. In summary, the appropriate management of symptomatic patients with both asthma and VCD usually includes a combination of speech therapy, continued medication for asthma, and treatment of both GERD and rhinitis. This typically enables subsequent cautious reduction of asthma medications.

Allergic bronchopulmonary aspergillosis is an airway disease that involves an immunologic reaction to growth of *Aspergillus fumigatus* in the bronchi. Patients typically present with episodes of refractory asthma and recurrent pulmonary infiltrates, and a diagnostic work-up reveals an elevated total serum immunoglobulin E (IgE) level and both specific IgE and IgG precipitins to *Aspergillus*. High-resolution CT of the chest often reveals proximal upper lobe bronchiectasis.

Table 5-7. DIFFERENTIAL DIAGNOSIS OF ASTHMA IN INFANTS AND CHILDREN

Upper airway diseases
  Allergic rhinitis and sinusitis
Obstruction involving large airways
  Foreign body in trachea or bronchus
  Vocal cord dysfunction
  Vascular rings or laryngeal webs
  Laryngotracheomalacia, tracheal stenosis, or bronchostenosis
  Enlarged lymph node or tumor
Obstruction involving small airways
  Viral bronchiolitis or obliterative bronchiolitis
  Cystic fibrosis
  Bronchopulmonary dysplasia
  Heart disease
Other causes
  Recurrent cough not caused by asthma
  Aspiration from swallowing mechanism dysfunction or GERD

GERD—gastroesophageal reflux disease.
Adapted from *National Heart, Lung, and Blood Institute [7•].*

REFERENCES AND RECOMMENDED READING

Papers of particular interest, published recently, have been highlighted as:
•   *Of importance*
••   *Of major importance*

1. Maier WC, Arrighi M, Morray B, *et al.*: The impact of asthma and asthma-like illness in Seattle school children. *J Clin Epidemiol* 1998, 51:557–568.

2. Siersted HC, Boldsen J, Hansen HS, *et al.*: Population-based study of risk factors for underdiagnosis of asthma in adolescence: Odense schoolchild study. *Br Med J* 1998, 316:651–657.

3. Bauer BA, Reed CE, Yunginger JW, *et al.*: Incidence and outcomes of asthma in the elderly. *Chest* 1997, 111:303–310.

4. Parameswaran K, Hildreth AJ, Chadha D, *et al.*: Asthma in the elderly: underperceived, underdiagnosed and undertreated; a community survey. *Respir Med* 1998, 92:573–577.

5. Newman KB, Dubester SN: Vocal cord dysfunction: masquerader of asthma. *Semin Respir Crit Care Med* 1994, 15:161–167.

6.••Newman KB, Mason UG, Schmaling KB: Clinical features of vocal cord dysfunction. *Am J Respir Crit Care Med* 1995, 152:1382–1386.
This landmark article describes the common features of vocal cord dysfunction presenting in adults previously diagnosed with refractory asthma.

7.• National Heart, Lung, and Blood Institute, National Asthma Education and Prevention Program: *Expert Panel Report 2: Guidelines for the Diagnosis and Management of Asthma.* Bethesda, MD: National Institutes of Health, Pub. No. 97-4051; 1997.
This authoritative document outlines the preferred approach to both diagnosis and treatment of asthma, including differential diagnostic considerations.

8. American Thoracic Society: lung function testing: selection of reference values and interpretive strategies. *Am Rev Respir Dis* 1991, 144:1202–1218.

9. Wantanabe S, Renzetti AD, Begin R, Bigler AH: Airway responsiveness to a bronchodilator aerosol. *Am Rev Respir Dis* 1974, 109:530–537.

10. Meslier N, Racineux JL, Six P, *et al.*: Diagnostic value in of chronic airway obstruction to separate asthma from chronic bronchitis: a statistical approach. *Eur Respir J* 1989, 2:497–505.

11. Tilles SA, Nelson HS: Differential diagnosis of adult asthma. *Immunol Allergy Clin North Am* 1996, 16:19–43.

12. Ryan G, Latimer KM, Dolovich J, *et al.*: Bronchial responsiveness to histamine: relationship to diurnal variation of peak flow rate, improvement after bronchodilator, and airway caliber. *Thorax* 1982, 37:423–429.

13. Webb J, Clark TJH, Chilvers C: Time course of response to prednisolone in chronic airflow obstruction. *Thorax* 1981, 36:18–21.

14.• Sont JK, Willems LN, Bel EH, *et al.*: Clinical control and histopathologic outcome of asthma when using airway hyperresponsiveness as an additional guide to long-term treatment. *Am J Respir Crit Care Med* 1999, 159:1043–1051.
This is an important demonstration of the relationship between bronchial hyperresponsiveness and asthma control.

15. Ramsdale EH, Morris MM, Roberts RS: Bronchial responsiveness to methacholine in chronic bronchitis: relationship to airflow obstruction and cold air responsiveness. *Thorax* 1984, 39:912–918.

16. Landwehr LP, Wood RP, Blager FB, *et al.*: Vocal cord dysfunction mimicking exercise-induced bronchospasm in adolescents. *Pediatrics* 1996, 98:971–974.

17. Morris MJ, Deal LE, Bean DR, *et al.*: Vocal cord dysfunction in patients with exertional dyspnea. *Chest* 1999, 116:1676–1682.

18. Bucca C, Rolla G, Brussino L *et al.*: Are asthma-like symptoms due to bronchial or extrathoracic airway dysfunction? *Lancet* 1995, 346:791–795.

19. Powell DM, Karanfilov BJ, Beechler KB, *et al.*: Paradoxical vocal cord dysfunction in juveniles. *Arch Otolaryngol Head Neck Surg* 2000, 126:29–34.

20. Heatley DG, Swift E: Paradoxical vocal cord dysfunction in an infant with stridor and gastroesophageal reflux. *Int J Pediatr Otolaryngol* 1996, 34:149–151.

21. Reisner C, Nelson HS: Vocal cord dysfunction with nocturnal awakening. *J Allergy Clin Immunol* 1997, 99:843–846.

22. Newman LJ, Platts-Mills TAE, Phillips CD, *et al.*: Chronic sinusitis: relationship of computed tomographic findings to allergy, asthma, and eosinophilia. *JAMA* 1994, 271:363–367.

23. Pfister R, Lutolf M, Schapowal A, *et al.*: Screening for sinus disease in patients with asthma: a computed tomography-controlled comparison of A-mode ultrasonography and standard radiography. *J Allergy Clin Immunol* 1994, 94:804–849.

24. Bresciani M, Paradis L, Des Roches, *et al.*: Rhinosinusitis in severe asthma. *J Allergy Clin Immunol* 2001, 107:73–80.

25. Braunstahl GJ, Overbeek SE, Kleinjan A, *et al.*: Nasal allergen provocation induces adhesion molecule expression and tissue eosinophilia in upper and lower airways. *J Allergy Clin Immunol* 2001, 107:469–476.

26. Braunstahl G, Kleinjan A, Overbeek SE, *et al.*: Segmental bronchoprovocation induces nasal inflammation in allergic rhinitis patients. *Am J Respir Crit Care Med* 2000, 161:2051–2057.

27. Braunstahl G, Overbeek SE, Fokkens WJ, *et al.*: Segmental bronchoprovocation in allergic rhinitis patients affects mast cell and basophil numbers in nasal and bronchial mucosa. *Am J Respir Crit Care Med* 2001, 164:858–865.

28. Corren J, Adinoff AD, Irvin CG: Changes in bronchial responsiveness following nasal provocation with allergen. *J Allergy Clin Immunol* 1992, 89:611–618.

29. Corren J, Adinoff AD, Buchmeier AD, *et al.*: Nasal beclomethasone prevents the seasonal increase in bronchial responsiveness in patients with allergic rhinitis and asthma. *J Allergy Clin Immunol* 1992, 90:250–256.

30. Adams RJ, Fuhlbridge AL, Finkelstein JA, *et al.*: Intranasal steroids and the risk of emergency department visits for asthma. *J Allergy Clin Immunol* 2002, 109:636–642.

31.• ten Brinke A, Grootendorst DC, Schmidt JT, *et al.*: Chronic sinusitis in severe asthma is related to sputum eosinophilia. *J Allergy Clin Immunol* 2002, 109:621–626.
This important study demonstrates the intimate relationship between chronic hyperplastic sinusitis and asthma. Neglecting sinusitis in patients with severe asthma is a mistake because these diagnoses seem to be different clinical manifestations of the same disease process.

32. Borish L: Sinusitis and asthma: entering the realm of evidence-based medicine. *J Allergy Clin Immunol* 2002, 109:606–608.

33.•• Harding SM: Gastroesophageal reflux and asthma: insight into the association. *J Allergy Clin Immunol* 1999, 104:251–259.
The majority of patients with refractory asthma also have gastroesophageal reflux disease. This is an excellent review of the relationship between these two common diseases. It includes a practical guide to management.

34. Lodi U, Harding SM, Coghlan HC, *et al.*: Autonomic regulation in asthmatics with gastroesophageal reflux. *Chest* 1997, 111:65–70.

35. Schan CA, Harding SM, Haile JM, *et al.*: Gastroesophageal reflux-induced bronchoconstriction: an intraesophageal acid infusion study using state of the art technology. *Chest* 1994, 106:731–737.

36. Field SK, Sutherland LR: Does medical antireflux therapy improve asthma in asthmatics with gastroesophageal reflux: a critical review of the literature. *Chest* 1998, 114:275–283.

37. Johnson WE, Hagen JA, Demeester TR, *et al.*: Outcome of respiratory symptoms after anti-reflux surgery on patients with gastroesophageal reflux disease. *Arch Surgery* 1996, 131:489–492.

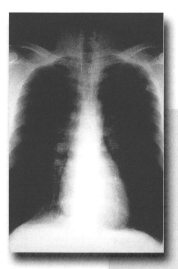

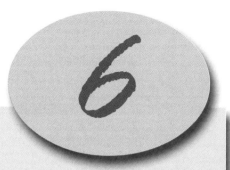

Allergy and Asthma

Elizabeth A. Erwin and
Thomas A. E. Platts-Mills

The association between allergy and asthma has long been recognized. More precise links for a causal role of allergens in asthma have been proposed with data from case-control, cross-sectional, and prospective studies, including birth cohort studies. Separately, the Bradford-Hill criteria were proposed to evaluate proof of causality between environmental exposure and noninfectious illness. However, when translated to evaluate the relationship between allergen exposure and asthma, these criteria include 1) a strong and consistent association between sensitization to allergens and asthma [1,2]; 2) exposure to allergen should precede asthma symptoms; 3) avoidance of the allergen should reverse the effect; 4) the mechanism must be biologically plausible; and 5) there must be evidence of a dose–response relationship between level of exposure and severity. The last criterion has been the most challenging, and it varies among allergens.

Nevertheless, confusing issues remain concerning the issue of why sensitization but not asthma occurs with outdoor pollens. It has been suggested that the periodicity of exposure may play a role, with daily exposure causing more persistent inflammation and subsequent asthma [3]. Particle size may also be important because of the resulting area of deposition. Most pollen deposits in the nose. *Alternaria* spores, although they are long, have an oblong shape that in the proper orientation is believed to be of respirable size. A more recent concern is the difference in immune response among even indoor allergens, which seems dependent on the level of exposure. An immune response to cats that includes IgG and IgG$_4$ antibodies without IgE that is not related to lung symptoms or asthma has been described [4].

This chapter addresses these issues and details the role of allergens in asthma (Fig. 6-1). Asthma seems to be a complex interaction of genetics and environment, which is variable depending on the nature of each allergen considered. Other factors such as viral infections or air pollution can affect the outcome as well, ultimately resulting in the different phenotypes of disease that are observed.

GENETICS

Allergy develops in a genetically predisposed population. Genome-wide studies have been done in different populations, including the Dutch, Hutterites, French, Australians, Germans, Japanese, and the Americans [5–11]. The Collaborative Study on the

Genetics of Asthma (CSGA) [11] compared phenotypes, including asthma and bronchial hyperreactivity, total IgE, specific IgE, skin tests, and eosinophils. Evidence for linkage to atopy was observed in at least two studies on chromosomes 2q, 6p, 7q, 11q, 13q, and 17q [5]. A 20-cM region on 11p has been linked to asthma or atopy in at least four populations [6]. Separate analysis for three ethnic groups in the study of the United States showed linkage to different chromosomes [11]. Those of European descent mapped to 6p, those of African-American ethnicity linked most strongly to 11q, and those of Hispanic heritage linked to 1p. Candidate genes for some of the chromosomal regions and their phenotypes have been proposed. The gene for FcεR1 is located on 11q [5]. The region on 13q contains the gene for endothelin receptor B. A broad region on 17q has been implicated, and several candidates have been suggested, including the transcription factor signal transducer and activator of transcription 5A, chemokine receptor 7, and the small inducible cytokines subfamily A. Several investigators have observed differences in linkages between maternal and paternal alleles [8,12]. The findings of Daniels *et al.* [8] included differences at three loci, supporting a role for immunologic interactions between mother and child rather than imprinting or anticipation.

Although a genetic contribution to asthma has long been accepted, there are several problems with genetic linkage studies [5]. First, heritability estimates of atopic phenotypes vary. Second, the number of contributing genes is unknown. If each gene involved makes a modest contribution, the ability to find linkage produced by one

gene may not be high. Third, environmental risk factors cause a confounding effect. Finally, parent-of-origin effects have not been evaluated in most studies.

ALLERGEN EXPOSURE

In those at risk, exposure to allergens leads to an immune response of IgE and IgG$_4$ that has traditionally been described as a Th2 response. The T cells associated with these responses can produce both interleukin (IL)-4 and -5. This response is dependent on the degree of exposure and the immunogenic properties of the allergen. Exposure measurements for dust mites and cockroaches are based on allergen concentrations in dust (µg/g) [13•]. These measurements are quite reproducible. However, most investigators have been unable to detect airborne mite allergens in the absence of disturbance. In contrast, allergens such as cat and dog dander that are consistently airborne are more difficult to measure and are dependent on such variables as disturbance and ventilation. Nevertheless, most studies to date have reported exposure to these allergens as the concentration of major allergen measured in reservoir dust (Table 6-1).

Dust Mites

Several studies have demonstrated a dose–response relationship between exposure to dust mites and the development of sensitization, asthma, or both. In an early study, Korsgaard [14] used dust mite counts to determine exposure. He consistently found a greater relative risk than when comparing a higher exposure group to a lower

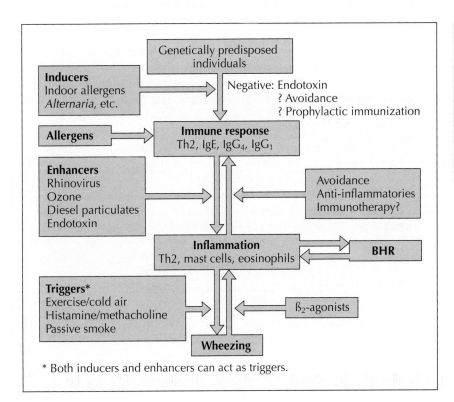

Figure 6-1.
A model for the role of allergens in asthma. In genetically predisposed individuals, sensitization to allergen results in an immune response that, if unchecked by intervention or if enhanced by air pollution or viral infection, leads to persistent inflammation and wheezing. BHR—bronchial hyperreactivity.

one. Also, the population-attributable risk was 60% when the concentration of dust mites was compared in patients with asthma and healthy patients. Thus, it was suggested that a large proportion of the occurrence of asthma in dust mite–sensitive patients was attributable to high exposure to dust mites. Direct measurement of mite allergen confirmed a dose–response relationship. Lau *et al.* [15] demonstrated a significant correlation between dust mite allergen exposure and sensitization. They suggested that a concentration of 2 µg/g or more of dust is a high-risk environment for development of specific IgE to dust mites. Furthermore, comparing atopic subjects with low dust mite exposure with atopic subjects with high exposure, the risk of becoming sensitized was seven- to elevenfold higher for atopic subjects with high exposure. In the United Kingdom, where 80% of children with asthma have a positive skin test result for house dust mites, Sporik *et al.* [16] found that at 11 years of age, their patients had a relative risk for asthma of 14.6 if they were allergic compared with those who were nonallergic. The relative risk increased to 19.7 if the child was sensitized to dust mites. Although correlation between exposure and sensitivity did not reach significance ($P = 0.062$), none of the children exposed to less than 2 µg Der p 1 per gram of dust were sensitized. This finding provided further evidence that 2 µg Der p 1 per gram of dust was an approximate threshold for exposure required for those at risk to become sensitized.

A description of mites is useful at this point because of their unique role in asthma [17]. Mites are classified in the phylum Arthropoda, subphylum Chelicerata. Their chelicerae are pincer-like. They are in the class Arachnida, order Acari. Astigmatid mites such as house dust mites exchange O_2 and CO_2 over their body surface rather than by an organized respiratory system. They feed on many different organic substrates, although they thrive on fungi and skin scales. In fact, they require fungi to be grown in culture. Although 20 or more species have been found in house dust, the three most common are *Dermatophagoides farinae*, *Dermatophagoides pteronyssinus*, and *Euroglyphus maynei* in temperate climates. *Blomia tropicalis* is an important species in tropical and subtropical areas. *D. farinae* and *D. pteronyssinus* are the most prevalent and often coinhabit homes with one species usually predominating, although variably in the same geographic area. The life cycle of mites is extremely sensitive to humidity because they achieve their water balance (with water providing 70% to 75% of their body weight) by absorbing water from water vapor in the air. The critical humidity for *D. farinae* ranges from 55% to 75% relative humidity over the temperature range 65°F to 85°F. Many of the allergens associated with mite fecal matter are enzymes from the digestive tract. Thus, the group 1 allergens are glycoproteins with cysteine protease activity.

Cockroaches

Perhaps some of the strongest evidence is found in communities where a high prevalence of asthma is associated with indoor allergens other than dust mites [13]. In some North American cities, sensitization to allergens from the German cockroach, *Blattella germanica*, is commonly associated with asthma among inner-city populations presenting to the emergency room [18,19]. In Baltimore, it was demonstrated that 33% of 81 children with moderate to severe asthma had a positive skin test result to cockroach [20]. The occurrence of positive skin test response increased with cockroach allergen levels in bedroom dust samples. Sensitization was 100% in those exposed to 10 U Bla g 1 per gram of dust and 5 U Bla g 2 per gram of dust. Risk factors for cockroach sensitization were being black, low socioeconomic status, age over 11 years, and

Table 6-1. PROPERTIES OF INDOOR ALLERGENS

Source	Airborne Particles, *µm*	Allergen, *kD*	Function/Homology
Dust mite (*Dermatophagoides pteronyssinus*)	Feces, 10–40	Der p 1, 25 Der p 2, 13	Cysteine protease Epididymal protein
German cockroach (*Blattella germanica*)	Frass saliva, > 5	Bla g 2, 36 Bla g 5, 23 Fel d 1, 36	Aspartic protease Glutathione transferase
Cat (*Felis domesticus*) } Dog (*Canis familiaris*) }	Dander particles, 2–15	Can f 1, 21 Mus m 1, 22	Uteroglobin Lipocalin
Mouse (*Mus domesticus*) } Rat (*Rattus norwegicus*) }	Urine on bedding, etc., 2–20	Rat n 1, 19 Lol p 1, 29	Major urinary protein Pheromone binding
Grass	Pollen, 30		Cysteine proteinase

*Data from *www.allergen.org*.

cockroach allergen exposure. The rate of sensitization among low socioeconomic status black patients was 75%. Rosenstreich *et al.* [21] found greater positive skin test result responses to cockroach (36.8%) than dust mite (34.9%) in eight inner-city areas. The majority of bedrooms had detectable cockroach allergen, 85%, with high levels exceeding 8 U Bla g 1 per gram of dust in 50%. In those who were sensitive to cockroach and exposed to high levels, the rate of hospitalization was 3.4 times higher. The group also had more unscheduled visits to health care providers for asthma and noted more day and nocturnal symptoms.

Alternaria

In the dry areas of the southwestern United States and Australia, *Alternaria* spp has been reported to be the dominant allergen associated with asthma. Examination of two regions of Australia, coastal and inland, revealed a variable prevalence of sensitivity to different allergens [3]. Although dust mite exposure was significantly lower inland, the prevalence of sensitivity was not different. However, more children were sensitized to *Alternaria* spp and rye grass in the inland region. *Alternaria* spp was the most important risk factor of current asthma in that region. In another study in Tucson, Arizona, sensitivity to

Alternaria spp showed a significant association with asthma [22]. Circumstantial evidence supporting exposure to *Alternaria* spp as a risk factor for respiratory arrest has also been reported from the Midwest portion of the United States [23].

Alternaria spp molds are found in temperate regions worldwide [24]. They are most common inland, in grain-growing areas, where they can grow on dead vegetation. Their spores are larger than those of other common fungi. Spore release is most often triggered by conditions that occur on summer and autumn mornings. Spore levels peak in autumn because of increased growth of fungi on rotting leaves. Alt a 1 is a heat-stable dimer of 28 kD. It is present in both spores and mycelia. This protein has been shown to play an important role in sensitization to *Alternaria* spp [25].

Cats

Cat allergens are a paradox. In mite-free environments, cat sensitization can be strongly associated with asthma (Table 6-2). Among school children in New Mexico, the odds ratio for a child who was cat-sensitized and exposed to cat allergen having asthma was 6.2 [29]. In northern Sweden, where it is too dry for dust mite growth, there is a high prevalence of sensitization to cats, dogs, and birch

Table 6-2. SENSITIZATION TO INDOOR ALLERGENS AND ASTHMA

Study	Country	Dominant Allergens	Odds Ratio	Pollen
Sporik *et al.* [1] (prospective)	United Kingdom	Mite (cat)	19.7*	NS
Sears *et al.* [26] (prospective)	New Zealand	Mite (*Aspergillus* spp)	6.6*	NS
Ronmark *et al.* [27] (population)	Sweden	Cat, dog	3.9*	Birch*
Peat *et al.* [2] (schools)	Australia	Mite	≥ 10*	NS
Lau *et al.* [15] (birth cohort)	Germany	Mite, cat	—	NS
	United States			
Squillace *et al.* [28] (schools)	Virginia	Mite (cat, cockroach)	6.6*	NS
Call *et al.* [19] (acute [ER])	Atlanta, GA	Mite, cockroach	8.2*	NS
Halonen *et al.* [22] (prospective)	Arizona	*Alternaria* spp	—	NS
Sporik *et al.* [29] (school)	New Mexico	Cat, dog	6.2*	NS
Lewis *et al.* [30] (birth cohort)	Boston, MA	Mite, cat	3.8*	NS

Significant.
ER—emergency room; NS—not significant.

trees [27••,31,32]. There was also a significant association with asthma for sensitization to cat allergen. However, the presence of a cat at home was not found to be a risk factor for asthma or sensitization. In fact, presence of a cat at home decreased the risk of sensitization. Only 17% of the children with IgE to cat had a cat at home, and 36% of the children without IgE had a cat at home. By contrast, the presence of a cat at home was associated with IgG to Fel d 1. In the United States, a decreased risk of sensitization was noted among school children exposed to more than 20 μg Fel d 1 per gram of dust [4••]. Although the prevalence of IgE to cat allergen was decreased in the high exposure group, IgG to Fel d 1 increased with exposure. Overall, the prevalence of IgG antibody without IgE was 20%. On average, 20% of the IgG antibody to Fel d 1 was IgG_4. Unlike IgE antibody, IgG antibody was not associated with asthma. We have described this phenotype as a modified Th2 response. This response has been demonstrated in a study from Boston as well as in the Virginia and Swedish cohorts [4,31]. The important feature is that the presence of IgG or IgG_4 without IgE is not related to asthma.

Mice and Rats

The relationship of mouse exposure to asthma has not yet been determined. A recent study investigated the prevalence and clinical importance of mouse allergen in eight major inner-city areas [33]. They found detectable mouse allergen in at least 1 room in 95% of homes. The highest levels (median, 1.6 μg/g dust) were measured in kitchens. Mean levels varied in different cities from a low of 0.3 to 7.87. Mouse sensitivity was reported in 89 (18%) of 499 children. Those with mouse allergen levels greater than the median had a higher risk of mouse sensitization than those with levels below the median. However, there was no significant relationship between mouse sensitization and asthma morbidity. In another study in Atlanta, sensitization was found in only 2% of 85 inner-city children with asthma [34].

Exposure to occupational allergens such as rat urinary proteins (RUPs) by laboratory workers can serve as a model to study the relationship of exposure to sensitization. Heederik *et al.* [35] pooled the results of three studies to increase the power of their analysis. Surprisingly, they found an increased sensitization risk in atopic patients at low exposure levels, but the highest exposure group had a risk of sensitization that was four times greater.

Immune Response

The relationship between asthma and sensitivity to specific allergens can be observed indirectly through total serum IgE levels. Asthma rates have been shown to increase with increasing serum IgE [36,37]. A linear relation between the odds ratio of having asthma and increasing IgE has been demonstrated. In one study [37], no asthma was reported in children with IgE less than 32

IU/mL, but 36% of those with IgE of greater than 1000 reported asthma. Furthermore, airway hyperresponsiveness also correlated with serum IgE, even in asymptomatic children.

When an increase in asthma was noted in one traditional village community in Papua New Guinea, investigation for the etiology was begun [38]. Despite relatively late age of onset, most of the patients demonstrated reactions to house dust mite and had elevated serum IgE antibody levels to *D. pteronyssinus*. It was also found that recently acquired cotton blankets had very high levels of dust mites. Although this is not proof of a causal relationship, it provides further evidence for the link between exposure, sensitization, and asthma.

INTERVENTIONS

The efficacy of various antiallergic therapies, including avoidance, immunotherapy, and now anti-IgE in prevention and treatment of asthma, provides direct evidence for a relationship between allergen exposure and asthma.

Trials of allergen avoidance have been done in two main groups: those in which patients are removed from their home environment, and those in which the home environment is modified (Table 6-3). Platts-Mills *et al.* [45] admitted nine patients with asthma who were sensitized to inhalant allergens, including *D. pteronyssinus*, to a mite-free hospital room. They observed decreased symptoms, improved peak flows, decreased medication use, and increased PD_{30} histamine. Boner *et al.* [46] admitted 14 patients with asthma on alternate-day oral corticosteroids to a sanatorium at a high altitude in Italy. They found improvement in pulmonary function, improved exercise tolerance, cessation of the need for oral steroids, and overall decrease in medication usage. Attempts to duplicate these results in home environments have been variable, but most trials for 6 months or longer have shown decreased symptoms. In one trial of 70 children with asthma, although successful mite allergen reduction was achieved, clinical improvement was modest [42]. There was a significant increase in FEV_1 (forced expiratory volume in 1 second) in the actively treated group at 6 months. Additionally, only 50% of the actively treated group took medications compared with 80% of the placebo-treated group, suggesting a decrease in symptoms. van der Heide *et al.* [47] obtained similar results with a large reduction in exposure but a small decrease in airway hyperresponsiveness. In several other trials in which mite allergen reduction was achieved, bronchial hyperreactivity was reduced significantly [41,44].

The successful controlled trials provide extensive evidence about effective methods of mite allergen avoidance [48,49]. Because of the realization that mattresses contained large numbers of mites, recommendations have evolved from vacuuming to the use of plastic covers to the current allergen-proof fabrics. In general, a pore size of 6 to 10 µm allows little to no leakage of allergen and completely prevents live dust mites from getting into the mattress or pillow. Interestingly, synthetic pillows have demonstrated greater amounts of mite allergens than feather pillows, emphasizing the importance of pillow covers. Studies have found that washing in hot water ($\geq 130°F$) is necessary to kill mites but because of pediatric safety issues regarding home water temperature, outside drying or drying in a tumble dryer for 20 minutes are good alternatives. Controlling humidity through air conditioning and dehumidifiers is an important feature of avoidance. If carpet removal is not an option, a double-thickness vacuum bag is the most important feature of a vacuum. The role of chemical agents and air filters for dust mites is not clear.

If allergen exposure plays a significant role in asthma, we might predict that treatment with immunotherapy could improve or even prevent the development of disease. In a multicenter study [50••], 208 children with rhinoconjunctivitis, positive skin prick test results, and conjunctival challenge were randomly assigned to treatment with specific immunotherapy to grass pollen, birch pollen, or both for 3 years. Although there was variation among the centers, for patients who did not have asthma, the common odds ratio was 2.5 in support of the finding that specific immunotherapy can prevent the development of asthma. Also among children with asthma, significantly more children in the control group experienced increased asthma symptoms after 2 and 3 years. In 1968, Johnstone and Dutton [51] published a 14-year placebo-controlled prospective study in 130 young children with asthma treated with desensitization. At 16 years of age, 22% of placebo-treated children were free of symptoms and 72% of children who were desensitized were free of symptoms. Children with either mild or severe asthma before the study experienced signifi-

cantly fewer days of wheezing with desensitization. Jacobsen *et al.* [52] reported on 50 patients, 19 of whom also had asthma, who were treated with specific immunotherapy for birch or a birch, alder, and hazel mixture for 3 years. All but two (89%) of the patients with asthma reported improvement in asthma symptoms. At 6-year follow-up, 68% of patients maintained this improvement. Perhaps more important, none of the patients with allergic rhinitis alone who had received immunotherapy developed asthma during the follow up period.

Anti-IgE, a recombinant, humanized monoclonal antibody that prevents binding of IgE to FcεR1, is currently being used in clinical trials to treat allergic disease. Busse *et al.* [53••] treated 400 patients with severe asthma and found the drug to be superior to placebo in all parameters, including number, severity, and duration of exacerbations. Furthermore, 40% of the patients treated with anti-IgE were able to discontinue inhaled corticosteroids compared with 20% of those receiving placebo.

INFLAMMATION

The depth of information regarding inflammation in asthma is extensive and is discussed in other chapters. However, it is necessary to mention a few details in brief here as further evidence in support of a relationship between allergens and asthma. The first factor is the response to anti-inflammatory nasal treatment in the form of intranasal corticosteroids. Watson *et al.* [54] evaluated 21 patients with allergic rhinitis and asthma in a randomized, controlled trial with intranasal beclomethasone dipropionate (BDP) or placebo for 4 weeks. The mean PC_{20} methacholine significantly improved with intranasal corticosteroids. Asthma symptom scores were lower in

Table 6-3. DECREASE IN BRONCHIAL HYPERREACTIVITY: EVIDENCE FROM SIX CONTROLLED TRIALS

Reference	Time	Patients, *n/n*	Intervention	Decrease in Mite	Primary Outcome
Murray and Ferguson [39]	1 y	10/10	Physical barriers	++	BHR
Walshaw and Evans [40]	1 y	22/20	Physical barriers	++	PEFR/BHR
Ehnert *et al.* [41]	1 y	8/16	Physical barriers, acaricide	++	BHR
Carswell *et al.* [42]	6 mo	24/25	Physical barriers, acaricide, washing, vacuuming	+	PEFR/BHR
van der Heide *et al.* [43]	6 mo	15/15	Physical barriers, air cleaner	++	BHR
Htut *et al.* [44]	6–12 mo	7/8	Hot air, ventilation steam cleaning	++	BHR

+—significant; ++—highly significant.
BHR—bronchial hyperreactivity; PEFR—peak expiratory flow rate.

those who were actively treated, but the improvement did not reach statistical significance.

The key inflammatory cells involved are considered part of the Th2 immune response [55]. Th2 lymphocytes are linked directly to eosinophilic inflammation by production of IL-4 and IL-5. IL-5 is the major eosinophil growth factor, and IL-4 causes upregulation of eosinophil adhesion and attraction. Eosinophils are a defining feature of asthma. Recent evidence has suggested that mast cells are increased in airway smooth muscle of individuals with asthma as well [56].

Finally, the maintenance of such inflammation may be integral in the asthmatic response to triggers such as viral infection. In a recent study [57], the combination of sensitization with high allergen exposure and viral infection was associated significantly with increased hospital admissions.

Enhancers

A thorough examination of the role of the environment includes consideration of air pollution. Although it is not a new problem, recent years have seen increases in air pollutants generated by motor vehicles [58,59]. These pollutants relevant in airway disease exacerbation include ozone and particulate matter such as diesel exhaust particles that include nitrogen oxides and aldehydes. In Europe, diesel exhaust is the principle source of particulate matter, but in the United States, sea spray and agricultural activity are important contributors. Ozone is a byproduct of atmospheric reactions that occur with nitrogen oxide species, volatile organic compounds, and ultraviolet light; therefore, its production occurs variably depending on the environment. Elevated levels of particulate air pollution have been associated with an increased mortality rate [60]. Both ozone and diesel exhaust particles have been shown to alter allergic inflammation. Extrinsic asthmatic patients experienced an increase in neutrophils and eosinophils after exposure to ozone [61]. Diesel exhaust particles have been shown to enhance ongoing IgE production [62]. Both also show enhancement of responses to natural allergens on allergen challenge. Nasal challenge with ozone and dust mites increased eosinophilic cationic protein levels significantly and showed a trend toward increased eosinophils and polymorphonuclear cells [63]. Nasal challenge with diesel exhaust particles and ragweed resulted in higher ragweed-specific IgE and IgG$_4$ levels [64].

Endotoxin, a contaminant of ambient air primarily in agricultural settings, has been identified in particulate matter. Parodoxically, endotoxin has been suggested to exacerbate asthma in individuals already sensitized to allergens but suppresses development of IgE responses to allergens and development of asthma at a young age [65–68].

Exposure to tobacco smoke is another environmental risk factor for wheezing, although it is most likely to be a cofactor rather than an initiator. The data are somewhat confusing. Studies of incidence and prognosis suggest an association of parental smoking with early nonatopic wheezing that is usually mild and transient [69]. However, studies of prevalence and severity suggest that exposure increases occurrence of more severe symptoms, clinic visits, and hospital admissions. Smoking does seem to affect immune responses, though, because levels of total IgE have been shown to be higher in smokers. In contrast, specific IgE levels vary such that current smoking is an important risk factor for sensitization to dust mites, but it is negatively associated with sensitization to grass and cats [70].

ATYPICAL ALLERGEN EXPOSURE

Intrinsic Asthma

Another whole subtype of asthma has been recognized and labeled "intrinsic" asthma. The precise definition varies, but traditionally inhalant skin test results are negative, total serum IgE is normal, and no specific IgE is found [71]. However, eosinophilia and extensive sinus disease are common among these individuals. Prevalence estimates vary from less than 5% to 20% in adults. There is debate about the relationship of this type of asthma to atopy. Humbert *et al.* [71] argued for more similarities than differences. Serologically, they cited IgE levels in the normal range, but higher than those observed in normal controls and higher eosinophil counts. Bronchial biopsy revealed eosinophils, increased IL-4 and IL-5 production, increased expression of FcϵR1, presence of cells positive for mRNA for the ϵ germline transcript, and ϵ heavy chain in both groups of asthmatic patients.

Trichophyton

Somewhere between the two classifications of asthma, although it has traditionally been considered intrinsic, is a category of severe cases of asthma that are related to hypersensitivity to allergens from fungi colonizing the patient. Wise and Sulzberger [72] first noted that some cases of late-onset asthma might be related to dermatophyte colonization of the feet and sensitization to extracts of *Trichophyton* spp. More recently, immediate hypersensitivity to *Trichophyton tonsurans* was demonstrated in a series of male patients with asthma and fungal infection of the skin and nails [73]. Their immune response was characterized by IgE and IgG, with IgG$_4$ to *Trichophyton* antigens consistent with a Th2-type immune response. This implies that infection caused by *Trichophyton* spp on the feet can be absorbed systemically and lead to IgE antibody production, sensitization of the airway, and development of allergic symptoms. In a second study [74], 11 patients were treated with 5 months of antifungal treatment using fluconazole. The patients showed improvement by decrease in bronchial hyperreactivity to *Trichophyton* spp and decrease in steroid dose. In many cases, improvement persisted with

3 years of treatment. Purified antigens Tri t 1 and Tri t 4 have revealed both immediate hypersensitivity and delayed-type hypersensitivity responses [75]. Through cloning and sequencing, a homology with serine proteases has been reported. The important principle is that the studies appear to establish that an intrinsic allergen can give rise to asthma.

Aspergillus

Other fungi have been implicated in severe asthma because of their presence in the lungs. *Aspergillus fumigatus*, which causes allergic bronchopulmonary aspergillosis (ABPA), has been the best described [76]. The associated immune response includes production of IgE to aspergillus and often IgG production with increased total IgE levels and peripheral eosinophilia. Production of multiple IgE-binding proteins variably expressed has resulted in discordant skin test results. The availability of a standardized extract would still challenge the diagnostician to distinguish sensitization to *Aspergillus* spp from ABPA. Recent research has focused on identifying ABPA-specific allergens. Hemmann *et al.* [77] demonstrated ABPA-specificity and skin test reactivity with rAsp f 4 and rAsp f 6, but suggested serum diagnosis with ImmunoCAP (Pharmacia, Peapack, NJ) because recombinant allergens are not yet approved for skin testing. If untreated, ABPA can lead to irreversible changes in lung function and end-stage pulmonary fibrosis [76]. The mainstay of treatment is corticosteroids, but in some cases, itraconazole has been an effective corticosteroid-sparing agent. Again, the results support the view that an allergen source on the body can play an important role in asthma.

CONCLUSIONS

There is little debate that allergens are relevant to asthma, but many questions remain to be answered. The important issue in each situation is to provide information that is helpful in the management of allergic individuals and at-risk families. The evidence is consistent that allergic individuals who have symptoms of rhinitis or asthma should decrease exposure. However, it is clear that the avoidance measures recommended for dust mites, cockroaches, and domestic animals are not the same. Thus, defining sensitization is essential for education about avoidance measures or immunotherapy. The evidence about primary prevention is less clear. For dust mites and cockroaches, there is a direct dose–response relationship between exposure and sensitization; however, this is not true for cat and dog allergens. Thus, we are not in a position to give strong advice about the conditions in a home that would decrease the risk of a young child's developing sensitization or asthma. In particular, it is not clear that avoiding keeping animals prevents or even decreases the risk of sensitization to domestic animals. On the other hand, the available data

are very confusing about whether exposure to an animal at home has nonspecific effects on sensitization or asthma symptoms. The evidence about the fungal allergens provides compelling evidence that "intrinsic" allergens can contribute to disease. The practical issue is that the newer antifungal medications are much better accepted that the older ones. Overall, the evidence strongly argues that the management of asthma requires defining sensitization in the majority of cases, and that allergen-specific measures play a major role in optimal management.

REFERENCES AND RECOMMENDED READING

Papers of particular interest, published recently, have been highlighted as:
- *Of importance*
- *Of major importance*

1. Sporik R, Chapman MD, Platts-Mills TAE: House dust mite exposure as a cause of asthma. *Clin Exp Allergy* 1992, 22:897–906.

2. Peat JK, Tovey E, Toelle BG, *et al.*: House dust mite allergens: a major risk factor for childhood asthma in Australia. *Am J Respir Crit Care Med* 1996, 153:141–146.

3. Peat JK, Tovey CM, Mellis CM, *et al.*: Importance of house dust mite and *Alternaria* allergens in childhood asthma: an epidemiological study in two climatic regions of Australia. *Clin Exp Allergy* 1993, 23:812–820.

4.•• Platts-Mills TAE, Vaughan J, Squillace S, et al.: Sensitisation, asthma, and a modified Th2 response in children exposed to cat allergen: a population-based cross-sectional study. Lancet 2001, 357:752–756.
A paper introducing evidence for the presence of IgG and IgG4 to Fel d 1 without IgE to cats in a subset of individuals with high exposure.

5. Koppelman GH, Stine OC, Xu J, *et al.*: Genome-wide search for atopy susceptibility genes in Dutch families with asthma. *J Allergy Clin Immunol* 2002, 109:498–506.

6. Ober C, Tsalenko A, Parry R, Cox NJ: A second-generation genome wide screen for asthma-susceptibility alleles in a founder population. *Am J Hum Genet* 2000, 67:1154–1162.

7. Dizier MH, Besse-Schmittler C, Guilloud-Bataille M, *et al.*: Genome screen for asthma and related phenotypes in the French EGEA study. *Am J Respir Crit Care Med* 2000, 162:1812–1818.

8. Daniels SE, Bhattacharrya S, James A, *et al.*: A genome-wide search for quantitative trait loci underlying asthma. *Nature* 1996, 383:247–250.

9. Wjst M, Fischer G, Immervoll T, *et al.*: A genome-wide search for linkage to asthma. *Genomics* 1999, 58:1–8.

10. Yokouchi Y, Nukaga Y, Shibasaki M, *et al.*: Significant evidence for linkage of mite-sensitive childhood asthma to chromosome 5q31-q33 near the interleukin 12 b locus by a genome-wide search in Japanese families. *Genomics* 2000, 66:152–160.

11. Xu J, Meyers DA, Ober C, *et al.*: Genome wide screen and identification of gene-gene interactions for asthma-susceptibility loci in three U.S. populations: Collaborative Study on the Genetics of Asthma. *Am J Hum Genet* 2001, 68:1437–1446.

12. Moffat ME, Cookson WOCM:. Maternal effects in atopic disease. *Clin Exp Allergy* 1998, 28(suppl):56–61.

13.• Platts-Mills TAE, Vervloet D, Thomas WR, *et al.*: Indoor allergens and asthma: report of the Third International Workshop. *J Allergy Clin Immunol* 1997, 100(suppl):1–24.
A thorough review of indoor allergens and asthma.

14. Korsgaard J: Mite asthma and residency: a case-control study on the impact of exposure to house-dust mites in dwellings. *Am Rev Resp Dis* 1983, 128:231–235.

15. Lau S, Falkenhorst G, Weber A, *et al.*: High mite-allergen exposure increases the risk of sensitization in atopic children and young adults. *J Allergy Clin Immunol* 1989, 84:718–725.

16. Sporik R, Holgate ST, Platts-Mills TAE, Cogswell JJ: Exposure to house dust mite allergen (Der p 1) and the development of asthma in childhood: a prospective study. *N Eng J Med* 1990, 323:502–507.

17. Arlian LG, Platts-Mills TAE: The biology of dust mites and the remediation of mite allergens in allergic disease. *J Allergy Clin Immunol* 2001, 107(suppl):406–413.

18. Gelber LE, Seltzer LH, Bouzoukis JK, *et al.*: Sensitization and exposure to indoor allergens as risk factors for asthma among patients presenting to hospital. *Am Rev Respir Dis* 1993, 147:573–578.

19. Call RS, SmithTF, Morris E, *et al.*: Risk factors for asthma in inner city children. *J Pediatr* 1992, 121:862–866.

20. Sarpong SB, Hamilton RG, Eggleston PA, Adkinson NF Jr: Socioeconomic status and race as risk factors for cockroach allergen exposure and sensitization in children with asthma. *J Allergy Clin Immunol* 1996, 97:1393–1401.

21. Rosenstreich DL, Eggleston P, Kattan M, *et al.*: Cockroaches in the asthma morbidity of inner-city children. *N Engl J Med* 1997, 336:1356–1363.

22. Halonen M, Stern DA, Wright AL, *et al.*: Alternaria as a major allergen for asthma in a desert environment. *Am J Respir Crit Care Med* 1997, 155:1356–1361.

23. O'Hallaren MT, Yunginger J, Offord KP, *et al.*: Exposure to an aeroallergen as a possible precipitating factor in respiratory arrest in young patients with asthma. *N Engl J Med* 1991, 324:359–363.

24. Perzanowski MS, Sporik R, Squillace AP, *et al.*: Association of sensitization to *Alternaria* allergens with asthma among school-age children. *J Allergy Clin Immunol* 1998, 101:626–632.

25. Kleine-Tebbe J, Worm M, Jeep S, *et al.*: Predominance of major allergen (Alt a 1) in *Alternaria*-sensitized patients. *Clin Exp Allergy* 1993, 23:211–218.

26. Sears MR, Herbison GP, Holdaway MD, *et al.*: The relative risks of sensitivity to grass pollen, house dust mite and cat dander in the development of childhood asthma. *Clin Exp Allergy* 1989, 19(4):419–424.

27.•• Ronmark E, Jonsson E, Platts-Mills TAE, Lundback B: Incidence and remission of asthma in schoolchildren: report from the obstructive lung disease in northern Sweden studies. *Pediatrics* 2001, 107(suppl E):37.
Evidence in a large population that the presence of a cat at home decreases the risk for asthma.

28. Squillace SP, Sporik RB, Rakes G, *et al.*: Sensitization to dust mites as a dominant risk factor for asthma among adolescents living in central Virginia. Multiple regression analysis of a population-based study. *Am J Respir Crit Care Med* 1997, 156(6):1760–1764.

29. Sporik R, Ingram JM, Price W, *et al.*: Association of asthma with serum IgE and skin test reactivity to allergens among children living at high altitude: tickling the dragon's breath. *Am J Respir Crit Care Med* 1995, 151:1388–1392.

30. Lewis SA, Weiss ST, Platts-Mills TA, *et al.*: Association of specific allergen sensitization with socioeconomic factors and allergic disease in a population of Boston women. *J Allergy Clin Immunol* 2001, 107(4):615–622.

31. Perzanowski MS, Ronmark E, Nold B, *et al.*: Relevance of allergens from cats and dogs to asthma in the northernmost province of Sweden: schools as a major site of exposure. *J Allergy Clin Immunol* 1999, 103:1018–1024.

32. Hesselmar B, Aberg N, Aberg B, *et al.*: Does early exposure to cat or dog protect against later allergy development? *Clin Exp Allergy* 1999, 29:611–617.

33. Phipatanakul W, Eggleston PA, Wright EC, Wood RA: Mouse allergen: I. The prevalence of mouse allergen in inner-city homes. The National Cooperative Inner-City Asthma Study. *J Allergy Clin Immunol* 2000, 106:1070–1074.

34. Carter MC, Perzanowski MS, Raymond A, Platts-Mills TAE: Home intervention in the treatment of asthma among inner-city children. *J Allergy Clin Immunol* 2001, 108:732–737.

35. Heederik D Venables KM, Malmberg P, *et al.*: Exposure-response relationships for work-related sensitization in workers exposed to rat urinary allergens: results from a pooled study. *J Allergy Clin Immunol* 1999, 103:678–684.

36. Burrows B, Martinez FD, Halonen M, *et al.*: Association of asthma with serum IgE levels and skin-test reactivity to allergens. *N Engl J Med* 1989, 320:271–276.

37. Sears MR, Burrows B, Flannery EM, *et al.*: Airway hyper-responsiveness in children is related to serum total IgE even in the absence of asthma and atopic disease. *Am Rev Respir Dis* 1991, 143(suppl A):19.

38. Dowse GK, Turner KJ, Stewart GA, *et al.*: The association between *Dermatophagoides* mites and the increasing prevalence of asthma in village communities within the Papua New Guinea highlands. *J Allergy Clin Immunol* 1985, 75:75–83.

39. Murray AB, Ferguson AC: Dust-free bedrooms in the treatment of asthmatic children with house dust or house dust mite allergy: a controlled trial. *Pediatrics* 1983,71:418–422.

40. Walshaw MJ, Evans CC: Allergen avoidance in house dust mite-sensitive adult asthma. *Q J Med* 1986, 58:199–215.

41. Ehnert B, Lau-Schadendorf S, Weber A, *et al.*: Reducing domestic exposure to dust mite allergen reduces bronchial hyperreactivity in sensitive children with asthma. *J Allergy Clin Immunol* 1992, 90:135–138.

42. Carswell F, Birmingham K, Oliver J, *et al.*: The respiratory effects of reduction of mite allergen in the bedrooms of asthmatic children: a double-blind controlled trial. *Clin Exp Allergy* 1996, 26:386–396.

43. van der Heide S, Kauffman HF, Dubois AE, de Monchy JG: Allergen reduction measures in houses of allergic asthmatic patients: effects of air-cleaners and allergen-impermeable mattress covers. *Eur Respir J* 1997, 10:1217–1223.

44. Htut T, Higenbottam TW, Gill GW, *et al.*: Eradication of house dust mite from homes of atopic asthmatic subjects: a double-blind trial. *J Allergy Clin Immunol* 2001, 107:55–60.

45. Platts-Mills TAE, Tovey ER, Mitchell EB, *et al.*: Reduction of bronchial hyperreactivity during prolonged allergen avoidance. *Lancet* 1982, 2:675–678.

46. Boner AL, Niero E, Antolini I, *et al.*: Pulmonary function and bronchial hyperreactivity in asthmatic children with house dust mite allergy during prolonged stay in the Italian Alps (Misurina, 1756 m). *Ann Allergy* 1985, 54:42–45.

47. van der Heide S, Kauffman HF, Dubois AEJ, deMonchy JGR: Allergen avoidance measures in homes of house dust mite allergic asthmatic patients: effects of acaricides and mattress encasing. *Allergy* 1997, 52:921–927.

48. Platts-Mills TAE, Vaughan JW, Carter MC, *et al.*: The role of intervention in established allergy: avoidance of indoor allergens in the treatment of chronic allergic disease. *J Allergy Clin Immunol* 2000, 106:787–804.

49. Tovey E, Marks G: Methods and effectiveness of environmental control. *J Allergy Clin Immunol* 1999, 103:179–191.

50.•• Moller C, Dreborg S, Ferdousi HA, *et al.*: Pollen immunotherapy reduces the development of asthma in children with seasonal rhinoconjunctivitis (the PAT study). *J Allergy Clin Immunol* 2002, 109:251–256.
A paper suggesting that immunotherapy may prevent asthma.

51. Johnstone DE, Dutton A: The value of hyposensitization therapy for bronchial asthma in children. *Pediatrics* 1968, 42:793–802.

52. Jacobsen L, Nuchel PB, Wihl JA, *et al.*: Immunotherapy with partially purified and standardized tree pollen extracts: IV. Results from long-term (6-year) follow-up. *Allergy* 1997, 52:914–920.

53. Busse W, Corren J, Lanier BQ, *et al.*: Omalizumab, anti-IgE recombinant humanized monoclonal antibody, for the treatment of severe allergic asthma. *J Allergy Clin Immunol* 2001, 108:184–190.
A paper describing the success of an immunologic therapy in asthma.

54. Watson WTA, Becker AB, Simons FER: Treatment of allergic rhinitis with intranasal corticosteroids in patients with mild asthma: effect on lower airway responsiveness. *J Allergy Clin Immunol* 1993, 91:97–101.

55. Wardlaw AJ, Brightling C, Green R, *et al.*: Eosinophils in asthma and other allergic diseases. *Br Med Bull* 2000, 56:985–1003.

56. Brightling CE, Bradding P, Symon FA, *et al.*: Mast-cell infiltration of airway smooth muscle in asthma. *N Engl J Med* 2002, 346:1699–1705.

57. Green RM, Custovic A, Sanderson G, *et al.*: Synergism between allergens and viruses and risk of hospital admission with asthma: case-control study. *Br Med J* 2002, 324:763–766.

58. Peden DB: Air pollution in asthma: effect of pollutants on airway inflammation. *Ann Allerg Asthma Immunol* 2001, 87(suppl):12–17.

59. Parnia S, Frew AJ: Is diesel the cause for the increase in allergic disease? *Ann Allerg Asthma Immunol* 2001, 87(suppl):18–23.

60. Dockery DW, Pope CA III, Xu XP, *et al.*: An association between air pollution and mortality in six US cities. *N Engl J Med* 1993, 329:1753–1759.

61. Peden DB, Boehlecke B, Horstman D, Devlin R: Prolonged acute exposure to 0.16 ppm ozone induces eosinophilic airway inflammation in asthmatic subjects with allergies. *J Allergy Clin Immunol* 1997, 100:802–808.

62. Takenaka H, Ahang K, Diaz-Sanchez D, *et al.*: Enhanced human IgE production results from exposure to the aromatic hydrocarbons form diesel exhaust: direct effects on B-cell IgE production. *J Allergy Clin Immunol* 1995, 95:103–115.

63. Peden DB, Setzer RW, Devlin RB: Ozone exposure has both a priming effect on allergen-induced responses and an intrinsic inflammatory action in the nasal airways of perennially allergic asthmatics. *Am J Respir Crit Care Med* 1995, 151:1336–1345.

64. Diaz-Sanchez D, Tsien A, Fleming J, Saxon A: Combined diesel exhaust particulate and ragweed allergen challenge markedly enhances human in vivo nasal ragweed-specific IgE and skews cytokine production to a T-helper cell 2-type pattern. *J Immunol* 1997, 158:2406–2413.

65. Gereda JE, Leung DY, Thatayatikom A, *et al.*: Relation between house dust endotoxin exposure, type 1 T-cell development, and allergen sensitisation in infants at high risk of asthma. *Lancet* 2000, 355:1680–1683.

66. Tulic MK, Wale JL, Holt PG, Sly PD: Modification of the inflammatory response to allergen challenge after exposure to bacterial lipopolysaccharide. *Am J Respir Cell Mol Biol* 2000, 22:604–612.

67. Michel O, Kips J, Duchateau J, *et al.*: Severity of asthma is related to endotoxin in house dust. *Am J Respir Crit Care Med* 1996, 154:1641–1646.

68. Park JH, Gold DR, Spiegelmen DL, *et al.*: House dust endotoxin and wheeze in the first year of life. *Am J Respir Crit Care Med* 2001, 163:322–328.

69. Strachan DP, Cook DG: Parental smoking and childhood asthma: longitudinal and case control studies. *Thorax* 1998, 53:204–212.

70. Jarvis D, Chinn S, Luczynska C, Burney P: The association of smoking with sensitization to common environmental allergens: results from the European Community Respiratory Health Survey. *J Allergy Clin Immunol* 1999, 104:934–940.

71. Humbert M, Menz G, Ying S, *et al.*: The immunopathology of extrinsic (nonatopic) asthma: more similarities than differences. *Immunol Today* 1999, 20:528–533.

72. Wise F, Sulzberger MB: Urticaria and hay fever due to *Trichophyton* (*Epidermophyton interdigital*). *JAMA* 1930, 95:1504–1508.

73. Ward GW Jr, Karlsson G, Rose G, Platts-Mills TAE: *Trichophyton* asthma: sensitization of bronchi and upper airways to dermatophyte antigen. *Lancet* 1989, 1:859–862.

74. Ward GW, Woodfolk JA, Hayden ML, *et al.*: Treatment of late-onset asthma with fluconazole. *J Allergy Clin Immunol* 1999, 104:541–546.

75. Woodfolk JA, Slunt JB, Duell B, *et al.*: Definition of a *Trichophyton* protein associated with delayed hypersensitivity in humans: evidence for immediate (IgE and IgG4) and delayed hypersensitivity to a single protein. *J Immunol* 1996, 156:1695–1701.

76. Vlahakis NE, Aksamit TR: Diagnosis and treatment of allergic bronchopulmonary aspergillosis. *Mayo Clinic Proc* 2001, 76:930–938.

77. Hemmann S, Menz G, Ismail C, *et al.*: Skin test reactivity to 2 recombinant *Aspergillus fumigatus* allergens in A. *fumigatus*-sensitized asthmatic subjects allows diagnostic separation of allergic bronchopulmonary aspergillosis from fungal sensitization. *J Allergy Clin Immunol* 1999, 104:601–607.

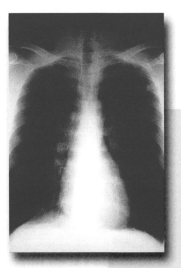

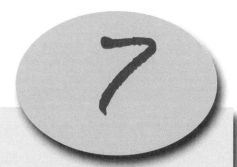

Sinusitis and Asthma

Cori Copilevitz and Raymond Slavin

The term "sinusitis" should be replaced by "rhinosinusitis," which is more accurate and descriptive of this condition because 1) sinusitis typically follows rhinitis, 2) it is unusual to have sinusitis without rhinitis, 3) the mucosa of the nose and sinuses are contiguous, and 4) nasal symptoms such as congestion and discharge are prominent features in sinusitis [1•].

Rhinosinusitis is an important topic for primary care physicians because it is both an extremely common and costly condition. In fact, it affects 14.7% of the population and is the most commonly reported chronic disease in the United States. It accounts for 11.6 million office visits per year and the fifth highest antibiotic use of all diseases [2].

DIAGNOSIS

Clinical clues to the diagnosis of acute rhinosinusitis include failure of typical cold symptoms to resolve after 7 to 10 days, change in character of nasal discharge from clear to purulent, and facial pain. The facial pain is usually most prominently felt in the cheeks and is worsened with bending or straining. The patient may also complain of teeth pain in the area of the back molars. Fevers and chills may also be present. On physical examination, thick green or yellow nasal discharge may be noted in the middle meatus, which is the draining site of the maxillary sinuses.

If the acute episode of rhinosinusitis is not addressed, the patient may proceed into a subacute or chronic phase of the disease. In this case, the patient generally presents complaining of nasal congestion, purulent postnasal drip, sore throat, foul breath, and fatigue. It is helpful for the physician to have a high diagnostic index of suspicion for this subtle presentation. In chronic rhinosinusitis, physical examination generally reveals an edematous and hyperemic nasal mucosa bathed in purulent mucus. If available, nasal endoscopy is useful for visualizing the middle meatus and the flow of the infected mucus. If sinus imaging is necessary to make a diagnosis of rhinosinusitis, a noncontrast limited coronal CT scan of the sinuses is the modality of choice over both plain radiographs and MRI. Standard radiographs inadequately visualize the ethmoid sinuses and have limited value in evaluating patients with chronic sinus disease. However, they are still the most commonly used imaging modality for evaluating sinus disease and may be the only one available in emergency situations.

It has been suggested that the traditional sinus symptom scoring system is not very accurate in predicting either the presence of actual sinus disease or its severity. In a recent study, 30% of asthmatic patients without any symptoms of nasal congestion, olfactory disturbance, headache, or facial pain had extensive sinus disease on CT. Nasal endoscopy did differ between patients with and without sinus disease with respect to detecting post-nasal drip and nasal secretions. This implies that, for an accurate estimation of the presence and severity of sinus disease, nasal endoscopy and CT scanning of the sinuses are more or less obligatory diagnostic procedures [3••].

ASSOCIATION OF RHINOSINUSITIS AND ASTHMA

The association between bronchial asthma and paranasal sinusitis has been noted for many years. A number of clinical studies performed as early as the 1920s and 1930s emphasized rhinosinusitis as a trigger for worsening asthma [4,5]. This relationship was eventually disputed because of the prevailing thought that sinus changes simply reflected a disease of the entire respiratory membrane and that management of rhinosinusitis would be expected to have little effect on the course of lower respiratory tract disease. In the past two decades, however, the relationship between the upper and lower airways has been reexamined.

One piece of evidence that demonstrates a strong relationship between rhinosinusitis and asthma is a study from the Los Angeles Children's Hospital that showed that 75% of pediatric patients admitted with status asthmaticus had abnormal sinus radiographs [6]. Another study from Finland that was done in adults reported abnormal sinus films in 87% of adults with asthma exacerbations [7]. In a report from the Netherlands, 84% of adults with severe asthma showed sinus CT abnormalities [3••]. A more recent study [8•] looked at 35 patients with severe asthma taking daily corticosteroids and 34 patients with mild to moderate asthma. The authors found that all the subjects with severe asthma had abnormalities in the CT scans of the sinuses compared with 88% of the individuals with mild to moderate asthma [8•].

There has been a suggestion that the association between chronic rhinosinusitis and asthma was strong only in the group with extensive sinus disease. It appears that peripheral blood eosinophil level is a good marker for extensive rhinosinusitis. In a study done by Newman *et al.* [9], 104 patients undergoing sinus surgery had CT scans reviewed for extent of disease, total serum IgE as well as specific IgE antibodies to common inhalant antigens measured, and a peripheral blood sample analyzed for total eosinophil count. The authors found that among the patients with peripheral eosinophilia, 87% had extensive sinus disease as seen by CT scan [9].

A recent study [3••] showed that the vast majority of patients with severe asthma not only had sinus CT abnormalities but that the extent of sinus disease was positively related to airway inflammation. This was reflected by increased eosinophils in induced sputum and peripheral blood, as well as the level of NO in exhaled air. This is indicative of an association between sinonasal and lower airway inflammation in patients with severe asthma [3••].

The overriding question is whether the association between rhinosinusitis and asthma represents an epiphenomenon—that is, are rhinosinusitis and asthma manifestations of the same underlying disease process in different parts of the respiratory tract, or is there a causal relationship? Can rhinosinusitis trigger bronchial asthma?

Although more clinical evidence is needed, some data suggest that difficult-to-treat asthma can be better controlled if coexisting rhinosinusitis is addressed, either with medications or surgery. This indicates evidence for an etiologic role of rhinosinusitis in lower airway disease.

RESULTS OF MEDICAL THERAPY OF RHINOSINUSITIS ON ASTHMA

Currently, there is no controlled study in adults that demonstrates improvement in asthma symptoms by medically treating patients with rhinosinusitis. There are, however, a number of studies in children that show a significant improvement in the asthmatic state with appropriate antibiotic treatment for coexistent rhinosinusitis. In one study by Rachelefsky *et al.* [10], 79% of the children were able to discontinue bronchodilator medication after the rhinosinusitis was medically treated. Pulmonary function test results were normal in 67% of patients who had demonstrated pretreatment abnormalities. Similar results were reported in another group of children from the University of Pittsburgh [11].

Another similar study done by Oliveira and Sole [12] looked at improvement of bronchial hyperresponsiveness (BHR) in children treated for sinusitis. The authors studied 46 atopic and 20 normal children. Methacholine challenges were done both before and 30 days after the sinusitis was treated with nasal saline, antibiotics, antihistamine or decongestant, and 5 days of prednisone. The authors found that the only patients who showed a decrease in their sensitivity to methacholine after treatment were patients with rhinitis and asthma with opacified maxillary sinuses at entry and those who had normal sinus radiographs at 30 days into the study. Therefore, the authors concluded that children with allergic rhinitis and sinusitis with asthma improved their BHR to methacholine and decreased their symptoms with appropriate response of their sinuses to medical therapy [12].

RESULTS OF SURGICAL THERAPY OF RHINOSINUSITIS ON ASTHMA

There is evidence in the literature that patients with medically resistant rhinosinusitis demonstrate improvement in their asthma after definitive nasosinus surgery. One study looked at 205 adult patients with the aspirin triad, all of whom were steroid dependent [13]. The aspirin triad, sometimes called the Samters triad, consists of nasal polyps, asthma, and aspirin sensitivity. These patients underwent functional endoscopic sinus surgery (FESS). After the procedure, 40% of the patients were able to discontinue their daily steroids for asthma control, and another 44% were able to decrease the dose of steroids to either every other day or only bursts. This study is particularly notable because patients with the Samters triad have notoriously difficult-to-treat asthma [14]. Another study looked at 20 patients between 16 and 72 years of age with asthma and chronic rhinosinusitis. These patients also underwent FESS. After the procedure, 70% reported the frequency of asthma to be less, and 65% reported less severe asthma. Notably, there was a 75% reduction in hospitalizations and an 81% reduction in emergency room and urgent care clinic visits in the year after FESS [14].

In children, the effect of FESS on chronic rhinosinusitis and asthma is also promising. Parsons and Phillips [15] reported a reduction of 89% in chronic cough and a 96% decrease in asthma after FESS in 52 children 7 months to 17 years of age. Additionally, the number of asthma exacerbations per month decreased from 6.7 to 2.5 and emergency room visits declined 79% [15]. Manning *et al.* [16] studied 14 steroid-dependent childhood asthmatic patients, six of whom were immune deficient. After FESS, 11 of the children showed improvement in their asthma, and there was decrease in lost school days from 22.3 to 14.5 as well as a decrease in hospital days from 21.4 to 6.

A study by Dunlop [17] looked at 50 patients with asthma who had endoscopic surgery. A total of 20% had reduction in the amount of inhaled corticosteroids required, and there were significant decreases in the use of oral corticosteroids and hospitalizations in the year after the surgery. Similarly, Dhong *et al.* [18] observed 19 patients who underwent endoscopic sinus surgery for rhinosinusitis. These patients demonstrated significant improvements in diurnal and nocturnal asthma symptoms and had improvements in asthma medication scores. No changes were noted in pulmonary function tests [18]. In an adult outcome study by Gliklich and Metson [19], it was noted that patients with preexisting asthma had the greatest improvement in overall health measures after sinus surgery. However, Goldstein *et al.* [20] did a retrospective medical record analysis on 13 patients with asthma who underwent FESS for medically refractory chronic rhinosinusitis and found no significant change in group mean asthma symptoms, asthma medication usage, pulmonary function test results, and number of emergency room visits or hospitalizations.

Okayama *et al.* [21] looked at 42 patients with chronic rhinosinusitis, 50 patients with stable asthma, 50 patients with chronic bronchitis, and 40 patients with allergic rhinitis and compared methacholine BHR. They found that BHR in subjects with chronic rhinosinusitis was less than that of the subjects with asthma but was similar to those with chronic bronchitis or allergic rhinitis in both its prevalence and degree. The authors then further examined patients with chronic rhinosinusitis and bronchial asthma who underwent endoscopic surgery. They noted that after the surgical treatment for chronic rhinosinusitis, the patients had a significant decrease in their BHR with improvements in both nasal symptoms and sinus lesions. Therefore, adequate therapy of chronic rhinosinusitis appeared to reduce BHR [21].

MECHANISMS RELATING RHINOSINUSITIS TO ASTHMA

Although the exact mechanism that links rhinosinusitis to asthma is unknown, a number of possibilities have been suggested. Four such theories involve the eosinophil, inflammatory mediators, neural reflexes, and circulating factors.

Eosinophils

It is well known that the eosinophil has a role in mediating injury to bronchial epithelium in patients with chronic asthma. The role of the eosinophil in chronic inflammatory disease of the paranasal sinuses has been evaluated by examining tissue from patients undergoing surgery for chronic rhinosinusitis. In one such study, it was shown that whereas sinus tissue from patients with sinusitis and concomitant asthma, allergic rhinitis, or both had a large number of eosinophils infiltrated in the tissue, patients with a history of chronic sinusitis alone did not [22].

Immunofluorescent studies have demonstrated a remarkable association between the presence of extracellular deposition of major basic protein and damage to sinus mucosa. The large amount of tissue eosinophilia seen in patients with chronic hyperplastic sinusitis has been shown to correlate with local cytokine production, particularly granulocyte-macrophage colony-stimulating factor (GM-CSF) and interleukin-2 (IL-2). The histopathologic examination of the paranasal sinus epithelium also appeared similar to that described in bronchial asthma. The suggestion is that the eosinophil acts as an effector cell in chronic inflammatory disease in paranasal respiratory epithelium, which points to the possibility that sinus disease in patients with bronchial asthma may have the same underlying mechanism of damage to the epithelial tissue.

Inflammatory Mediators

Another theory in which rhinosinusitis may act as an aggravator of bronchial asthma is by local stimulation of irritant receptors by inflammatory mediators and resulting bronchospasm. One study looked at the fluid obtained from maxillary sinus lavage in patients undergoing surgery for chronic sinusitis compared with nasal lavage fluid of patients with allergic rhinitis [23]. The levels of inflammatory mediators such as leukotrienes, prostaglandin D_2 (PGD_2), and histamine were significantly elevated in patients with chronic rhinosinusitis and were in the range associated with local inflammation and irritant receptor stimulation [23].

Another study, which used a radionucleotide technique, failed to demonstrate pulmonary aspiration of purulent nasal secretions. This indicates that the seeding of the lower airways with mucopurulent secretions is an unlikely cause of concomitant pulmonary disease. Therefore, it also seems unlikely that local mediators of inflammation would be aspirated into the lungs. There is the possibility that the sinus secretions could set off reflexes in other parts of the respiratory tract that could worsen bronchial asthma.

Neural Reflexes

The postulated neuroanatomic pathways that may reflexly connect the paranasal sinuses to the lungs are as follows: receptors in the nose, pharynx, and presumably in the paranasal sinuses give rise to afferent fibers that, in turn, form part of the trigeminal nerve. The trigeminal nerve passes to the brain stem, where it can connect via the reticular formation with the dorsal vagal nucleus. From the vagal nucleus, parasympathetic efferent fibers travel in the vagus nerve to the bronchi. The cholinergic parasympathetic nervous system plays a role in maintaining resting bronchial muscle tone as well as in mediating acute bronchospastic responses. The vagus nerve provides the cholinergic motor supply to airway smooth muscle.

Further insights into the mechanism of sinusitis-induced asthma have recently emerged. In a study of 106 patients with chronic sinusitis, histamine challenge to the lower airway before and after medical treatment was performed. Forced expiratory volume in 1 second (FEV_1) was measured as an index of bronchial narrowing and mid-inspiratory flow (MIF_{50}) was measured as an index of extrabronchial airway narrowing. Both intrabronchial and extrabronchial hyperreactivity decreased after treatment, with the reduction in extrabronchial hyperreactivity being more pronounced and preceding the intrabronchial hyperreactivity decline. The changes in intrabronchial and extrabronchial reactivity were strongly associated with pharyngitis, as determined by medical history, physical examination, and nasal lavage. The authors propose that airway hyperresponsiveness in rhinosinusitis might depend on pharyngobronchial reflexes triggered by seeding of the inflammatory process into the pharynx through postnasal drip of mediators and infected material from affected sinuses.

In a later study, these same authors demonstrated actual damage of pharyngeal mucosa in patients with chronic rhinosinusitis marked by epithelial thinning and a striking increase in pharyngeal nerve fiber density. This favors increased access of irritants to submucosal nerve endings inducing the release of sensory neuropeptides via axon reflexes with activation of a neural arch, resulting in reflex airway constriction.

Circulating Factors

As previously noted, the extent of sinus disease seen on CT was correlated with peripheral blood and sputum eosinophilia. This suggests not simply a local phenomenon, but rather a systemic process. Patients with chronic hyperplastic rhinosinusitis have an intense inflammatory process of the upper airway. It could be hypothesized that the inflamed sinus tissue not only releases mediators and cytokines into the circulation, which would directly affect the lower airways, but also releases chemotactic factors that recruit eosinophils from the bone marrow and direct them to the upper and lower airways [24••].

CONCLUSIONS

The diagnostic index of suspicion for rhinosinusitis must be high in any case of difficult-to-control asthma. Although the precise mechanism for the relationship is not known, strongly suggestive clinical evidence exists in both children and adults that rhinosinusitis not only occurs in association with bronchial asthma but may also play a role in its pathogenesis. This is based on multiple studies that indicate that appropriate medical or surgical treatment of rhinosinusitis significantly improves asthma symptomatology.

REFERENCES AND RECOMMENDED READING

Papers of particular interest, published recently, have been highlighted as:
• Of importance
•• Of major importance

1.• Kaliner M, Osguthorpe J, Fireman P, *et al.*: Sinusitis: bench to bedside. Current findings, future directions. *J Allergy Clin Immunol* 1997, 99:829–848.
A complete overview of sinusitis resulting from a consensus conference of allergists and otorhinolaryngologists.

2. McCuig L, Hughes J: Trends in antimicrobial drug prescribing among office based physicians in the United States. *JAMA* 1995, 273:214–219.

3.•• ten Brinke A, Grootendorst D, Schmidt JT, *et al.*: Chronic sinusitis in severe asthma is related to sputum eosinophilia. *J Allergy Clin Immunol* 2002, 109:621-626.
An excellent study implicating the eosinophil as the common denominator in airway inflammation in the sinuses and the lungs.

4. Gottlieb MS: Relation of intranasal sinus disease in the production of asthma. *JAMA* 1925, 85:105–109.

5. Bullen SS: Incidence of asthma in 400 cases of chronic sinusitis. *J Allergy* 1932, 4:402–408.

6. Fuller C, Richards W, Gilsanz V, *et al.*: Sinusitis in status asthmaticus. *J Allergy Clin Immunol* 1990, 85:222.

7. Rossi OVJ, Pirila T, Laitinen J, *et al.*: Sinus aspirates and radiographic abnormalities in severe attacks of asthma. *Int Arch Allergy Immunol* 1994, 103:209–216.

8.• Bresciani M, Paradis L, Des Roches A, *et al.*: Rhinosinusitis in severe asthma. *J Allergy Clin Immunol* 2001, 107:73–80.
A recent study showing the extraordinary incidence of CT abnormalities of the sinuses in patients with asthma.

9. Newman L, Platts-Mills T, Phillips CD, *et al.*: Chronic sinusitis: relationship of computed tomography findings in allergy, asthma, and eosinophilia. *JAMA* 1994, 271:363–367.

10. Rachelefsky G, Katz R, Siegel SC: Chronic sinus disease with associated reactive airway disease in children. *Pediatrics* 1984, 73:526–529.

11. Friedman R, Ackerman M, Wald E: Asthma and bacterial sinusitis in children. *J Allergy Clin Immunol* 1984, 74:185–189.

12. Oliveira C, Sole D: Improvement of bronchial hyperresponsiveness in asthmatic children treated for concomitant sinusitis. *Ann Allergy Asthma Immunol* 1997, 79:70–74.

13. English GM: Nasal polypectomy and sinus surgery in patients with asthma and aspirin idiosyncrasy. *Laryngoscope* 1986, 96:374–380.

14. Nishioka GJ, Cook PR, Davies WE, *et al.*: Functional endoscopic sinus surgery in patients with chronic sinusitis and asthma. *Otolaryngol Head Neck Surg* 1994, 110:494–500.

15. Parsons D, Phillips S: Functional endoscopic surgery in children. *Larynoscope* 1993, 103:899–903.

16. Manning S, Wasserman R, Silver R, Phillips DL: Results of endoscopic sinus surgery in pediatric patients with chronic sinusitis and asthma. *Arch Otolaryngol Head Neck Surg* 1994, 120:1142–1145.

17. Dunlop G, Scadding GK, Lund VJ: The effect of endoscopic sinus surgery on asthma: management of patients with chronic rhinosinusitis, nasal polyposis, and asthma. *Am J Rhinol* 1999, 13:261–265.

18. Dhong H, Jung YS, Chung SK, Choi DC: Effect of endoscopic sinus surgery on asthmatic patients with chronic rhinosinusitis. *Otolaryngol Head Neck Surg* 2001, 124:99–104.

19. Gliklich R, Metson R: Effect of sinus surgery on quality of life. *Otolaryngol Head Neck Surg* 1997, 117:12–17.

20. Goldstein M, Grundfast S, Dunsky EH, *et al.*: Effect of functional endoscopic sinus surgery on bronchial asthma outcomes. *Arch Otolaryngol Head Neck Surg* 1999, 125:314–319.

21. Okayama M, Iijima H, Shimura S, *et al.*: Methacholine bronchial hyperresponsiveness in chronic sinusitis. *Respiration* 1998, 65:450–457.

22. Harlin BL, Ansel DG, Lane SR, *et al.*: A clinical and pathologic study of chronic sinusitis: the role of the eosinophil. *J Allergy Clin Immunol* 1988, 81:867–875.

23. Georgitis JW, Matthews BL, Stone B: Chronic sinusitis: characterization of cellular influx and inflammatory mediators in sinus lavage fluid. *Int Arch of Allergy Immunol* 1995, 106:416–421.

24.•• Denburg J, Sehmi R, Saito H, *et al.*: Systemic aspects of allergic disease: bone marrow responses. *J Allergy Clin Immunol* 2000, 196(suppl):242–246.
An excellent review of the concept that rhinosinusitis may represent a systemic process rather than simply a local one.

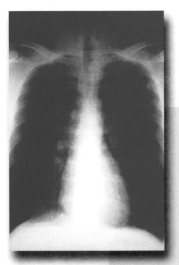

The Role of Gastroesophageal Reflux Disease in Asthma

Mark R. Stein

Gastroesophageal reflux disease (GERD) is a common disorder that affects between 7% and 20% of the adult population, depending on the reported frequency and the severity of symptoms [1,2]. The significant increase in the prevalence of GERD symptoms in adult asthmatic patients, about 72% [3•], suggests that there is something unique about the relationship between GERD and asthma.

Astute physicians have recognized the clinical relevance of this relationship since the Middle Ages, when Maimonides noted that asthma worsened after feasting [4]. Almost 100 years ago, Sir William Osler also noted a worsening of asthma after large meals, and he suggested a larger lunch and smaller dinner to avoid nocturnal asthma. He appears to be the first physician to have suggested that "reflex influences from the stomach" lead to worsening asthma [5]. This chapter reviews the prevalence of GERD in asthma and the mechanisms that explain this relationship. It provides an approach to diagnosis and reviews both medical and surgical treatment.

PREVALENCE OF GASTROESOPHAGEAL REFLUX DISEASE IN ASTHMATIC PATIENTS

The prevalence of GERD in individuals with asthma has been studied by symptom questionnaires, barium studies, pH probe studies, and endoscopic evidence of mucosal injury. One large retrospective study [3•] looked at this relationship from the standpoint of prevalence of asthma in patients with severe GERD.

Although more than 200 articles have been published on this subject, in his review of the literature, Sontag [3•] narrowed this number to 18 articles with adequate information to provide prevalence data. Three studies in adults showed percentage of patients with GERD symptoms. The first study, which was done by Perrin-Foyalle *et al.* [6], demonstrated reflux symptoms in 65% of the 150 consecutive asthmatic patients. The second study, done by O'Connell *et al.* [7], found that 72% of 189 consecutive asthmatics had heartburn. In the third study, Field *et al.* [8] noted that 77% of asthmatic patients had heartburn. If these three studies are reviewed together, then the total number of patients is 443, and the total with GERD symptoms is 318. This would yield a 72% prevalence of GERD symptoms in asthmatic patients. Is the figure too high or too low? Harding *et al.* [9] prospectively studied a group of asthmatic patients without symptoms of GERD and found 62% to have GERD on pH probe studies, suggesting that the 72% figure may actually be too low. In children, the prevalence in nine studies ranged from 47% to 75% [3•,4–11].

The prevalence of abnormal acid reflux on pH probe in six studies reviewed by Sontag [3•] ranged from 33% to 90% [12]. When averaged together, 69% of asthmatic patients have pH probe evidence of GERD. Looking for endoscopic evidence of esophageal mucosal injury in asthmatic patients, Sontag *et al.* [13] found that 39% had esophageal erosions or ulcerations and 13% had Barrett's esophagus. The prevalence of hiatal hernia in asthmatic patients has been reported to range from 59% to 64% [13,14].

In a large retrospective review [15•] of all Veterans Affairs hospitals admissions between 1981 and 1994, all cases with a primary or secondary discharge diagnosis of GERD-related esophagitis or esophageal stricture were reviewed. These 101,366 cases and an identical number of unmatched control patients, randomly selected, were analyzed for comorbidity of respiratory diseases. There was an impressive difference in the comorbidity of sinusitis, pharyngitis, laryngeal stenosis, chronic bronchitis, bronchial asthma, chronic obstructive pulmonary disease, pulmonary fibrosis, pulmonary collapse, and pneumonia (*P*< 0.0001) [15•]. The odds ratio of 1.5 for the presence of asthma was the highest of all pulmonary disorders reviewed [15•]. A large European study by Gislason *et al.* [16] found that young adults with symptoms of GERD after bedtime had a strong association with asthma and other respiratory disorders.

PATHOPHYSIOLOGY

Microaspiration

When considering the relationship of GERD and asthma, it is easy to envision refluxate spilling into the airway. Macroaspiration may lead to pneumonia, lung abscess, or bronchiectasis. Because these disorders are rarely found in asthmatic patients, microaspiration has been postulated as a mechanism for bronchoconstriction and airway remodeling. Acute microaspiration can be appreciated clinically when the patient develops dyspnea, exercise-induced hypoxemia, and localized rales or wheezing with no other pathologic processes to explain these findings. The chest radiographs are usually normal but may demonstrate atelectasis.

Initial attempts to look for microaspiration involved isotope studies. These studies had the patient ingest the isotope in a liquid or solid (incorporated in egg) form, or the isotope was instilled by nasogastric tube. Because the liquid form could lead to upper airway isotope labeling, it might result in false-positive studies with aspiration of isotope from the upper airway instead of the stomach [17,18]. The isotope ^{99}Tc sulfur colloid is given in the evening with a scintigraphic study the next morning. This technique was first successfully used to document microaspiration in 1977 [19]. In studies by other investigators, the results have varied widely, from 0% to 75% (Table 8-1) [19–24].

If all of the isotope studies from Table 8-1 were added together, there would be 148 patients studied, with 46 (31%) having positive study results. If only the studies in which isotope was instilled by nasogastric tube were analyzed, then there would be 109 patients with 20 (18%) positive studies. The low rate of positive studies may reflect a low sensitivity of the test technique or may reflect the fact that microaspiration does not occur on a daily basis. The most accurate results are obtained by instilling isotope in the stomach by nasogastric tube or by ingestion of isotope in a solid form. Positive study results are more likely to occur with ingestion of alcoholic beverages and a large fatty meal, but such indulgences are not likely to occur when the patient is being closely observed.

Microaspiration has also been proven by a second technique using simultaneous esophageal and tracheal pH

Table 8-1. ISOTOPE STUDIES SHOWING ASPIRATION

Author	Date	Route	Dose	Patients, *n*	Positive Studies, *n* (%)
Reich *et al.* [18]	1977	O, L	3–5 mCi	7	2 (29)
Ghaed and Stein [19]	1979	NG, L	5 mCi	20	0
Chernow *et al.* [21]	1979	NG, L	10 mCi	6	50 (3)
Ducolone *et al.* [20]	1987	O, L+S	2 mCi	28	21 (6)
		NG, L	10 mCi		
Crausaz and Faver [22]	1988	O, L+S	0.5 MCi		75 (24)
			4.5 mCi	32	
Ruth *et al.* [23]	1993	NG, L	200 MBq	55	20 (11)

L—liquid; NG—nasogastric tube; O—oral; S—solid.
Adapted from Stein [24].

monitoring [25,26]. An esophageal pH drop must precede the tracheal pH drop for the latter to be considered significant. In these studies, if only esophageal reflux was present, the peak expiratory flow rates (PEFRs) were lower by an average of 8 L/min. When esophageal acidification was followed by a fall in tracheal pH, the PEFRs fell an average of 84 L/min.

Additional indirect evidence for microaspiration comes from studies of pharyngeal reflux in patients with posterior laryngitis or sinusitis. Multiple studies have used pH probes 2 and 5 cm above the upper esophageal sphincter to provide evidence of significant pharyngeal pH drops [27–32]. Criteria for a positive study result include esophageal acidification preceding the pharyngeal pH drop to at least 5 [30]. This evidence is indirect because acid in the pharynx does not prove aspiration but suggests the possibility of aspiration [17,18].

Tuchman *et al.* [33] used a cat model to investigate aspiration of acid. Airway mechanics were measured in 13 animals while infusing 0.9% saline or 0.2 NHCl into the esophagus or trachea. Esophageal infusion of acid resulted in a 1.42-fold increase of total airway resistance; however, tracheal acidification with 0.05 mL of 0.2 NHCl resulted in a 4.65-fold increase in total airway resistance. This increased airway resistance was blocked with vagotomy. Instilling 0.05 mL of ^{99m}Tc sulfur colloid in the trachea did not result in any scintigraphic evidence of microaspiration. This study indicates that even when aspiration occurs, there is a significant vagally mediated response.

Vagal Reflexes

Although a vagal reflex explaining the relationship between GERD and asthma had been suggested first by Osler [5] and later by Bray [34], it was not until 1978 that Mansfield and Stein [35] first produced evidence of this relationship in humans. A Bernstein acid infusion test was used to precipitate reflux symptoms. The reflux symptoms were associated with an increase in total airway resistance (Rrs; $P = 0.01$), which was statistically different from the preceding saline infusion and the post–acid neutralization values [35]. Mansfield *et al.* [36] went on to measure airway resistance in an anesthetized dog model with induced esophagitis. In this model, either infusing the esophagus with 0.1 NHCl or distending the lower esophagus with a 60-mL air-filled balloon could elicit a bronchoconstrictive response. This response could be blocked with bilateral vagotomy.

Wright *et al.* [37] studied 136 subjects who were referred for manometry. Each patient underwent sequential esophageal infusions with sterile water, normal saline, and 0.1 NHCl at 6 mL/min rate for 15 minutes. Careful cardiopulmonary monitoring was performed. After both the normal saline (pH 5.5 to 6) [38] and the HCl infusions, there was a decrease in the forced expiratory volume in 1 second (FEV$_1$; $P < 0.001$). There was no statistical difference between the two stimuli. The heart rate decreased significantly after both the normal saline and the HCl

infusion ($P < 0.001$). The oxygen saturation also decreased after both the normal saline and the HCl infusions ($P < 0.001$). There were no statistical differences in those patients who had heartburn with HCl infusions and those who did not. The pretreatment of a subgroup of patients with atropine (0.6 mg given intramuscularly) blocked the changes noted previously. The study provides evidence for a vagal nerve–mediated esophagobronchial-cardiac reflex [37]. There is a suggestion in this study that the differences between water and normal saline or 0.1 NHCl are both osmotic as well as pH related. The use of atrial pacing in sleep apnea emphasizes the importance of the esophago-bronchial-cardiac vagally mediated reflexes [39].

Several other studies have used the acid infusion technique to demonstrate similar changes in airway function [20,38,40]. Saito and Okazawa [41] found in a guinea pig model that vagally induced bronchoconstriction was accompanied by eosinophils in the inner wall of the airway. This eosinophilic accumulation was blocked by atropine [41].

Hyperreactivity Airway

Several studies have demonstrated that asthmatic patients have widespread cholinergic hyperresponsiveness [42–44]. Herve *et al.* [45] studied 12 asthmatic patients without symptoms of GERD and seven normal control subjects. Using pH probe studies in the asthmatic patients, seven of them were found to have GERD. All asthmatic patients were studied on 3 successive days using a protocol of three randomized challenges: esophageal perfusion of isotonic saline followed by 0.1 NHCl; esophageal perfusion of isotonic saline followed by isocapnic hyperventilation of dry air; or esophageal perfusion of 0.1 NHCl followed by isocapnic hyperventilation of dry air. In five patients, the procedure was repeated using methacholine challenge in place of isocapnic hyperventilation. The seven asthmatic patients with GERD on pH probe were found to have a decrease in maximal expiratory flows at 50% of vital capacity (MEF$_{50}$) with $P < 0.01$. In three of these patients, pretreatment with atropine (2 mg given intramuscularly) was successful in blocking the decrease in MEF$_{50}$. When comparing the effects of 0.1 NHCl perfusion versus isotonic saline perfusion, there were significant differences using 0.1 NHCl for isocapnic hyperventilation ($P < 0.001$) and for methacholine challenge ($P < 0.01$). This has been the definitive study demonstrating airway hyperresponsiveness in patients with GERD who were asymptomatic. Vincent *et al.* [46] found that a methacholine provocative dose producing a 20% decrease in FEV$_1$ (PC$_{20}$) correlated with the number of reflux episodes during a 24-hour pH probe study. The studies of airway hyperreactivity indicate that GERD primes the airway to be more responsive to irritants and odors. Extreme odor and irritant sensitivity can be found in some of these patients with GERD-primed asthma.

Neurogenic Inflammation

There is a growing body of literature addressing the role of neuroinflammation in airway disease. Undem *et al.* [47,48•] recently reviewed these relationships. Neurokinin receptors are present in human nasal membranes, and neurokinin-1 (NK1) and neurokinin-2 (NK2) receptors have been found in human central airways [49]. Increased expression of NK1 and NK2 receptors has been found in asthmatic airways [50,51]. Stimulation of these receptors has been associated with bronchoconstriction (NK2) as well as vascular and proinflammatory effects (NK1) [52•]. Vagal afferents containing substance P have been identified as innervating the epithelium of the guinea pig trachea [53]. Canning [54] reviewed the axon reflex that leads to the release of tachykinins, including substance P and neurokinin A (Fig. 8-1). These capsaicin-sensitive nerve fibers have been triggered by acid reflux in animal models leading to neurogenic airway inflammation [55,56]. These fibers appear sensitive to both hydrogen ions and changes in osmolality [57,58]. In human studies of patients with allergic rhinitis, there is evidence that allergen challenge in the nose results in an increase in nerve growth factor (NGF) [59]. NGF has been found to induce increased substance P expression in airway neurons with rapid adapting receptors and leads to phenotypic switching so that fast-conducting, large capsaicin-insensitive nodose neurons ("A" fibers) become tachykinin-releasing fibers [60,61]. Baraniuk *et al.* [57] used a unilateral hypertonic saline nasal provocative challenge in humans. This resulted in unilateral dose-dependent increases in sensations or pain, blockage, and rhinorrhea. There was increased release of substance P and increased glandular secretion.

The role of neuroinflammation in asthma and in GERD-induced asthma is expanding. Viral infection, an asthma-triggering factor, has also been found to stimulate expression of substance P and neurokinin A in nonnociceptive vagal afferents (similar to the effect of NGF) in the guinea pig [62]. Neurokinins provide additional factors for direct tissue inflammation. They also appear to have significant effects on vagal tone, both through the central nervous system (CNS) effects of neurokinins and their peripheral effects, which are partly related to NGF. These responses may be even more significant in patients with an allergic component to their asthma [59–61]. Figure 8-2 demonstrates some of the relationships among GERD, microaspiration, vagal reflexes, and axon reflexes.

DIAGNOSIS

History

Although not every asthmatic patient with GERD has GERD symptoms, symptoms are a good clue in the majority of patients with GERD and asthma [3•,6–8]. A detailed questionnaire has been validated for the diagnosis of GERD [64]. A modified questionnaire, with 19 questions, has been found helpful in clinical practice (Table 8-2) [65]. The initial questions focus on the presence and frequency of dyspepsia, regurgitation, and use of

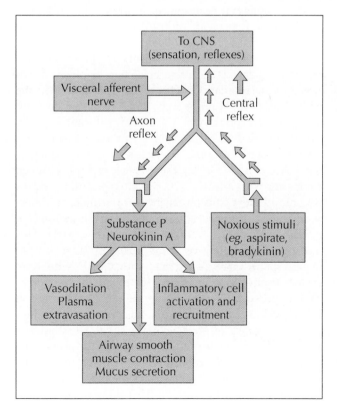

Figure 8-1.

An afferent nerve–mediated axon reflex. These capsaicin-sensitive fibers are highly sensitive to a variety of mechanical and chemical stimuli. They release proinflammatory neurotransmitters such as the tachykinins substance P and neurokinin A. CNS—central nervous system. (*Adapted from* Canning [54].)

antacids. Other related symptoms and conditions are also addressed. This questionnaire helps to quickly identify patients with GERD or laryngopharyngeal reflux.

Physical

The physical findings are usually sparse unless microaspiration has been occurring. Whereas wet rales may suggest recent aspiration, dry rales may indicate fibrosis from old aspiration. Epigastric or subxiphoid tenderness may suggest esophagitis. A stool sample that is positive for occult blood may suggest severe erosive esophagitis, among other diagnoses. Clubbing of fingers and increased anteroposterior chest diameter may be two late findings in cases with significant recurrent microaspiration.

Most of the significant physical findings can only be found on direct laryngoscopy, which can be an extension of the office physical examination. These findings are found in Table 8-3 [66–68,69•]. Carr *et al.* [67] indicated that severe arytenoid edema, postglottic edema, or enlargement of the lingual tonsil were pathognomonic of GERD in their cases. Otolaryngologists have differed on exactly which findings in the larynx are most significant in correlating with laryngopharyngeal reflux [66–68, 69•]. A scoring system has been suggested to grade changes found on laryngoscopy, which may help to improve the interpretation of what is seen and avoid variance among clinicians [70].

Diagnostic Studies

The appropriate evaluation of GERD has been reviewed elsewhere [71,72]. Studies that demonstrate the presence of microaspiration have already been reviewed. Most physicians do not use isotope studies for aspiration because of the low yield of positive test results. Most patients would refuse the invasiveness of simultaneous esophageal and tracheal pH monitoring. Barium swallows and endoscopic studies are helpful in documenting the presence of reflux, hiatal hernia, and esophagitis, but negative results do not rule out GERD. If a patient has good esophageal clearance of acid, there may be no esophageal tissue injury seen. The esophageal mucosal nerve plexus can still be stimulated by acid or distention [35–38,40], leading to both vagal and axon reflexes. The 24-hour dual pH probe is currently the best available test for the diagnosis of GERD and associated supraesophageal manifestations of GERD. Although some have reported on the use of pharyngeal pH probes, they are not currently available in clinical practice [28–32]. Even a negative pH probe result does not completely rule out GERD. A pH probe in the nasopharynx, esophagus, or both will discourage the type of activities most likely to cause GERD, such as eating a large high-fat meal, accompanied by plenty of alcohol, followed by coffee and a chocolate after-dinner mint.

Although the 24-hour pH probe is the most accurate test available, many patients are unwilling to undergo the discomfort of the study. For most patients and clinicians, the test of choice is a therapeutic trial of proton pump inhibitor (PPI) therapy. This usually involves a twice-daily pre-meal dose of PPI therapy for 2 to 3 months. This approach is based on information from the work of Harding *et al.* [73••], describing successful treatment of

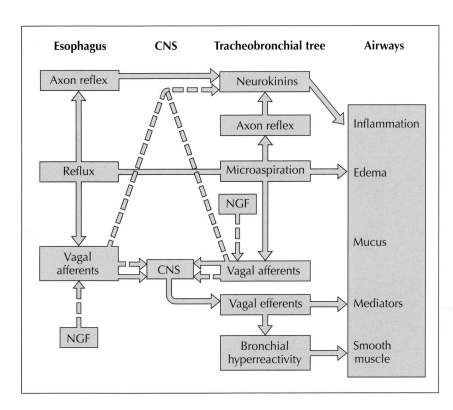

Figure 8-2.
Relationships between gastroesophageal reflux disease (GERD), microaspiration, vagal reflexes, and axon reflexes. GERD leads to microaspiration, and it also initiates axon reflexes and stimulation of vagal afferents both in the esophagus and airways. The addition of nerve growth factor (NGF) leads to switching of vagal afferent "A" fibers to neurokinin releasing fibers, which leads to additional neurokinin release, both in the central nervous system (CNS) and airways. The net result of this neural stimulation is both hyperreactive airways and airway inflammation. (*Adapted from* Harding [63].)

GERD-associated asthma through complete acid suppression. Eubanks *et al.* [32] suggested a 3-month trial of twice-daily PPI therapy for patients with pharyngeal reflux with respiratory symptoms. With a good response, the PPI dose may be decreased to once daily. If a poor response is seen, then it becomes important to obtain a pH probe study while on PPI therapy to assure adequate acid suppression. When acid reflux is still present, a higher dose of PPI and consideration of surgical treatment are needed. If there is adequate acid suppression and no improvement in asthma, it may be time to consider other factors contributing to airway inflammation. However, non-acid reflux occurs, and it may also trigger vagal and axon reflexes. Studies using intraluminal electrical impedance techniques are being used to measure the movement of refluxed gas and liquid in the esophagus [74]. This technique should prove useful in evaluating the role of non-acid reflux in airway diseases [75].

TREATMENT

Medical Therapy

Good therapy starts with initiation of appropriate asthma therapy, using medications that will not aggravate GERD. This includes avoidance of high-dose theo-phylline [76,77••]. Avoidance of all medications that aggravate GERD should be a consideration. This group of drugs includes calcium channel blockers, narcotics, benzodiazepines, dopamine, α-adrenergic agonists, progesterone, isoproterenol, nitroglycerine, and anti-cholinergics (especially atropine). Patients older than 50 years of age are frequently prescribed one or more of these medications.

In view of two recent studies [78,79•], there is a need to consider prophylactic therapy for GERD in asthmatic patients with severe exacerbations or status asthmaticus. Crowell *et al.* [78] demonstrated that inhaled albuterol produced a dose-dependent reduction in lower esophageal sphincter basal tone. Prednisone, when used at a dose of 60 mg/d for 7 days, increased esophageal acid contact times [79•]. Because continuous nebulized albuterol and high-dose intravenous corticosteroids are often part of the initial treatment of status asthmaticus, it is important to plan for control of GERD.

The cornerstone of therapy for GERD is lifestyle changes [80,81]. Because these changes include avoidance of nicotine, caffeine, chocolate, and alcohol, and a return to ideal body weight, most patients are not completely compliant. In fact, many patients complain that these changes take all the fun out of life!

Table 8-2. QUESTIONNAIRE FOR PATIENTS WITH AIRWAY DISEASE			
Do You Have	**Yes**	**No**	**Not Sure**
Heartburn or indigestion			
How often			
Regurgitation of stomach contents coming into your mouth			
How often?			
Use of antacids (Rolaids, Tums, Maalox)			
How often?			
Vomiting that occurs easily or frequently			
Frequent burps or hiccups			
Chronic cough worse after meals			
Chronic cough worse after lying down			
Chronic sinus disease			
Chest pain			
Stomach pain			
Neck pain			
Feelings of throat closing or something stuck in throat			
Adult-onset asthma			
Asthma not relieved with usual treatments			
Asthma worse after meals, alcohol, lying down, bending to tie shoes, or after onset of heartburn			
Worse heartburn after taking theophylline			
Anemia			

Adapted from *Stein [65]*.

Weight loss is often the most important factor in controlling GERD. Significant weight loss has resulted in remarkable improvement of GERD and asthma. This improvement is accompanied by dramatic reduction in medications required for both conditions. Changes in the volume and timing of meals are important. Liquids of low pH or high osmolality, such as citrus juices, may aggravate GERD symptoms, most notably when esophagitis is present. Fatty foods and chocolate have adverse effects on lower esophageal sphincter pressure (LESP) and delay gastric emptying. Carminatives, peppermint and spearmint, and onion and garlic have been found to decrease LESP. Avoidance of large meals and carbonated beverages is important to avoid increasing gastric volume, which results in increasing reflux. This is most important in the 3 hours before going to sleep. Elevation of the head of the bed is important for those with nocturnal reflux. Many patients with supraesophageal reflux leading to upper airway disease without asthma only have upright reflux and do not need to elevate the head of the bed [69•].

There are a variety of medications available to treat patients with GERD. Most patients have already used over-the-counter (OTC) antacids or alginic acid (Gaviscon; SmithKline Beecham Consumer Healthcare, Pittsburgh, PA) before seeking medical assistance. Now that H_2-receptor antagonists are also available OTC (usually at 50% of the prescription dose), patients may have also tried this group of medications at subtherapeutic doses. A detailed review is available looking at four placebo-controlled crossover studies using H_2-receptor antagonists in treating GERD-associated asthma [81]. Some improvement of asthma was noted in two studies [82,83], but technical problems with each study limited the ability to arrive at conclusions regarding effectiveness.

Medical therapy has dramatically improved since the availability of PPIs. These drugs block the final common pathway in the secretion of hydrochloric acid by binding with the H^+/K^+-ATPase enzyme, which activates the acid pump in the parietal cells. This group of drugs is generally well tolerated and easy to use in either a once- or twice-daily dosage before meals. Side effects are infrequent but include headaches, dry mouth, diarrhea, nausea, dizziness, weakness, numbness, and hair loss. Omeprazole has drug interactions based on inhibitory effects on selective cytochrome P-450 isoenzymes. This cytochrome P-450 inhibition influences the metabolism of phenytoin, warfarin sodium, and benzodiazepines. Other PPI drugs have different effects on the cytochrome P-450 isoenzymes with differing patterns of drug interactions. All PPI drugs are extremely effective in reducing acid secretion and may interfere with the absorption of some drugs, which depend on the presence of gastric acid.

Studies of the effectiveness of PPI therapy in treating asthmatic patients with GERD were reviewed previously [81,84]. There is a growing consensus concerning what constitutes an appropriate study and study group. The results may be biased by several factors, which are added or deleted. The patient population should include asthmatic patients who are classified as having moderately severe or severe asthma. This ensures the ability to measure improvement of symptoms, decreases in medication use, and changes in pulmonary functions. Ideally, other variables should be controlled, including active sinus disease and level of allergen or irritant exposure. The length of study should be at least 90 days to permit time for healing of esophagitis, laryngeal inflammation, and any other airway inflammation. This tissue repair will be needed to reduce vagal reflexes. The dose of medication used is quite important. If acid suppression is not achieved, there is low probability of finding improvement of asthma. Measuring adequate acid suppression may require multiple pH probe studies.

There has been only one study that meets most of the criteria noted above. In 1996, Harding *et al.* [73••] described the largest and longest study using omeprazole in asthmatic patients with GERD. In this study, acid control was documented with serial pH probe studies, and omeprazole dose was titrated between 20 and 60 mg/d. The 30 adult moderate asthmatic patients with GERD were followed for 3 months of therapy using acid suppressive doses. All patients had at least weekly reflux symptoms and increased distal acid reflux. With acid suppressive therapy, there was improvement of asthma control. Asthma symptom scores improved, with 66% having at least a 20% improvement in asthma symptoms. PEFRs increased 20% from baseline with treatment in 20% of patients. Asthma medication use was lowered in 17%, and prednisone dose was reduced by greater than 40% in 27% of asthmatic patients. It is important to note that 27% of patients required a dose of omeprazole greater than 20 mg/d, with six patients requiring 40 mg and two patients requiring 60 mg. Data analysis revealed that regurgitation greater than once per week or excessive proximal esophageal reflux on pH probe predicted which asthmatic

Table 8-3. LARYNGOSCOPIC FINDINGS THAT SUGGEST GASTROESOPHAGEAL REFLUX DISEASE

Posterior glottic edema (and erythema) or subglottic edema

Arytenoid edema (and erythema of medial wall)

Vocal cord nodules or granulomas

Vocal fold edema (and erythema) or ventricular obliteration

Large lingual tonsils

Data from *Hicks* et al. [66], *Carr* et al. [67,68], and *Koufman* [69•].

patients would respond to omeprazole therapy at 100% sensitivity and with a positive predictive value of 79%. This study provides a useful landmark in defining parameters that need to be considered in properly evaluating PPI therapy for GERD-associated asthma. Expectations of a response to PPI therapy without adequate acid suppression are unrealistic. The lack of a control group in the study has been the main deficiency.

Although some newer promotility agents, cisapride and domperidone, have been useful in treating GERD, neither agent is currently available in the United States. Cisapride had proven helpful in healing mild esophagitis, and it was found to be comparable with cimetidine and ranitidine in symptom relief [85]. It also showed benefit in one pediatric study [10] with GERD and asthma. The older promotility agents, metoclopramide and bethanechol, were not as effective, and metoclopramide is associated with CNS side effects [86].

Comparison studies using either H$_2$-receptor antagonists or PPIs to treat GERD demonstrate superiority for PPI [87]. It appears that the same is true in GERD-related asthma [88].

In summary, medical therapy is much more than just prescribing a pill. Excellent outlines have been devised to approach patients with asthma and GERD symptoms [72,77••,81,84]. One of the most useful is seen in Figure 8-3 [77••]. Effective therapy requires educating patients on lifestyle modification and making sure they follow through on making appropriate changes. The most cost-effective therapy is using a PPI [88]. Starting with twice-daily therapy is an approach with the best chance for success [83]. If there is good relief of GERD symptoms and improvement of asthma, then the dose can be reduced to once daily after 2 to 3 months. Inadequate response to PPIs has led to the additional use of H$_2$-receptor antagonist at bedtime. It is not yet clear whether this approach leads to long-term benefits. The addition of metoclopramide has also been tried with varying degrees of success. Failure of asthma to respond to twice-daily therapy requires reevaluation with a pH probe study with the patient on PPI therapy to check for adequate acid suppression. If there is adequate suppression of acid and no evidence of continued reflux (*ie*, alkaline reflux), then it is important to consider other causes for persistent

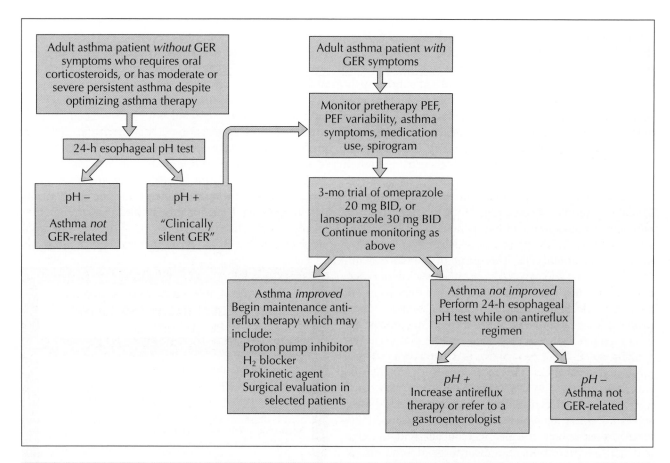

Figure 8-3.
Proposed management approach to gastroesophageal reflux (GER) disease in adult patients with asthma. BID—twice a day; PEF—peak expiratory flow;

pH+—positive esophageal pH test result;
pH- —negative esophageal pH test result.
(*Adapted from* Harding [77••].)

asthma. GERD is a chronic condition and requires long-term therapy, which is expensive. Fortunately, the safety record in long-term use of omeprazole has been good [89].

Concern has been raised that, despite a 69% improvement in asthma symptoms, there is a lack of effectiveness of medical treatment of GERD in terms of improvement in pulmonary function scores [90]. Field and Sutherland [90], who reviewed all English studies in the Medline database concerning the effectiveness of medical therapy for GERD in relieving asthma, suggested that GERD stimulates pain and an increase in minute volume, which could trigger bronchospasm in some patients. This could explain why the degree of change in pulmonary function seems related to the severity of the GERD and the degree of esophagitis present [91]. However, Wright *et al.* [37] indicated vagal reflex effects on the airway with acid infusion even in patients with no pyrosis or chest pain during this acid infusion. Herve *et al.* [45] demonstrated airway hyperreactivity in asthmatic patients with GERD but without reflux symptoms. It may be that there is a preponderance of studies in the literature that do not measure up to currently accepted criteria for research in this field. Based on Harding's work [73••], studying only asthmatic patients with frequent regurgitation would likely provide different results than studying a group with no regurgitation. The lack of improvement in pulmonary function tests could also be caused by airway remodeling as a result of even occasional episodes of microaspiration in this group of asthmatic patients.

Surgical Therapy

Surgical therapy compared to medical therapy was reviewed both by gastroenterologists [81] and surgeons [92–94]. Field *et al.* [95] surveyed the literature and found 417 surgically treated asthmatic patients with GERD. After surgery, there were decreased asthma symptoms in 79% of patients, decreased asthma medication use in 88%, and improved pulmonary functions in 27%. However, it has been noted that "most of the surgical trials have a variety of design flaws including lack of a control group, poor documentation of airflow obstruction both preoperatively and postoperatively, poor documentation of baseline asthma severity and baseline asthma therapy, and lack of objective documentation of GERD control in the postoperative state" [81]. Despite these design flaws, the surgical literature documents the significant improvement of asthma and upper airway symptoms after fundoplication [92–94].

Gastroenterologists, otolaryngologists, and surgeons agree that some patients need surgical intervention for the supraesophageal manifestations of GERD. Although PPI therapy has been able to control GERD symptoms and heal esophagitis in most patients, not all patients respond, and not all tolerate PPI therapy. Those who respond best to PPI therapy appear to be the best surgical candidates because there is already documented improvement of asthma or respiratory symptoms with acid control. Long-term therapy with PPIs and other medications is expensive, and side effects are possible. Antireflux surgery should be considered for those who need long-term treatment. Surgery may be required when medical therapy fails to control aspiration with recurrent pneumonia or pulmonary fibrosis, intractable asthma, persistent hoarseness in a singer, paroxysmal laryngospasm [96], vocal cord dysfunction (VCD) syndrome [97], recurrent vocal cord nodules, and glottic or subglottic stenosis. Some advantages of surgery are the ability to eat a normal diet and sleep flat in bed. Even with adequate acid control, reflux is still present without surgery. Alkaline reflux and microaspiration may still contribute to respiratory problems.

A good surgical outcome requires a surgeon who is highly skilled in fundoplication techniques. There is more than one type of fundoplication technique that can be used to prevent reflux [92–94]. Experienced surgeons match the procedure to the patient based on the presence of hiatal hernia, shortened esophagus, and whether a laparoscopic approach is appropriate [92–94]. There is the need for a thorough preoperative assessment, including esophageal manometry. DeMeester *et al.* [92,98] found that fundoplication is not likely to be effective in controlling asthma if an esophageal body motor abnormality is present. Factors predictive of a good response to fundoplication in asthmatic patients with GERD include weekly regurgitation, proximal reflux, presence of nocturnal asthma, pH probe evidence of an acid event preceding the onset of wheeze or cough, and normal esophageal manometry results.

Use of laparoscopic fundoplication has greatly reduced hospital stays and leads to an early return to work or full activity. Although short- and long-term results seem to be as good as with open fundoplication, the same complications may occur. These surgical complications include gastroparesis, dysphagia, recurrent reflux, and gas bloat syndrome [92–94]. Surgeons with significant experience with fundoplication should be ready to deal with these potential complications.

OVERLAPPING CONDITIONS

Sleep apnea can significantly worsen GERD by increasing negative intrathoracic pressure [99] and has also been associated with an impaired swallowing reflex [100]. Sleep apnea may worsen asthma even without GERD, partially by increased vagal tone [37,39,101,102]. GERD has also been found to aggravate sleep apnea [103,104], which can lead to a vicious cycle. Nasal continuous positive airway pressure (CPAP) can help to prevent sleep apnea and improve the associated GERD [104]. Surgery may be needed if the patient is unable to tolerate nasal CPAP.

Geriatric patients tend to have more severe GERD [105,106]. Treatment of these patients is more difficult because of concomitant diseases and medications, as well as changes in swallowing function and airway protective mechanisms [65], poor tolerance for medications, poor compliance with lifestyle modification, and inability to pay for expensive medications (Table 8-4) [107]. When omeprazole is available as a generic drug, the cost of treating patients with GERD should decrease significantly. The geriatric population may also have obstructive sleep apnea as a significant factor aggravating GERD [108]. Laparoscopic surgery remains an option in these patients when there is severe respiratory disease and no significant contraindications.

Paroxysmal laryngospasm is a condition that can mimic asthma [96]. This disorder, which is triggered by an acid-initiated reflex, leads to transient laryngospasm with airway obstruction and an inability to inspire air. Patients with asthma usually have more difficulty exhaling. This condition can cause extreme anxiety and even panic until it is successfully diagnosed and treated. It usually responds well to twice daily PPI therapy [69•].

Vocal cord dysfunction syndrome may mimic asthma, but the two conditions may occur together. Perkner *et al.* [97] examined two groups of patients with VCD and found GERD in 70% of patients with irritant-induced VCD versus 59% in patients with vocal cord dysfunction not induced by irritants. Treating for GERD, if present, may be of value in decreasing the vagal stimulation of the larynx. This group of patients develops inspiratory stridor with only a small posterior chink of vocal cord opening. This leads to increased negative intrathoracic pressure, which in turn increases GERD.

CONCLUSIONS

Abundant evidence has been reviewed showing GERD as a significant factor contributing to the severity of asthma through microaspiration, vagally mediated reflexes, increased airway hyperreactivity, and neuroinflammation. Prevalence figures suggest that 70% to 90% of individuals with asthma also have GERD. Even asthmatic patients without reflux symptoms are found to have GERD. Why is this prevalence rate so high? Autonomic dysfunction may be the answer. New information suggests increasing complexity to autonomic regulation of airway caliber [109]. This information, coupled with a better appreciation of the role of neuroinflammation, may help provide better answers. Clinicians who look for GERD in patients with asthma will find that their patients benefit. Although most patients with asthma may have GERD, it is most important to consider the possibility of GERD in patients with severe asthma [107,110•]. A need still exists for better studies assessing the most appropriate use of PPI therapy for asthmatic patients of differing severity with associated GERD of varying severity. Good study design can help prevent dubious results from confusing the literature [111]. The future will include a study comparing the effectiveness of long-term PPI therapy with laparoscopic fundoplication.

Table 8-4. THE DAILY COST OF THERAPY FOR GASTROESOPHAGEAL REFLUX DISEASE

Drug Name	Dose	Average Cost Per Day, US $*
Cimetidine	800 mg BID	4.47
Generic	800 mg BID	1.39
Ranitidine	150 mg BID	2.59
Generic	150 mg BID	1.37
Famotidine	20 mg BID	2.83
Nizatidine	150 mg BID	3.15
Sucralfate	1 g QID	2.42
Generic	1 g QID	1.42
Omeprazole	20 mg/d	3.87
Esomeprazole	40 mg/d	3.80
Lansoprazole	30 mg/d	3.88
Pantoprazole	40 mg/d	2.93
Rabeprazole	20 mg/d	3.65

*The daily cost of medications for gastroesophageal reflux disease was based on once-daily use of proton pump inhibitor (PPI) drugs. Twice-daily PPI therapy significantly raises this cost. Cost calculations are based on the average retail price of 100 tablets in the Palm Beach County, Florida area, April 2001 [107].
BID—twice a day; QID—four times a day.

ACKNOWLEDGMENTS

The author thanks Jennifer Haylett for assistance in the preparation of this manuscript. He thanks his friend and colleague, Louis Mark, MD, for his assistance with editing. Above all, he thanks his loving wife, Phyllis, for her patience and support.

REFERENCES AND RECOMMENDED READING

Papers of particular interest, published recently, have been highlighted as:
• *Of importance*
•• *Of major importance*

1. Greenberger NJ: Update in gastroenterology. *Ann Intern Med* 1997, 126:221–225.

2. Locke GR, Talley NJ, Fett SL, *et al.*: Prevalence and clinical spectrum of gastroesophageal reflux: a population-based study in Olmstead County, Minnesota. *Gastroenterology* 1997, 112:1448–1456.

3.• Sontag SJ: The prevalence of GERD in asthma. In *Gastroesophageal Reflux Disease and Airway Disease*. Edited by Stein MR. New York: Marcel Dekker; 1999:115–138.
This chapter provides the best in-depth review of prevalence of GERD in asthmatic patients.

4. Maimonides M: Treatise on asthma. In *Medical Writings of Moses Maimonides*. Edited by Munther S. Philadelphia: JB Lippincott; 1963:1135–1204.

5. Osler WB: *The Principles and Practice of Medicine*, edn 8. New York: Appleton; 1912.

6. Perrin-Foyalle M, Bel A, Kofman J, *et al.*: Asthma and gastroesophageal reflux: results of a survey of over 150 cases. *Poumon Coeur* 1980, 36:225–230.

7. O'Connell S, Sontag SJ, Miller T, *et al.*: Asthmatics have a high prevalence of reflux symptoms regardless of the use of bronchodilators [abstract]. *Gastroenterology* 1990, 98:97.

8. Field SK, Underwood M, Brant R, *et al.*: Prevalence of gastroesophageal reflux symptoms in asthma. *Chest* 1996, 109:316–322.

9 Harding SM, Guzzo MR, Richter JE: The prevalence of gastroesophageal reflux in asthma patients without reflux symptoms. *Am J Respir Crit Care Med* 2000, 162:34–39.

10. Tucci, J, Resti M, Fontana R, *et al.*: Gastroesophageal reflux and bronchial asthma: prevalence and effect of cisapride therapy. *J Pediatr Gastroenterol Nutr* 1993, 17:265–270.

11. Cinquetti M, Micelli S, Voltolina C, *et al.*: The pattern of gastroesophageal reflux in asthmatic children. *J Asthma* 2002, 39:135–142.

12. Sontag S, O'Connell S, Khandelwal S, *et al.*: Most asthmatics have gastroesophageal reflux with or without bronchodilator therapy. *Gastroenterology* 1990, 99:613–620.

13. Sontag SJ, Schnell TG, Miller TQ, *et al.*: Prevalence of oesophagitis in asthmatics. *Gut* 1992, 33:872–876.

14. Mays EE: Intrinsic asthma in adults, association with gastroesophageal reflux. *JAMA* 1976, 236:2626–2628.

15.• El-Serag HB, Sonnenberg A: Comorbid occurrence of laryngeal or pulmonary disease with esophagitis in United States military veterans. *Gastroenterology* 1997, 113:755–760.
With 101,366 cases of severe GERD examined for associated respiratory disease and compared with a control group of equal size, this powerful retrospective study is not likely to be repeated. The P values and odds ratios are impressive.

16. Gislason T, Jamson C, Vermeire P, *et al.*: Respiratory symptoms and nocturnal gastroesophageal reflux: a population-based study of young adults in three European countries. *Chest* 2002, 121:158–163.

17. Gleeson K, Eggli DF, Maxwell SL: Quantitative aspiration during sleep in normal subjects. *Chest* 1997, 111:1266–1272.

18. Reich SB, Earley WC, Ravin TH, *et al.*: Evaluation of gastropulmonary aspiration by a radioactive technique: concise communication. *J Nucl Med* 1977, 18:1079–1081.

19. Ghaed N, Stein MR: Assessment of a technique for scintigraphic monitoring of pulmonary aspiration of gastric contents in asthmatics with gastroesophageal reflux. *Ann Allergy* 1979, 42:306–308.

20. Ducolone A, Vandevenne A, Jouin H, *et al.*: Gastroesophageal reflux in patients with asthma and chronic bronchitis. *Am Rev Respir Dis* 1987, 135:327–332.

21. Chernow B, Johnson L, Janowitz WR, *et al.*: Pulmonary aspiration as a consequence of gastroesophageal reflux, a diagnostic technique. *Dig Dis Sci* 1979, 24:639–844.

22. Crausaz FM, Faver F: Aspiration of solid food particles into the lungs of patients with gastroesophageal reflux and chronic bronchial disease. *Chest* 1988, 93:376–378.

23. Ruth M, Carlsson S, Mansson I, *et al.*: Scintigraphic detection of gastro-pulmonary aspiration in patients with respiratory disorders. *Clin Physiol* 1993, 13:19–33.

24. Stein MR: Simplifying the diagnosis and treatment of gastroesophageal reflux and airway disease. *J Asthma* 1995, 32:167–172.

25. Jack CIA, Calverley PMA, Connelly RJ, *et al.*: Simultaneous tracheal and esophageal pH measurements in asthmatics with gastro-esophageal reflux. *Thorax* 1995, 50:201–204.

26. Connelly RJ, Berrisford RG, Jack CI, *et al.*: Simultaneous tracheal and esophageal pH monitoring: investigating reflux-associated asthma. *Ann Thorac Surg* 1993, 56:1029–1033.

27. Ulualp SO, Toohill RJ, Hoffmann R, *et al.*: Pharyngeal pH monitoring in patients with posterior laryngitis. *Otolaryngol Head Neck Surg* 1999, 120:672–677.

28. Ulualp SO, Toohill RJ, Shaker R: Pharyngeal acid reflux in patients with single and multiple otolaryngologic disorders. *Otolaryngol Head Neck Surg* 1999, 121:725–730.

29. Ulualp SO, Toohill RJ, Hoffman R, Shaker R: Possible role of gastroesophagopharyngeal acid reflux in the pathogenesis of chronic sinus disease. *Am J Rhinol* 1999, 13:197–202.

30. Ulualp SO, Toohill RJ: Laryngopharyngeal reflux: state of the art diagnosis and treatment. *Otolaryngol Clin North Am* 2000, 33:785–801.

31. Shaker R, Gu C, Torrico L, *et al.*: A new technique for determining the intra-pharyngeal distribution of gastric acid refluxate. *Gastroenterology* 2000, 118:A409.

32. Eubanks TR, Omelanczuk P, Hillel A, *et al.*: Pharyngeal pH measurements in patients with respiratory symptoms before and during proton pump inhibitor therapy. *Am J Surg* 2001, 181:466–470.

33. Tuchman DN, Boyle JT, Pack AI: Comparison of airway responses following tracheal or oesophageal acidification in the cat. *Gastroenterology* 1984, 87:872–881.

34. Bray GW: Recent advances in the treatment of asthma and hayfever. *Practitioner* 1934, 34:342–348.

35. Mansfield LE, Stein MR: Gastroesophageal reflux and asthma: a possible reflex mechanism. *Ann Allergy* 1978, 41:224–226.

36. Mansfield LE, Hameister HH, Spaulding HS, *et al.*: The role of the vagus nerve in airway narrowing caused by intraesophageal hydrochloric acid provocation and esophageal distention. *Ann Allergy* 1981, 47:431–434.

37. Wright RA, Miller SA, Corsello BF: Acid-induced esophago-bronchial-cardiac reflexes in humans. *Gastroenterology* 1990, 99:71–73.

38. Schan CA, Harding SM, Haile JM, *et al.*: Gastroesophageal reflux-induced bronchoconstriction: an intraesophageal acid infusion study using state-of-the-art technology. *Chest* 1994, 106:731–737.

39. Garrigue S, Bordier P, Jais P, *et al.*: Benefit of atrial pacing in sleep apnea. *N Engl J Med* 2002, 346:404–412.

40. Harding SM, Schan CA, Guzzo MR, *et al.*: Gastroesophageal reflux-induced bronchoconstriction: is microaspiration a factor? *Chest* 1995, 108:1220–1227.

41. Saito Y, Okazawa M: Eosinophilic leukocyte accumulation during vagally induced bronchoconstriction. *Am J Resp Crit Care Med* 1997, 156:1614–1620.

42. Lodi U, Harding SM, Coghlan HC, *et al.*: Autonomic regulation in asthmatics with gastroesophageal reflux. *Chest* 1997, 111:65–70.

43. Smith L, Shelhamer J, Kaliner M: Cholinergic nervous system and immediate hypersensitivity: II. An analysis of papillary responses. *J Allergy Clin Immunol* 1980, 66:374–378.

44. Kaliner M, Shelhamer JH, Davis PB, Smith LJ, Venter JC: Autonomic nervous system abnormalities and allergy [clinical conference]. *Ann Intern Med* 1982, 96:349–357.

45. Herve P, Denjean A, Jian R, *et al.*: Intraesophageal perfusion of acid increases the bronchomotor response to methacholine and to isocapnic hyperventilation in asthmatic subjects. *Am Rev Respir Dis* 1986, 134:986–989.

46. Vincent D, Cohen-Jonathan AM, Leport J, *et al.*: Gastro-oesophageal reflux prevalence and relationship with bronchial reactivity in asthma. *Eur Respir J* 1997, 10:2255–2259.

47. Undem BJ, Kajekar R, Hunter DD, *et al.*: Neural integration and allergic disease. *J Allergy Clin Immunol* 2000, 106:5213–5220.

48.• Undem BJ, Carr MJ: The role of nerves in asthma. *Curr Allergy Asthma Rep* 2002, 2:159–165.
This current review of nerves in asthma explores the role of neuroinflammation.

49. Mapp CE, Miotto D, Braccioni F, *et al.*: The distribution of neurokinin-1 and neurokinin-2 receptors in human central airways. *Am J Respir Crit Care Med* 2000, 161:207–215.

50. Adcock IM, Peters M, Gelder C, *et al.*: Increased tachykinin receptor gene expression in asthmatic lung and its modulation by steroids. *J Mol Endocrinol* 1993, 11:1–7.

51. Bai TR, Zhou D, Weir T, *et al.*: Substance P (NK1)- and neurokinin A (NK2)-receptor gene expression in inflammatory airway diseases. *Am J Physiol* 1995, 269:L309–L317.

52.• Joos GF, Germonpre PR, Pauwels RA: Role of tachykinins in asthma. *Allergy* 2000, 55:321–337.
This is an excellent review of the role of tachykinins (neuroinflammation) in asthma.

53. Hunter DD, Umdem BJ: Identification and substance P content of vagal afferent neurons innervating the epithelium of the guinea pig trachea. *Am J Respir Crit Care Med* 1999, 159:1943–1948.

54. Canning BJ: Inflammation in asthma: the role of nerves and the potential influence of gastroesophageal reflux disease. In *Gastroesophageal Reflux Disease and Airway Disease.* Edited by Stein MR. New York: Marcel Dekker; 1999:19–54.

55. Hamamoto J, Kohrogi H, Kawano O, *et al.*: Esophageal stimulation by hydrochloric acid causes neurogenic inflammation in the airways of guinea pigs. *J Appl Physiol* 1997, 82:738–745.

56. Martling CR, Lundberg JM: Capsaicin-sensitive afferents contribute to acute airway edema following tracheal instillation of hydrochloric acid or gastric juice in the rat. *Anesthesiology* 1988, 68:350–356.

57. Baraniuk JN, Ali M, Yuta A, *et al.*: Hypertonic saline nasal provocation stimulates nociceptive nerves, substance P release, and glandular mucous exocytosis in normal humans. *Am Rev Respir Crit Care Med* 1999, 160:655–662.

58. Pedersen KE, Meeker SN, Riccio MM, Undem BJ: Selective stimulation of jugular ganglion afferent neurons in guinea pig airways by hypertonic saline. *J Appl Physiol* 1998, 84:499–506.

59. Sanico AM, Stanisz AM, Gleeson TD, *et al.*: Nerve growth factor expression and release in allergic inflammatory disease of the upper airways. *Am J Respir Crit Care Med* 2000, 161:1631–1635.

60. Hunter DD, Myers AC, Undem BJ: Nerve growth factor-induced phenotypic switch in guinea pig airway sensory neurons. *Am J Respir Crit Care Med* 2000, 161:1985–1990.

61. Moore KA, Undem BJ, Weinreich D: Antigen inhalation unmasks NK-2 tachykinin receptor-mediated responses in vagal afferents. *Am J Respir Crit Care Med* 2000, 161:232–236.

62. Carr MJ, Hunter DD, Jacoby DB, *et al.*: Expression of tachykinins in non-nociceptive vagal afferent neurons during respiratory viral infection in guinea pigs. *Am J Respir Crit Care Med* 2002, 165:1071–1075.

63. Harding SM: Pulmonary abnormalities in gastroesophageal reflux disease. In *Ambulatory Esophageal pH Monitoring. Practical Approach and Clinical Applications.* Edited by Richter JE. Baltimore: Williams and Wilkins; 1997:149–164.

64. Locke GR, Talley NJ, Weaver AL, *et al.*: A new questionnaire for gastroesophageal reflux disease. *Mayo Clin Proc* 1994, 69:539–547.

65. Stein MR: Odds and ends and the state of the art. In *Gastroesophageal Reflux Disease and Airway Disease.* Edited by Stein MR. New York: Marcel Dekker; 1999:303–322.

66. Hicks DM, Ours TM, Abelson TI, *et al.*: The prevalence of hypopharynx findings associated with gastroesophageal reflux in normal volunteers. *J Voice*, 2002 (in press).

67. Carr MM, Nguyen A, Poje C, *et al.*: Correlation of findings on direct laryngoscopy and bronchoscopy with presence of extraesophageal reflux disease. *Laryngoscope* 2000, 110:1560–1562.

68. Carr MM, Nagy ML, Pizzuto M, *et al.*: Correlation of findings of direct laryngoscopy and bronchoscopy with gastroesophageal reflux disease in children. *Arch Otolaryngol Head Neck Surg* 2001, 127:369–374.

69.• Koufman JA: The otolaryngologic manifestations of GERD. In *Gastroesophageal Reflux Disease and Airway Disease.* Edited by Stein MR. New York: Marcel Dekker; 1999:69–88.
This chapter provides an excellent review of the many supra-esophageal complications of GERD and indicates differences between GERD and laryngopharyngeal reflux.

70. Belafsky PC, Postma GN, Koufman JA: The validity and reliability of the reflux finding score (RFS). *Laryngoscope* 2001, 111:1313–1317.

71. Katz PO, Castell DO: Diagnosis of gastroesophageal reflux disease. In *Gastroesophageal Reflux Disease and Airway Disease.* Edited by Stein MR. New York: Marcel Dekker; 1999:55–68.

72. Theodoropoulos DS, Lockey RF, Boyce Jr, HW, *et al.*: Gastroesophageal reflux and asthma: a review of pathogenesis, diagnosis, and therapy. *Allergy* 1999, 54:651–661.

73.••Harding SM, Richter JE, Guzzo MR, *et al.*: Asthma and gastro-esophageal reflux: Acid suppressive therapy improves asthma outcome. *Am J Med* 1996, 100:395–405.
This study of the use of PPI therapy in GERD with asthma has become the model for all future studies. It clearly demonstrates that adequate acid suppression must be documented for a trial of therapy to be considered sufficient.

74. Sifrim D, Holloway R, Silny J, *et al.*: Acid, nonacid, and gas reflux in patients with gastroesophageal reflux disease during ambulatory 24-hour pH-impedance recordings. *Gastroenterology* 2001, 120:1588–1598.

75. Castell DO: Combined multichannel intraluminal impedance and pHmetry: an evolving technique to measure type and proximal extent of gastroesophageal reflux. *Am J Med* 2001, 111:S157–S159.

76. Harding SM: GERD, airway disease, and the mechanisms of interaction. In *Gastroesophageal Reflux Disease and Airway Disease.* Edited by Stein MR. New York: Marcel Dekker; 1999:139–178.

77.••Harding SM: Gastroesophageal reflux and asthma: insight into the association. *J Allergy Clin Immunol* 1999, 104:251–258.
This is an excellent review by a leading researcher in this field.

78. Crowell MD, Zayat EN, Lacy BE, *et al.*: The effects of an inhaled B2-adrenergic agonist on lower esophageal function. *Chest* 2001, 120:1184–1189.

79.• Lazenby JP, Guzzo MR, Harding SM, *et al.*: Oral corticosteroids increase esophageal acid contact times in patients with stable asthma. *Chest* 2002, 121:625–634.
This study provides new information on the role of prednisone in contributing to esophagitis and reviews the effects of other asthma therapies on GERD.

80. Katzku DA, Castell DO: Conservative therapy (phase 1) for gastroesophageal reflux disease (lifestyle modifications). In *The Esophagus.* Edited by Castell DO, Richter JE. Philadelphia: Lippincott Williams and Wilkins; 1999:437–445.

81. Kavuru MS, Richter JE: Medical treatment of gastroesophageal reflux disease and airway disease. In *Gastroesophageal Reflux Disease and Airway Disease.* Edited by Stein MR. New York: Marcel Dekker; 1999:179–207.

82. Goodall RJ, Earis JE, Cooper DN, Bernstein A: Relationship between asthma and gastro-oesophageal reflux. *Thorax* 1981, 36:116–121.

83. Ekstrom T, Lindgren BR, Tibbling L: Effects of ranitidine treatment on patients with asthma and a history of gastro-oesophageal reflux: a double blind cross over study. *Thorax* 1989, 44:19–23.

84. Harding SM, Sontag SJ: Asthma and gastroesophageal reflux. *Am J Gastroenterol* 2000, 95:523–532.

85. Vigneri S, Termini R, Leandro G, *et al.*: A comparison of five maintenance therapies for reflux esophagitis. *N Engl J Med* 1995, 333:1106–1110.

86. Miller LG, Jankovic J: Metoclopramide-induced movement disorders. *Arch Intern Med* 1989, 149:2486–2492.

87. Richter JE, Campbell DR, Kahrilas PH, *et al.*: Lansoprazole compared with ranitidine for the treatment of nonerosive gastro-esophageal reflux disease. *Arch Intern Med* 2000, 160:1803–1809.

88. O'Connor JFB, Singer MR, Richter JE: The cost-effectiveness of strategies to assess gastroesophageal reflux as an exacerbating factor in asthma. *Am J Gastroenterol* 1999, 94:1472–1480.

89. Klinekenberg-Knol EC, Nelis F, Dent J, *et al.*: Long-term omeprazole treatment in resistant gastroesophageal reflux disease: Efficacy, safety, and influence on gastric mucosa. *Gastroenterology* 2000, 118:661–669.

90. Field SK, Sutherland LR: Does medical anti-reflux therapy improve asthma in asthmatics with gastroesophageal reflux? A critical review of the literature. *Chest* 1998, 114:275–283.

91. Cuttitta G, Cibella F, Visconti A, *et al.*: Spontaneous gastro-esophageal reflux and airway patency during the night in adult asthmatics. *Am J Crit Care Med* 2000, 161:177–181.

92. DeMeester SR, DeMeester TR: Surgical treatment of gastro-esophageal reflux disease with emphasis on respiratory symptoms. In *Gastroesophageal Reflux Disease and Airway Disease.* Edited by Stein MR. New York: Marcel Dekker; 1999:209–236.

93. Branton SA, Hinder RA, Floch NR, *et al.*: Surgical treatment of gastroesophageal reflux disease. In *The Esophagus.* Edited by Castell DO, Richter JE. Philadelphia: Lippincott Williams and Wilkins; 1999:511–525.

94. Hinder RA, Branton SA, Floch NR: Surgical therapy for supra-esophageal reflux complications of gastroesophageal reflux disease. *Am J Med* 2000, 108:1785–1805.

95. Field SK, Gelfand GAJ, McFadden SD: The effects of antireflux surgery on asthmatics with gastroesophageal reflux. *Chest* 1999, 116:766–774.

96. Loughlin CJ, Koufman JA: Paroxysmal laryngospasm secondary to gastroesophageal reflux. *Laryngoscope* 1996, 106:1502–1505.

97. Perkner JJ, Fennelly KP, Balkissoon R, *et al.*: Irritant-associated vocal cord dysfunction. *J Occup Environ Med* 1998, 40:136–143.

98. DeMeester TR, Johnson WE: Outcome of respiratory symptoms after surgical treatment of swallowing disorders. *Semin Respir Crit Care Med* 1995, 16:514–519.

99. Ing AJ, Ngu MC, Breslin AB. Obstructive sleep apnea and gastroesophageal reflux. *Am J Med* 2000, 108(suppl 4a):120s–125s.

100. Teramoto S, Sudo E, Matsuse T, *et al.*: Impaired swallowing reflex in patients with obstructive sleep apnea syndrome. *Chest* 1999, 116:17–21.

101. Bohadana AB, Hannhart B, Teculesu DB: Nocturnal worsening of asthma and sleep-disordered breathing. *J Asthma* 2002, 39:85–100.

102. Bullard RD: Sleep disorders in severe asthma. In *Severe Asthma: Pathogenesis and Clinical Management.* Edited by Szefler SJ, Leung DY. New York: Marcel Dekker; 2001:323–341.

103. Kerr P, Shoenut JP, Millar T, *et al.*: Nasal CPAP reduces gastro-esophageal reflux in obstructive sleep apnea syndrome. *Chest* 1992, 101:1539–1544.

104. Kerr P, Shoenut JP, Steens RD, *et al.*: Nasal continuous positive airway pressure: a new treatment for nocturnal gastroesophageal reflux? *J Clin Gastroenterol* 1993, 17:276–280.

105. Zhu H, Pace F, Sangaletti O, Bianchi Porro G: Features of symptomatic gastroesophageal reflux in elderly patients. *Scand J Gastroenterol* 1993, 28:235–238.

106. Collen MJ, Abdulian JD, Chen YK: Gastroesophageal reflux in the elderly: more severe disease that requires aggressive therapy. *Am J Gastroenterol* 1995, 90:1053–1057.

107. Stein MR: Gastroesophageal reflux disease and asthma in the adult. *Allerg Immunology Clin North Am* 2001, 21:449–417.

108. Teramoto S, Ohga E, Matsui H, *et al.*: Obstructive sleep apnea syndrome may be a significant cause of gastroesophageal reflux disease in older people. *J Am Geriatr Soc* 1999, 47:1273–1274.

109. Mazzone SB, Canning BJ: Evidence for differential reflex regulation of cholinergic and noncholinergic parasympathetic nerves innervating the airways. *Am J Respir Crit Care Med* 2002, 165:1076–1083.

110.•Bratton DL, Hanna PD: Gastroesophageal reflux in severe asthma. In *Severe Asthma Pathogenesis and Clinical Management.* Edited by Szefler SJ, Leung DY. New York: Marcel Dekker; 2001:239–269.
This chapter is an excellent concise review of GERD in severe asthma.

111. Field SK: Asthma and gastroesophageal reflux: another piece in the puzzle? *Chest* 2002, 121:1024–1027.

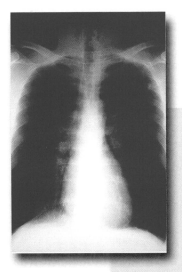

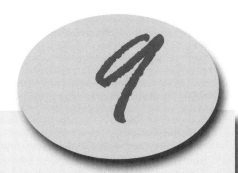

Bronchitis and Asthma

Esther L. Langmack and Richard J. Martin

Cough is the most common problem for which patients seek medical attention in the United States [1]. Asthma and bronchitis are important considerations in the diagnosis of acute and chronic cough. Sputum production is often a feature of cough in asthma and bronchitis, due to abnormalities in pulmonary mucus production and mucociliary clearance in both conditions. Distinguishing between asthma, bronchitis, and other diseases associated with acute or chronic cough can be challenging. This chapter describes the pathophysiology of sputum production in asthma, the work-up of asthma in the coughing patient, and an approach to refractory cough in the patient previously diagnosed with asthma.

COUGH AND SPUTUM IN ASTHMA

Cough and sputum production are frequent symptoms of asthma, especially during exacerbations of the disease. Factors contributing to cough and sputum production in asthma include mucus hypersecretion, abnormal mucus composition, decreased rates of mucociliary clearance, release of pro-inflammatory mediators, allergen and irritant exposure, and, when present, infection (Table 9-1). There is evidence that cough in asthma is more than an irritating symptom. Airway mucus production contributes to the morbidity and mortality of asthma by obstructing the airway lumen, thus worsening airflow limitation. In autopsy studies, patients dying of status asthmaticus have widespread plugging of the airways with highly viscous mucus [2]. Sputum production may also be a marker for more severe asthma. A history of sputum production has been independently associated with an accelerated rate of decline in FEV_1 (forced expiratory volume in 1 second) in asthmatic patients [3].

Airway mucus is a complex mixture of mucin glycoproteins, proteoglycans, lipids, secretory IgA immunoglobulins, lysozyme, peroxidase, lactoferrin, and surfactant [4]. Goblet cells and submucosal glands store and secrete mucin glycoproteins ("mucins"), the major ingredient of mucus and the primary determinants of its viscosity, elasticity, and adhesive properties. During bronchopulmonary infection, or when airway inflammation is increased, mucus may also contain cellular debris. The beating motion of cilia on columnar epithelial cells propels mucus from distal to more proximal bronchi, where it is expelled by coughing. The rate of mucociliary clearance, or the speed at which mucus is transported from the distal to more proximal airways, depends on the volume and physiochemical properties of mucus, the structural integrity of the airway epithelium, and the coordination and beating frequency of cilia [4]. Other factors that alter mucus composition and clearance include inflammatory mediators, neuropeptides, neural input to the airways, infection, and physical or chemical injury to the airways.

In asthmatic patients, airway mucus secretion is increased, the rate of mucociliary clearance is decreased, and mucus composition is altered, compared to normal, resulting in mucous plugging of the airways. Mucus hypersecretion and stasis trigger a complex reflex arc to produce cough [5••]. In the asthmatic airway, goblet cell hyperplasia and metaplasia and submucosal gland hypertrophy contribute to mucus hypersecretion by increasing the total volume of mucin-producing cells. The number of goblet cells in airway epithelium is 2.5 times greater in stable, mild-to-moderate asthmatic patients than in healthy controls [6]. Within the epithelium, asthmatic patients have three times more stored mucin glycoprotein than healthy subjects [6]. Disruption of ciliated epithelium, another characteristic structural abnormality of the asthmatic airway [2,7], impairs mucus clearance by reducing the number of functional cilia. Clumps of sloughed epithelial cells (Creola bodies) are sometimes observed in sputum. Sputum from asthmatic patients also contains higher than normal concentrations of DNA and mucin [8], substances that increase sputum viscosity. Increased mucin is thought to enhance mucous plugging of small airways and give rise to Curschmann's spirals, corkscrew-shaped casts of small airways found in sputum. The number of eosinophils and the amount of eosinophil lysophospholipase (the substance from which Charcot-Leyden crystals are formed) are also increased in the sputum of asthmatic patients. Goblet cell metaplasia, loss of functional ciliated columnar epithelial cells, abnormal

Table 9-1. FACTORS CONTRIBUTING TO COUGH AND SPUTUM IN ASTHMA

Mucus hypersecretion
  Goblet cell metaplasia and hyperplasia
  Submucosal gland hypertrophy
Abnormal mucus composition
  Increased mucin glycoproteins, DNA, plasma proteins
  Increased eosinophils and inflammatory mediators
Decreased rate of mucociliary clearance
  Disruption of airway ciliated columnar epithelial cells
Allergen-induced release of inflammatory mediators
  Cysteinyl leukotrienes
  Histamine
Exposure to irritants
Viral or bacterial infection

mucus composition, and decreased mucociliary clearance are also hallmarks of other airway diseases, including smoking-induced chronic bronchitis [9] and cystic fibrosis [10]. Whether the cellular mechanisms of goblet cell metaplasia and reduced mucociliary clearance in these diseases are similar to those in asthma is not known.

Mucociliary clearance in asthma is reduced during periods of stability and is further decreased during acute exacerbations [11]. Mucociliary clearance has been studied by measuring the rate of transport of radiolabeled particles or aerosols from the distal to more proximal tracheobronchial tree. In stable asthmatic patients, the rate of tracheal mucociliary clearance was roughly half that of normal controls in one study [12]. Several other studies have confirmed subtle impairment of mucociliary clearance in stable asthmatic patients compared to normal controls [13–15]. Patients with severe asthma may have decreased mucociliary clearance compared with patients with mild asthma [16]. In asthmatic patients hospitalized for acute exacerbations, mucociliary clearance was severely impaired (Fig. 9-1), but it improved significantly after recovery [17].

Allergen challenge has been shown to stimulate mucus hypersecretion in animal studies [4] and to increase mucin stores in human airway epithelium [18]. Inflammatory mediators associated with allergen exposure stimulate goblet cells and submucosal glands in asthmatic airways to release mucus. For example, cysteinyl leukotrienes (leukotrienes C_4, D_4, and E_4) increase mucus release from human airways in vitro [19,20]. Histamine increases active water transport toward the airway lumen [21], thus increasing mucus volume in animal models [22]. Other inflammatory cell products, including neutrophil elastase, eosinophil cationic protein, and mast chymase also stimulate goblet cell mucus secretion [4].

Allergen exposure has also been found to decrease mucociliary clearance in asthmatic patients. In stable, allergic patients with asthma, inhaled ragweed antigen decreased the rate of mucus clearance from the trachea by 53% 1 hour after exposure [12]. Pretreatment with inhaled cromolyn sodium [12] or a cysteinyl leukotriene antagonist [23] prevented allergen-induced decreases in tracheal mucus clearance. These findings suggest that, in addition to reducing mucus hypersecretion, mast cell mediators and leukotrienes play a role in allergen-mediated decreases in mucociliary clearance. Neutrophil elastase, eosinophil major basic protein, and reactive oxygen species impair ciliary activity, thus reducing mucociliary clearance [4].

ACUTE COUGH

Acute bronchitis is typically defined as a productive or nonproductive cough of less than 3 weeks duration. Viral infections are the most common cause of cough in patients without underlying lung disease ("uncomplicated acute bronchitis"), and they are the most common infectious cause of asthma exacerbations. New evidence suggests that infection with the "atypical" bacteria *Mycoplasma pneumoniae* or *Chlamydia pneumoniae* (TWAR), organisms that can cause acute bronchitis, may be more common in asthmatic patients. The clinician should be alert to the possibility that the patient with frequent episodes of acute bronchitis may have underlying asthma. In the asthmatic patient with acute cough, a thorough search for factors that exacerbate asthma should be undertaken.

Uncomplicated Acute Bronchitis

The vast majority of cases (≥ 90%) of acute bronchitis in otherwise healthy children and adults are caused by viral infections [24••]. Viruses that cause acute bronchitis include those that are responsible for lower respiratory tract symptoms (influenza B, influenza A, parainfluenza 3, and respiratory syncytial virus) and those that result primarily in upper respiratory tract symptoms (corona virus, adenovirus, rhinovirus) [24••]. Viral infections directly damage respiratory mucosa, increase mucus production, decrease mucociliary clearance, stimulate airway irritant receptors, and enhance airway reactivity. These inflammatory and physiologic changes give rise to symptoms of cough, sputum production and, in some cases, wheezing. Contrary to what many patients and physicians may believe, the presence of purulent sputum does not distinguish between viral and bacterial bronchitis. Sputum purulence results from the presence of inflammatory cells or sloughed mucosal epithelial cells in airway secretions, and can be associated with either viral or bacterial infection [25]. Fortunately, inflammation in acute viral bronchitis is usually transient and resolves as soon as the infection clears. It is unusual for the cough associated with acute viral bronchitis to last for more than 7 to 10 days, although in rare cases it can last for months.

The only bacterial causes of uncomplicated acute bronchitis that have been identified in otherwise healthy adults are *M. pneumoniae*, *C. pneumoniae*, and *Bordetella pertussis*. These organisms are estimated to cause 5% to 10% of all cases of uncomplicated acute bronchitis in adults [24••]. In adults without underlying lung disease, *Streptococcus pneumoniae*, *Haemophilus influenzae*, and *Moraxella catarrhalis* have *not* been identified as common pathogens.

Although viral infections are by far the most common cause of acute bronchitis, clinicians should consider the possibility that the patient with acute cough may have previously unrecognized asthma. In the primary care setting, it is estimated that between 19% [26] and 37% [27] of patients presenting with acute bronchitis symptoms have underlying asthma. In another study [28], patients with acute bronchitis were 6.5 times more likely to have been told they had asthma in the past, and were 9 times more likely to be diagnosed with asthma in the future, compared with patients without acute bronchitis. In patients with acute bronchitis, female gender, wheezing, dyspneic episodes over the preceding year, and symptoms provoked by allergens were associated with an underlying diagnosis of asthma [27]. It has been suggested that the diagnosis of asthma be considered in all patients with recurrent episodes of acute bronchitis [29].

Asthma may be difficult to diagnose in the setting of acute cough, however. Abnormal pulmonary function, manifested by transient airflow obstruction and increased bronchial hyperresponsiveness, is present in many patients with uncomplicated acute bronchitis of infectious origin who do not have a previous history of asthma [30,31]. Forty percent of nonasthmatic patients in one study had an FEV_1 less than 80% of that predicted during their episode of acute bronchitis [30]. Pulmonary function in patients with uncomplicated acute bronchitis usually returns to normal after 2 to 3 weeks, but abnormalities may persist for as long as 8 weeks [30,31]. Consequently, it is recommended that a comprehensive evaluation for asthma, including pulmonary function testing, be deferred until cough becomes chronic (at least 3 weeks in duration).

Routine administration of antibiotics for treatment of uncomplicated acute bronchitis has not been shown to have a beneficial effect, based on the results of several

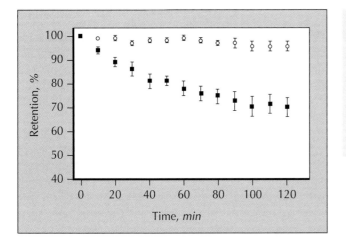

Figure 9-1.
Retention of an inhaled radiolabeled aerosol by patients hospitalized for an acute exacerbation of asthma (*open circles*) and by the same patients after discharge (*solid squares*). The rate of mucociliary clearance, which is inversely related to percentage of retention, was severely impaired in the hospitalized patients and improved after discharge.
(*Adapted from* Messina *et al.* [17].)

randomized, placebo-controlled trials [24••]. These findings are not surprising, given that viruses are the major pathogens in this disease. However, antibiotic treatment for suspected *B. pertussis* infection or antiviral treatment for suspected influenza A infection are recommended during outbreaks of these illnesses [24••]. For most patients, symptomatic therapy is sufficient. Inhaled albuterol has been shown in several studies to reduce the duration and severity of cough [32,33]. Antitussive agents may provide some relief until the infection has resolved.

Approach to the Asthmatic Patient with Acute Cough

When an asthmatic patient presents with acute cough, the primary diagnostic concern is whether the symptom of cough represents acute, infectious bronchitis or whether it is a prominent manifestation of an asthma exacerbation. These two possibilities are not mutually exclusive, as respiratory tract infections, particularly viral infections, are one of the most common triggers of asthma exacerbations [34,35]. Nonetheless, it is essential to consider all possible triggers for asthma (Table 9-2), as many of these are remediable. Conditions commonly diagnosed in asthmatic patients, such as postnasal drainage precipitated by sinusitis or rhinitis, or gastroesophageal reflux disease (GERD), may also cause acute cough without necessarily exacerbating asthma.

Viral infections are a significant and common trigger for asthma exacerbations in all age groups. In school-aged children, asthma exacerbations were associated with a respiratory virus infection in 80% to 85% of cases, and 50% of these were rhinoviruses [34]. In adult asthmatic patients, 44% of exacerbations were associated with viral infections, predominantly rhinoviruses [35]. Hospital admissions for asthma exacerbations in children and adults have been strongly linked to respiratory virus

infections [36]. As in healthy individuals, viral infection in asthmatic patients typically begins with a sore throat, followed by rhinorrhea, sneezing, and cough. Cough, sputum production, and reduced peak expiratory flow rates (PEFRs) begin soon after the onset of the infection and last about 2 weeks [34]. Compared to normal individuals, asthmatic patients are not at greater risk of rhinovirus infection, but they do develop lower respiratory tract symptoms, including cough, wheezing, and dyspnea, more frequently, and these symptoms are of greater severity and duration [37]. The mechanisms by which respiratory virus infections exacerbate asthma and airway inflammation, acutely and possibly chronically, are the focus of intensive investigation [38•].

Bacterial infections have also been shown to play a role in exacerbation of asthma. Bacterial sinusitis, a relatively common occurrence in asthmatic patients, may exacerbate lower airway disease. *S. pneumoniae* and *H. influenzae* are the most frequently cultured organisms in acute sinusitis, accounting for 76% of positive cultures [39]. Current evidence does not suggest, however, that asthmatic patients are any more likely than normal individuals to develop bronchitis caused by *S. pneumoniae*, *H. influenzae*, or *M. catarrhalis*.

Infections with *M. pneumoniae* and *C. pneumoniae*, bacteria that also cause acute bronchitis in otherwise healthy individuals, have been associated with exacerbations of asthma in multiple studies [40•]. How often *M. pneumoniae* or *C. pneumoniae* cause acute asthma exacerbations is difficult to determine, however, due to difficulties culturing these bacteria and controversy over what constitutes positive serologic evidence of infection. Interestingly, *M. pneumoniae* and *C. pneumoniae* infections have been implicated in the development and perpetuation of chronic, persistent asthma [41,42]. One or both organisms have recently been shown by the polymerase chain reaction (PCR) technique to be present in either the upper or lower airways of stable asthmatic patients more frequently than in healthy patients (Fig. 9-2) [43]. Asthmatic patients with positive PCR for one or both organisms had significantly greater mast cell tissue infiltration and a trend toward greater numbers of T lymphocytes in airway biopsies, compared to asthmatic patients who were PCR-negative [43]. These findings suggest that infection with these organisms may alter the chronic inflammatory process in asthmatic airways. It is not yet known whether asthma develops as a direct result of *M. pneumoniae* or *C. pneumoniae* infection in some patients, or whether individuals predisposed to asthma are simply more susceptible to infection.

Regardless of the cause of acute cough in the asthmatic patient, it must be determined whether asthma control is adequate, and, if it is not, the severity of the exacerbation must be assessed [44••]. In addition to worsening asthma symptoms, the clinician should always look for objective indicators of increased airflow limitation, such as a reduction in FEV_1 or FEV_1/FVC (forced vital capac-

Table 9-2. POSSIBLE CAUSES OF ASTHMA EXACERBATIONS

Allergen exposure

Irritant exposure

Occupational exposure

Rhinitis

Sinusitis

Gastroesophageal reflux disease

Viral respiratory tract infection

Medication nonadherence

Inadequate anti-inflammatory therapy

Aspirin or other NSAID exposure

Sulfite sensitivity

β-blocker use

ity) ratio by spirometry, or a decrease in PEFRs. If the patient is tracking PEFRs at home, an increase in diurnal PEFR variability is also evidence of worsening asthma. An increase in the frequency or severity of nighttime asthma symptoms may be one of the first signs of an acute asthma exacerbation [45].

The mainstays of treatment for acute asthma exacerbations are short-acting, inhaled β_2-agonists and systemic corticosteroids (for moderate-to-severe exacerbations) [44••]. Relevant exposures and other precipitating factors should be thoroughly addressed (Table 9-2). Despite concerns that corticosteroids might blunt the immune response to viral or bacterial infection, there is no evidence that withholding corticosteroids will accelerate recovery from infectious bronchitis.

Antibiotics are not generally recommended for acute exacerbations of asthma [44••], because lower respiratory tract infections triggering exacerbations are believed to be most often viral, rather than bacterial, in origin. Antibiotics are indicated, however, for acute bacterial sinusitis, for pneumonia, and for situations in which there is a high clin-

ical suspicion of bacterial bronchitis (fever, purulent sputum with increased neutrophils) [44••]. Suspicion of bacterial bronchitis increases in the patient who smokes or who has chronic obstructive pulmonary disease (COPD) [46••] rather than "pure" asthma. Although some studies suggest that chronic, stable patients with asthma may be more likely than normal subjects to be infected with *M. pneumoniae* or *C. pneumoniae* [43], it is not yet known how often these organisms are a cause of acute bronchitis in asthmatic patients. Consequently, empiric treatment with antibiotics effective against *M. pneumoniae* or *C. pneumoniae*, such as macrolide agents, cannot be generally recommended. Antibiotic treatment for suspected *B. pertussis* or antiviral treatment for suspected influenza A infection is recommended when clinical suspicion is high.

Because acute cough in the setting of asthma exacerbation may reflect alterations in mucus production or transport, drugs that impair mucociliary clearance (benzodiazepines, opiates, general anesthetics) should generally be avoided or, if necessary for some other condition, used with caution. β_2-adrenergic agonists and systemic

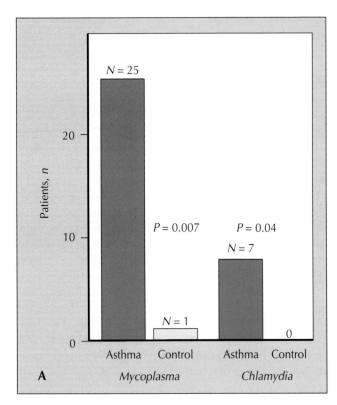
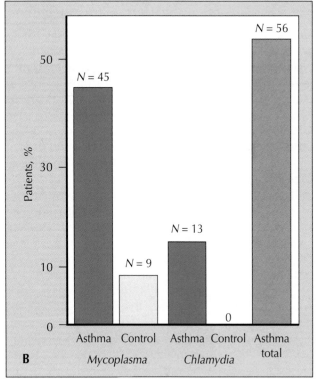

Figure 9-2.

Presence of *Mycoplasma* and *Chlamydia* species in stable asthmatics and healthy controls. **A,** Number of subjects with positive polymerase chain reaction results for *Mycoplasma* and *Chlamydia* species in the upper airway, lower airway, or peripheral blood mononuclear cells in asthmatic patients and control patients. Of the 25 asthmatic patients with positive results for *Mycoplasma*, 23 had *M. pneumoniae* and two had either *M. fermentans*

or *M. genitalium*. Of the seven asthmatic patients positive for *C. pneumoniae*, one was also positive for *M. pneumoniae*. **B,** Percentage of the total population of asthmatic patients and control patients with positive results for *Mycoplasma* and *Chlamydia* species, as well as the asthmatic population combined total percentage of positive results. (*Adapted from* Martin *et al.* [43].)

corticosteroids increase mucociliary clearance, as do methylxanthines [4]. Guaifenesin, an expectorant, has few side effects and may be helpful, as long as the preparation does not contain narcotics [44••]. Inhaled acetylcysteine and potassium iodide should be avoided, as they may precipitate acute bronchospasm [44••].

CHRONIC COUGH

Chronic cough is typically defined as a productive or nonproductive cough lasting more than 3 weeks in duration. Chronic bronchitis is often defined as the presence of a cough productive of 2 or more tablespoons of sputum per day for 3 or more successive months in each of 2 successive years, in the patient in whom other causes (*eg*, lung cancer, tuberculosis) have been excluded. A prospectively validated, diagnostic and therapeutic approach to the outpatient with chronic cough has been described in detail elsewhere [5••,47,48•]. Asthma as a cause of chronic cough and diagnostic considerations in the patient previously diagnosed with asthma will be the focus of the remainder of this chapter.

Asthma as a Cause of Chronic Cough

Undiagnosed asthma is one of the most common causes of chronic cough in all age groups [5••]. In immunocompetent, adult outpatients presenting to a pulmonary/allergy clinic, asthma was one of the top three causes of chronic cough, accounting for cough in 24% of patients [49]. Postnasal drainage (from rhinitis or sinusitis) and GERD were the two other most frequently encountered causes of chronic cough, accounting for 41% and 21% of patients, respectively, in the same study [49]. The clinical characteristics of cough due to asthma are not distinctive [50], and the cough in asthma may be productive or nonproductive. In one series of patients with chronic cough with excessive sputum production, 24% of patients had asthma [51]. The cough may also be of surprisingly long duration. In one report, asthmatic patients [49] complained of cough lasting for 4 years, on average.

Although most patients with asthma will have other symptoms (episodic wheezing, dyspnea), cough may be the only presenting symptom of asthma in some patients. Termed *cough-variant asthma*, this condition is present in 6.5% to 57% of patients with chronic cough due to asthma [52]. As in any patient with suspected asthma, the diagnosis of cough-variant asthma should be confirmed by documenting variable airflow limitation and/or bronchial hyperresponsiveness. A 12% or greater increase in FEV_1 by spirometry over baseline after inhaled β_2-agonist is evidence of significantly variable airflow limitation [53]. Because patients with cough-variant asthma often have normal spirometry, a methacholine challenge should be performed to evaluate bronchial hyperresponsiveness [5••]. In the setting of chronic cough, the methacholine challenge has as negative predictive value of 100%

[5••], essentially ruling out asthma when it is negative. A working diagnosis of cough-variant asthma can be made when the methacholine challenge test is positive, keeping in mind that a positive test has been observed in conditions other than asthma (*eg*, congestive heart failure, cystic fibrosis). The positive predictive value of methacholine challenge in the setting of chronic cough is estimated to be between 60% and 82% [5••].

The definitive diagnosis of cough related to asthma, including cough-variant asthma, is confirmed when the cough responds to asthma treatment. Treatment should include asthma education and assessment of the patient's home and work environments for allergens and irritants. Cough-variant asthma usually responds well to treatment with inhaled corticosteroids alone or in combination with an inhaled β_2-agonist for acute symptoms, although systemic corticosteroids may be necessary in some patients [5••]. Maximal benefit is often not seen for 6 to 8 weeks [54]. If cough persists despite attempts to maximize asthma therapy, then the possibility of an alternative diagnosis or a coexisting condition, such as postnasal drainage or GERD, should be considered. Empiric treatment of the patient with chronic cough with corticosteroids without confirmation of the diagnosis of asthma by physiologic testing is not recommended, as other conditions (*eg*, eosinophilic bronchitis [55], COPD) may also respond clinically to corticosteroids, resulting in a missed diagnosis.

Approach to the Asthmatic Patient with Chronic Cough

A patient who carries a diagnosis of asthma may present with a chronic, refractory cough. In this situation, the first step is always to verify the diagnosis of asthma by physiologic testing (spirometry pre- and post-bronchodilator, and in some cases, methacholine challenge). It may be necessary to repeat pulmonary function tests, because the quality of testing varies from institution to institution, and because the patient's illness may have changed over time. Physiologic testing is essential because other conditions may mimic asthma. For example, the patient with vocal cord dysfunction may complain of chronic cough, intermittent wheezing, and breathlessness [56], but a careful history, lung function test results, and laryngoscopy distinguish it from asthma. Particular concern is due the older patient who complains of chronic cough, has no prior history of asthma or allergies, and has been recently diagnosed as "asthmatic." Left ventricular heart failure (the cause of "cardiac asthma"), COPD, the entire range of interstitial lung diseases, and laryngeal or pulmonary neoplasms, among other causes, must be considered in this age group. If the patient does not have asthma, additional diagnostic testing may be necessary to establish the cause of cough, according to previously published guidelines [5••].

In some cases, the coughing patient previously diagnosed as "asthmatic" will be found to have an underlying or overlapping condition also characterized by airflow limitation, such as bronchiectasis. Bronchiectasis, a disease defined by the presence of permanently dilated of bronchi, has multiple causes, including various infections, α_1-antitrypsin deficiency, cystic fibrosis, allergic bronchopulmonary aspergillosis, certain rheumatologic diseases or immunodeficiency states, toxic inhalation, and chronic aspiration [57]. Most patients with bronchiectasis will have a cough chronically productive of mucoid or purulent sputum. High-resolution CT scanning of the chest is the most sensitive method for detecting bronchiectasis. Treatment is directed at effective airway clearance and at correcting the underlying cause, when possible.

Another disease that may be difficult to distinguish from asthma is COPD, which may present with chronic cough and airflow limitation. COPD is a progressive disease characterized by airflow limitation that is not fully reversible and an abnormal inflammatory response to inhaled toxins, particularly tobacco smoke [46••]. Patients with chronic bronchitis are most often considered a phenotypic subset of patients with COPD. In individuals susceptible to COPD, cigarette smoking impairs mucociliary clearance [4] and induces inflammatory and structural changes in the lungs distinct from those observed in asthma [58•]. COPD may also be caused by heavy exposure to occupational dusts and chemicals. Correctly diagnosing a patient as having COPD, rather than asthma, has important consequences for treatment. For example, inhaled corticosteroids are not considered first-line treatment for COPD [46••], as they are for persistent asthma, and an individual with COPD may respond best to anticholinergic bronchodilators, rather than β_2-agonists. A phenotypic subset of patients with smoking-related COPD have clinical and physiologic features of both chronic bronchitis and asthma ("asthmatic bronchitis"), including a significant response to inhaled β_2-agonists on pulmonary function testing. Some evidence suggests that patients with COPD who have a significant bronchodilator response to β_2-agonists [59] or more eosinophils in induced sputum [60], perhaps consistent with a more "asthmatic" phenotype, may be the most likely to benefit from inhaled corticosteroids. A history of 15 to 20 or more pack-years of cigarette smoking, a low diffusing capacity for carbon monoxide and largely fixed airflow limitation by pulmonary function testing, and the presence of emphysema by high-resolution CT scanning support a diagnosis of COPD rather than asthma. Comprehensive guidelines for the diagnosis and management of COPD have recently been published [46••].

If the diagnosis of asthma is confirmed, then the adequacy of asthma control should be carefully assessed and therapy increased, if necessary. Factors known to exacerbate asthma (Table 9-2) should be readdressed, with particular attention to possible environmental triggers and common coexisting conditions, such as postnasal drainage and GERD. It is not uncommon for persistent cough to be caused by more than one disease process. Cough may be caused by more than one condition up to 93% of the time [5••]. In one study, of 18 asthmatic patients found to have multiple causes of chronic cough, six had coexisting GERD and 13 had coexisting postnasal drainage [49]. Gastroesophageal reflux and/or chronic postnasal drainage should be considered as causes of chronic cough when cough persists after asthma treatment has been increased. Complete resolution of chronic cough after adequate therapy for GERD, rhinitis, and/or sinusitis confirms the diagnosis.

Gastroesophageal reflux disease may be "silent," without gastrointestinal symptoms, up to 75% of the time [5••]. The only evidence of GERD-related cough may be reflux-associated coughs on 24-hour esophageal pH monitoring performed without antacid medications; the total percentage of time with pH less than 4 may be normal [48•]. In some cases, barium esophagography is necessary to detect reflux when stomach contents have a relatively normal pH [48•], or 24-hour esophageal monitoring must be repeated to catch reflux-induced cough. Common pitfalls in the management of GERD-related cough include failure to address diet or exacerbating conditions, such as obstructive sleep apnea, and failure to continue diet, prokinetic, and acid suppressive therapy for an adequate period of time (at least 2 to 3 months) [5••].

Like GERD, postnasal drainage may be clinically silent. Routine sinus radiographs or CT scanning of the sinuses may be helpful in diagnosing the condition. For patients with cough caused by postnasal drainage, decongestant, antihistamine, and antibiotic therapy are indicated [5••]. First-generation histamine$_1$ (H$_1$)-antagonists have been shown to be superior to newer agents for controlling cough induced by postnasal drip, and should be used for at least 3 weeks [5••]. Intranasal ipratropium bromide is the agent of choice for patients in whom first-generation antihistamines are contraindicated [48•].

If cough persists in the asthmatic patient after the above measures have been taken, then the scope of diagnostic investigation should be widened to consider more unusual causes of chronic cough (Table 9-3). High-resolution CT scanning may be particularly helpful in detecting interstitial lung disease, neoplasm, emphysema, bronchiolitis, or bronchiectasis that is not visible on plain chest radiographs. Bronchoscopy is always indicated for the patient who has refractory cough despite a thorough diagnostic evaluation. Bronchoscopy may reveal laryngeal or endobronchial lesions not visualized by radiologic methods. Protected-specimen brush sampling in the airways can detect chronic bacterial infection not readily appreciated by noninvasive means in some patients with chronic, refractory cough [61]. Laryngoscopy and evaluation by an otorhinolaryngologist may also be valuable when an asthmatic paient has chronic, refractory cough.

Table 9-3. DIAGNOSTIC CONSIDERATIONS IN THE ASTHMATIC PATIENT WITH PERSISTENT COUGH

Postnasal drainage from rhinitis or sinusitis

Gastroesophageal reflux disease

Drug exposure (ACE inhibitors, β-blockers, aspirin, NSAIDs)

Ongoing allergen or irritant exposure, at home or work

Past heavy exposure causing bronchitis, *eg*, sulfur mustard gas

Inadequately treated asthma

Severe asthma

Bronchiolitis

Bronchiectasis

Chronic obstructive pulmonary disease

Recurrent aspiration

Interstitial lung disease

Airway foreign body

Pulmonary or laryngeal infection

Pulmonary or laryngeal neoplasm

Laryngeal inflammation

Pleural or pericardial infection or inflammation

Chronic pulmonary edema

Chronic external and middle ear disease

CONCLUSIONS

Abnormalities in mucus production, mucus composition, and mucociliary clearance contribute to cough and sputum production in asthma. The diagnosis of underlying asthma should be considered in all patients with recurrent episodes of acute bronchitis or with cough lasting more than 3 weeks. Addressing exacerbating factors, evaluating the adequacy of asthma control, and searching for overlapping or coexisting conditions comprise an effective approach to the asthmatic patient who complains of acute or refractory cough.

ACKNOWLEDGMENT

We would like to thank Mrs. Gaynelle Ivandick for her excellent technical support in the preparation of this manuscript.

REFERENCES AND RECOMMENDED READING

Papers of particular interest, published recently, have been highlighted as:
•   Of importance
•• Of major importance

1. Schappert SM: National Ambulatory Medical Care Survey: 1991 summary. *Adv Data* 1993, 29:1–16.

2. Benatar SR: Fatal asthma. *N Engl J Med* 1986, 314:423–429.

3. Lange P, Parner J, Vestbo J, *et al.*: A 15-year follow-up study of ventilatory function in adults with asthma. *N Engl J Med* 1998, 339:1194–1200.

4. Wanner A, Salathe M ,O'Riordan TG: Mucociliary clearance in the airways. *Am J Respir Crit Care Med* 1996, 154:1868–1902.

5.•• Irwin RS, Boulet LP, Cloutier MM, *et al.*: Managing cough as a defense mechanism and as a symptom. A consensus panel report of the American College of Chest Physicians. *Chest* 1998, 114:133S–181S.
Comprehensive, evidence-based recommendations on the topics of cough mechanisms, diagnosis of cough, and treatment of common causes of chronic cough.

6. Ordonez CL, Khashayar R, Wong HH, *et al.*: Mild and moderate asthma is associated with airway goblet cell hyperplasia and abnormalities in mucin gene expression. *Am J Respir Crit Care Med* 2001, 163:517–523.

7. Carroll N, Elliot J, Morton A, *et al.*: The structure of large and small airways in nonfatal and fatal asthma. *Am Rev Respir Dis* 1993, 147:405–410.

8. Fahy JV, Steiger DJ, Liu J, *et al.*: Markers of mucus secretion and DNA levels in induced sputum from asthmatic and from healthy subjects. *Am Rev Respir Dis* 1993, 147:1132–1137.

9. Goodman RM, Yergin BM, Landa JF, *et al.*: Relationship of smoking history and pulmonary function tests to tracheal mucous velocity in nonsmokers, young smokers, ex-smokers, and patients with chronic bronchitis. *Am Rev Respir Dis* 1978, 117:205–214.

10. Regnis JA, Robinson M, Bailey DL, *et al.*: Mucociliary clearance in patients with cystic fibrosis and in normal subjects. *Am J Respir Crit Care Med* 1994, 150:66–71.

11. Del Donno M, Bittesnich D, Chetta A, *et al.*: The effect of inflammation on mucociliary clearance in asthma: an overview. *Chest* 2000, 118:1142–1149.

12. Mezey RJ, Cohn MA, Fernandez RJ, *et al.*: Mucociliary transport in allergic patients with antigen-induced bronchospasm. *Am Rev Respir Dis* 1978, 118:677–684.

13. Pavia D, Bateman JR, Sheahan NF, *et al.*: Tracheobronchial mucociliary clearance in asthma: impairment during remission. *Thorax* 1985, 40:171–175.

14. Bateman JR, Pavia D, Sheahan NF, *et al.*: Impaired tracheobronchial clearance in patients with mild stable asthma. *Thorax* 1983, 38:463–467.

15. Foster WM, Langenback EG, Bergofsky EH: Lung mucociliary function in man: interdependence of bronchial and tracheal mucus transport velocities with lung clearance in bronchial asthma and healthy subjects. *Ann Occup Hyg* 1982, 26:227–244.

16. O'Riordan TG, Zwang J, Smaldone GC: Mucociliary clearance in adult asthma. *Am Rev Respir Dis* 1992, 146:598–603.

17. Messina MS, O'Riordan TG, Smaldone GC: Changes in mucociliary clearance during acute exacerbations of asthma. *Am Rev Respir Dis* 1991, 143:993–997.

18. Khashayar R, Zhao C, Wong HH, *et al.*: Effect of allergen challenge on airway epithelial mucin stores in asthmatic subjects. *Am J Respir Crit Care Med* 2000, 161:A204.

19. Marom Z, Shelhamer JH, Bach MK, *et al.*: Slow-reacting substances, leukotrienes C4 and D4, increase the release of mucus from human airways in vitro. *Am Rev Respir Dis* 1982, 126:449–451.

20. Coles SJ, Neill KH, Reid LM, *et al.*: Effects of leukotrienes C4 and D4 on glycoprotein and lysozyme secretion by human bronchial mucosa. *Prostaglandins* 1983, 25:155–170.

21. Marin MG, Davis B, Nadel JA: Effect of histamine on electrical and ion transport properties of tracheal epithelium. *J Appl Physiol* 1977, 42:735–738.

22. Webber SE, Widdicombe JG: The actions of methacholine, phenylephrine, salbutamol and histamine on mucus secretion from the ferret in-vitro trachea. *Agents Actions* 1987, 22:82–85.

23. Ahmed T, Greenblatt DW, Birch S, *et al.*: Abnormal mucociliary transport in allergic patients with antigen-induced bronchospasm: role of slow reacting substance of anaphylaxis. *Am Rev Respir Dis* 1981, 124:110–114.

24.•• Gonzales R, Bartlett JG, Besser RE, *et al.*: Principles of appropriate antibiotic use for treatment of uncomplicated acute bronchitis: background. *Ann Intern Med* 2001, 134:521–529.
Position paper for the American College of Physicians providing evidence-based recommendations for the evaluation and treatment of uncomplicated acute bronchitis, including a detailed discussion of the use of antibiotics.

25. Gonzales R, Barrett PH, Jr, Steiner JF: The relation between purulent manifestations and antibiotic treatment of upper respiratory tract infections. *J Gen Intern Med* 1999, 14:151–156.

26. Jonsson JS, Gislason T, Gislason D, *et al.*: Acute bronchitis and clinical outcome three years later: prospective cohort study. *BMJ* 1998, 317:1433.

27. Thiadens HA, Postma DS, de Bock GH, *et al.*: Asthma in adult patients presenting with symptoms of acute bronchitis in general practice. *Scand J Prim Health Care* 2000, 18:188–192.

28. Williamson HA Jr, Schultz P: An association between acute bronchitis and asthma. *J Fam Pract* 1987, 24:35–38.

29. Hueston WJ, Mainous AG 3rd: Acute bronchitis. *Am Fam Physician* 1998, 57:1270–1276, 1281–1272.

30. Williamson HA Jr: Pulmonary function tests in acute bronchitis: evidence for reversible airway obstruction. *J Fam Pract* 1987, 25:251–256.

31. Melbye H, Kongerud J, Vorland L: Reversible airflow limitation in adults with respiratory infection. *Eur Respir J* 1994, 7:1239–1245.

32. Hueston WJ: Albuterol delivered by metered-dose inhaler to treat acute bronchitis. *J Fam Pract* 1994, 39:437–440.

33. Melbye H, Aasebo U, Straume B: Symptomatic effect of inhaled fenoterol in acute bronchitis: a placebo-controlled double-blind study. *Fam Pract* 1991, 8:216–222.

34. Johnston SL, Pattemore PK, Sanderson G, *et al.*: Community study of role of viral infections in exacerbations of asthma in 9–11 year old children. *BMJ* 1995, 310:1225–1229.

35. Nicholson KG, Kent J, Ireland DC: Respiratory viruses and exacerbations of asthma in adults. *BMJ* 1993, 307:982–986.

36. Johnston SL, Pattemore PK, Sanderson G, *et al.*: The relationship between upper respiratory infections and hospital admissions for asthma: a time-trend analysis. *Am J Respir Crit Care Med* 1996, 154:654–660.

37. Corne JM, Marshall C, Smith S, *et al.*: Frequency, severity, and duration of rhinovirus infections in asthmatic and non-asthmatic individuals: a longitudinal cohort study. *Lancet* 2002, 359:831–834.

38.• Gern JE, Busse WW: The role of viral infections in the natural history of asthma. *J Allergy Clin Immunol* 2000, 106:201–212.
Evidence linking respiratory viral infections to the development, exacerbation, and persistence of asthma.

39. Senior BA, Kennedy DW: Management of sinusitis in the asthmatic patient. *Ann Allergy Asthma Immunol* 1996, 77:6–15; quiz 15–19.

40.• Kraft M: The role of bacterial infections in asthma. *Clin Chest Med* 2000, 21:301–313.
Detailed review of studies linking infection with Mycoplasma pneumoniae *and* Chlamydia pneumoniae *with the development of asthma.*

41. Hahn DL, Dodge RW, Golubjatnikov R: Association of *Chlamydia pneumoniae* (strain TWAR) infection with wheezing, asthmatic bronchitis, and adult-onset asthma. *JAMA* 1991, 266:225–230.

42. Gil JC, Cedillo RL, Mayagoitia BG, *et al.*: Isolation of *Mycoplasma pneumoniae* from asthmatic patients. *Ann Allergy* 1993, 70:23–25.

43. Martin RJ, Kraft M, Chu HW, *et al.*: A link between chronic asthma and chronic infection. *J Allergy Clin Immunol* 2001, 107:595–601.

44.•• National Heart, Lung, and Blood Institute, National Asthma Education and Prevention Program: *Expert Panel Report 2: Guidelines for the Diagnosis and Management of Asthma.* Bethesda, MD: National Institutes of Health, Pub. No. 97-4051; 1997.
Practice standards for the diagnosis and treatment of asthma in children and adults, in the clinic, emergency department and hospital. New NHLBI guidelines are anticipated in 2002.

45. Pincus DJ, Beam WR, Martin RJ: Chronobiology and chronotherapy of asthma. *Clin Chest Med* 1995, 16:699–713.

46.•• Pauwels RA, Buist AS, Ma P, *et al.*: Global strategy for the diagnosis, management, and prevention of chronic obstructive pulmonary disease: National Heart, Lung, and Blood Institute and World Health Organization Global Initiative for Chronic Obstructive Lung Disease (GOLD): executive summary. *Respir Care* 2001, 46:798–825.
Current recommendations for the diagnosis and management of chronic obstructive pulmonary disease. Also known as the "GOLD guidelines."

47. Irwin RS, Corrao WM, Pratter MR: Chronic persistent cough in the adult: the spectrum and frequency of causes and successful outcome of specific therapy. *Am Rev Respir Dis* 1981, 123:413–417.

48.• Irwin RS, Madison JM: The persistently troublesome cough. *Am J Respir Crit Care Med* 2002, 165:1469–1474.
Common pitfalls in the work-up of the patient with chronic cough, with particular attention to the diagnosis of eosinophilic bronchitis, postnasal drip syndrome, asthma, and GERD.

49. Irwin RS, Curley FJ, French CL: Chronic cough. The spectrum and frequency of causes, key components of the diagnostic evaluation, and outcome of specific therapy. *Am Rev Respir Dis* 1990, 141:640–647.

50. Mello CJ, Irwin RS, Curley FJ: Predictive values of the character, timing, and complications of chronic cough in diagnosing its cause. *Arch Intern Med* 1996, 156:997–1003.

51. Smyrnios NA, Irwin RS, Curley FJ: Chronic cough with a history of excessive sputum production. The spectrum and frequency of causes, key components of the diagnostic evaluation, and outcome of specific therapy. *Chest* 1995, 108:991–997.

52. Johnson D, Osborn LM: Cough variant asthma: a review of the clinical literature. *J Asthma* 1991, 28:85–90.

53. American Thoracic Society: Lung function testing: selection of reference values and interpretation strategies. *Am Rev Respir Dis* 1991, 144:1202–1218.

54. Cheriyan S, Greenberger PA, Patterson R: Outcome of cough variant asthma treated with inhaled steroids. *Ann Allergy* 1994, 73:478–480.

55. Brightling CE, Pavord ID: Eosinophilic bronchitis: an important cause of prolonged cough. *Ann Med* 2000, 32:446–451.

56. Christopher KL, Wood RP 2nd, Eckert RC, *et al.*: Vocal-cord dysfunction presenting as asthma. *N Engl J Med* 1983, 308:1566–1570.

57. Barker AF: Bronchiectasis. *N Engl J Med* 2002, 346:1383–1393.

58.• Jeffery PK: Comparison of the structural and inflammatory features of COPD and asthma. Giles F. Filley Lecture. *Chest* 2000, 117:251S–260S.
Review of airway tissue histopathology and cellular inflammation in COPD and asthma, pointing out important differences between these two common diseases.

59. Dompeling E, van Schayck CP, Molema J, *et al.*: Inhaled beclomethasone improves the course of asthma and COPD. *Eur Respir J* 1992, 5:945–952.

60. Pizzichini E, Pizzichini MM, Gibson P, *et al.*: Sputum eosinophilia predicts benefit from prednisone in smokers with chronic obstructive bronchitis. *Am J Respir Crit Care Med* 1998, 158:1511–1517.

61. Schaefer OP, Irwin RS: Chronic cough due to clinically "silent" suppurative disease of the airways: a new clinical entity. *Am J Respir Crit Care Med* 1999, 159:A830.

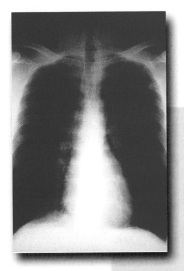

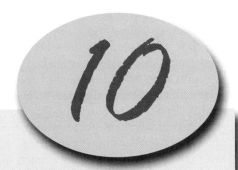

Respiratory Reactions to Nonsteroidal Anti-inflammatory Drugs

Jennifer A. Namazy and Ronald A. Simon

Aspirin, or acetylsalicylic acid (ASA), the first nonsteroidal anti-inflammatory drug (NSAID), has been used for more than 100 years by people around the world for its analgesic, anti-inflammatory, and platelet inhibitory properties [1•]. Within the past 40 years, a variety of NSAIDs have been introduced. Both ASA and NSAIDs are generally well tolerated; however, there are various side effects that can be life threatening. Through their effects on the enzyme cyclooxygenase-1 (COX-1), gastritis and peptic ulcer disease are frequent side effects. Other adverse effects include hepatitis, erythema multiforme, anemia, hepatotoxicity, interstitial nephritis, toxic epidermal necrolysis, and Stevens-Johnson syndrome. Several types of pseudoallergic and allergic reactions to ASA and NSAIDs have been described. Many of these reactions are dependent on their effects on COX-1 inhibition.

Samter and Beers [2] were the first to describe the classic triad of asthma, rhinitis and nasal polyps, and ASA sensitivity. This description has become more complicated over the years, and most recently it has been expanded to include chronic sinusitis. Various terms have been used to describe the respiratory reactions to NSAIDs, including ASA intolerance, ASA idiosyncrasy, pseudo-allergic reactions, or ASA sensitivity. It is important to remember that ASA respiratory disease, not ASA sensitivity, is the underlying problem. In patients with ASA-exacerbated respiratory disease (AERD), avoiding ASA and NSAIDs does not change the course of respiratory inflammation, which progresses over time.

PATHOGENESIS OF ASPIRIN-EXACERBATED RESPIRATORY DISEASE

Inflammatory Cells

In 1971, Vane [3] discovered the shared pharmacologic effects of ASA and NSAIDs on inhibition of COX enzymes in the metabolic cascade of arachidonic acid metabolism. The COX enzymes exist in at least two isoforms: COX-1 and COX-2. COX-1 is expressed in most mammalian cells, and COX-2 is induced during inflammation.

Both mast cells and eosinophils synthesize arachidonic acid products. All biochemical events related to AERD appear to occur in mast cells of nasal and bronchial mucosa. Along with eosinophils, they are important cells in inducing ongoing inflammation. Both types of cells have been observed in nasal cytograms and nasal tissue biopsy from ASA-sensitive asthmatic patients [4]. Sladek *et al.* [5] analyzed bronchoalveolar lavage (BAL) fluid from ASA-sensitive asthmatic patients and found elevation in number of eosinophils and eosinophil cationic protein compared with control subjects. Yamashita *et al.* [6] found numerous eosinophils and degranulated mast cells in immunohistochemically stained polyp tissue of ASA-sensitive asthmatic patients. Neutrophils and macrophages, which also synthesize arachidonic acid products, are found in BAL fluid from both ASA-sensitive and ASA-tolerant asthmatic patients. The fact that they are not increased in ASA-sensitive asthmatic patients does not exclude their participation in AERD.

In 1980, Samuelsson *et al.* [7] reported that a second metabolic pathway for arachidonic acid metabolism was also involved in inflammation. This pathway involves 5-lipoxygenase enzyme induction of leukotriene synthesis. Leukotrienes (LT) (C, D, E4) are potent mediators of chemotaxis of eosinophils, increased vascular permeability, mucous gland secretion, and bronchoconstriction. Interestingly, as the COX pathway is blocked, there is preferential diversion to the 5-lipoxygenase pathway.

There is evidence that ASA-sensitive asthmatic patients produce higher amounts of arachidonate products. Sladek *et al.* [5] measured higher concentrations of LTC4 and TXB4 in BAL fluid taken from ASA-sensitive asthmatic patients before ASA-lysine challenge. Christie *et al.* [8] and Smith *et al.* [9] reported higher urinary LTE4 and TXB2 in ASA-sensitive asthmatic patients compared with control subjects. This suggests that even before ASA challenge, ASA-sensitive asthmatic patients produce more leukotrienes and prostanoids.

What stimulates and propagates such an inflammatory response? Szczeklik and Stevenson [10] have suggested that AERD is the result of a chronic or latent viral infection of the respiratory tract with activation of T lymphocytes and secretion of cytokines followed by recruitment, activation, and stimulation of inflammatory cells.

Inflammatory Mediators

Clinical presentation of reactions to ASA and other NSAIDs are reminiscent of immediate hypersensitivity reactions. However, an antigen–antibody mechanism has never been demonstrated in patients with AERD.

Based on the cross-reactivity of patients with AERD to structurally distinct NSAIDs upon first exposure, it is thought that initiation of ASA-induced reactions is not based on antigen–antibody reactions but is caused by the inhibition in respiratory cells of intracellular COX enzymes [11•]. In vitro studies have shown that there may be a difference in function of COX enzymes when comparing ASA-sensitive asthmatic patients with ASA-tolerant patients [12]. This may be an explanation of why more reactions are not seen with ASA exposure.

A crucial event in the pathogenesis of ASA-induced respiratory reaction occurs as ASA or NSAIDs rapidly

bind COX-1. There is a subsequent decrease in the synthesis of COX products such as prostaglandin E_2 (PGE_2). Under normal circumstances, PGE_2 inhibits 5-lipoxygenase. Without the modulating effects of PGE_2, the 5-lipoxygenase pathway is preferentially stimulated, and there is an increase in the production of leukotrienes. Upregulated cysLT1 receptors augment the effects of leukotrienes and are considered as major mediators in ASA-induced asthmatic reactions [13].

Therefore, it is not surprising that most patients with ASA-sensitive asthma excrete two- to tenfold higher amounts of LTE4 in their urine than asthmatic patients who are tolerant to ASA. Christie *et al.* [8] found that after oral challenge in ASA-sensitive asthmatic patients, there was a significant elevation in urinary LTE4. Several studies have also shown elevated LTC4 and histamine in nasal lavage fluid after oral ASA challenge. Similar findings have been reported in studies of the lower respiratory tract. Sladek *et al.* [5] obtained BAL fluid after ASA inhalation challenges in ASA-sensitive asthmatic patients. The fluid contained elevated levels of LTC4 and histamine.

It remains unclear why there is a subset of patients who are ASA sensitive and why there is an overproduction of leukotrienes in these patients. As mentioned earlier, the modulating effect of PGE_2 on 5-lipoxygenase is an essential target in the development of ASA respiratory disease. Sestini *et al.* [14] pretreated ASA-sensitive asthmatic patients with PGE_2 by inhalation before ASA inhalation challenge. No reactions were reported. In addition, the urinary LTE4 levels did not increase.

During ASA desensitization, there is continued inhibition of COX-1 as well as phospholipase A2. This leads to a decrease in synthesis of leukotrienes and prostanoids. In addition, cysLT1 receptors are downregulated, further blunting the effects of available leukotrienes. Studies [15,16] have shown that during acute desensitization, there is a slight decrease in TXB2 and LTB4. In contrast, during chronic desensitization, LTB4 synthesis declines substantially.

CLASSIFICATION OF ASPIRIN AND NSAID SENSITIVITY

In an editorial, Stevenson and Sanchez-Borges [17•] offer a classification system of allergic and pseudoallergic reactions to ASA and NSAIDs (Table 10-1). Current literature is filled with terms that describe various reactions to ASA and NSAIDs. This runs the risk of leading to confusion when reading the literature and communicating with each other. Therefore, it is important to review the proposed classification when discussing ASA and NSAID sensitivity.

The term "NSAID-induced asthma and rhinitis in asthmatic patients" describes patients with AERD who, after ingesting ASA or NSAIDs, develop upper or lower respiratory tract symptoms, including rhinorrhea, nasal congestion, laryngospasm, and bronchospasm. These reactions tend to be dose dependent, in that although smaller doses of ASA or NSAIDs may not induce a significant reaction, larger and possibly therapeutic doses may induce severe reactions.

The term "blended reactions" refers to combinations of urticaria and asthma that occur in otherwise normal individuals. In essence, this type of reaction does not fit into any of the previously described reactions and was included in order to ensure accurate classification.

Other Presentations of Aspirin and NSAID Sensitivity

In hypersensitivity pneumonitis, which is rare, patients present with NSAID-induced cough, fever, pulmonary infiltrates, and eosinophilia [18]. The clinical course includes rapid resolution of infiltrates over several weeks with the use of systemic steroids. It appears to be an immune reaction, either delayed hypersensitivity or IgE mediated. In 1983, Nader and Schillaci [19] induced typical pulmonary infiltrates and eosinophilia in patients within 24 hours of challenge with naproxen. Lung biopsy specimens of infiltrates revealed interstitial lymphocytes and eosinophils. Subsequently, there have been three other controlled oral challenges with naproxen in sensitive patients with similar responses [20–22]. Hypersensitivity pneumonitis has been described for a number of different NSAIDs, but not for aspirin.

PREVALENCE OF ASPIRIN-EXACERBATED RESPIRATORY DISEASE

Aspirin-exacerbated respiratory disease, which is virtually only seen in adults, has a variable prevalence. Giraldo *et al.*
[23] noted that 5% of hospitalized adult asthmatic patients reported a history of ASA-induced respiratory reactions. In 1972, the Scripps Clinic and Research Foundation found 9% of challenged adult asthmatic patients to be ASA sensitive. The prevalence of ASA sensitivity in asthmatic patients with associated rhinitis or nasal polyps increases this number significantly to 30% to 40% [24].

The prevalence of ASA-sensitive asthma also appears to be higher in women. Of 300 ASA-sensitive asthmatic patients referred to the Scripps Clinic from 1995 to 2001, 174 (58%) were women, and 126 (42%) were men.

NATURAL HISTORY OF ASPIRIN-EXACERBATED RESPIRATORY DISEASE

Typically, ASA respiratory disease affects adults between age 20 and 40 years. In the Scripps Clinic study from 1995 to 2001, nasal polyps or asthma first developed in these patients around the age of 34 years. In the European Network study of aspirin-induced asthma, persistent rhinitis appeared at a mean age of 29.7 years followed by the development of asthma symptoms [25].

Respiratory inflammation frequently precedes the development of ASA- and NSAID-induced reactions. These patients, who were previously in good health, typically relate a story of developing an ordinary upper respiratory infection (URI). However, the clinical course is different than past URIs in that it appears to persist and, in some cases, develops into a pansinusitis with nasal polyps. Clinical symptoms commonly include headache, nasal congestion, and decreased sense of smell.

Radiographic abnormalities range from muco-periosteal thickening to complete opacification of the

Table 10-1. PROPOSED NSAID CLASSIFICATION*

Description of Reactions	Underlying Disease	Cross-reactions First Exposure	Current Terminology
NSAID-induced rhinitis and asthma	Asthma, nasal polyps, sinusitis	Yes	Intolerance, ASA induced, sensitivity
NSAID-induced urticaria or angioedema	Chronic idiopathic urticaria	Yes	Acute or chronic urticaria angioedema
Single-drug–induced urticaria or angioedema	None	No	Acute urticaria or angioedema
Multiple drug–induced urticaria or angioedema	None	Yes	Acute urticaria
Single drug–induced anaphylaxis	None	No	Anaphylactoid
Single drug– or NSAID-induced blended reaction	Asthma, rhinitis, urticaria, or none	Yes or no	Asthma and urticaria

Adapted from Stevenson and Sanchez-Borges [17•].
ASA—acetylsalicylic acid.

sinuses. At Scripps Clinic between 1991 and 1997, 234 patients with AERD were referred for ASA desensitization. A total of 200 patients were proven by challenge to be ASA sensitive. Prior sinus CT scans were not available for six patients; however, in the remaining 194 patients, 96% (187 patients) had abnormal sinus radiographs or CT scans [26•]. Inflammation may be limited to the upper respiratory tract, but more likely, lower respiratory tract inflammation develops as well.

There are no in vitro tests that can measure ASA sensitivity. Physicians should be suspicious of an asthmatic patient with nasal polyps and chronic pansinusitis. It is important to remember, however, that the majority of the patients with this clinical presentation will never have reactions to ASA or NSAIDs. Most of these patients actually have an IgE-mediated rhinitis with sensitivity to dust mites and, in some cases, sulfites. Conversely, some patients' symptoms appear idiopathic in nature. It is important to watch these patients because they may develop AERD in the future.

DIAGNOSIS OF ASPIRIN AND NSAID SENSITIVITY

Patients with ASA- and NSAID-induced asthma and rhinitis, urticaria, angioedema, or anaphylaxis cannot be identified with any known in vitro test. Because of this limitation, the only way to definitively make the diagnosis is through provocative challenge testing. ASA challenges include the oral, bronchial, or nasal routes.

In the United States, only oral ASA challenges are available. Reactions during ASA challenge include not only severe bronchospastic and nasal reactions, but also cutaneous, gastrointestinal, or vascular effects.

The more irritable the tracheobronchial tree, the more severe the bronchospastic reaction to ASA challenge. Therefore, oral and inhaled corticosteroids, intranasal corticosteroids, theophylline, and long-acting bronchodilators should be continued at the time of oral challenges. Discontinuing these medications may lead to worsening of patient's asthma and subsequent decline in

lung function. In these situations, ASA challenges cannot be safely and accurately performed. Despite continuing theophylline and intranasal and inhaled corticosteroids, ASA- and NSAID-induced respiratory reactions still occur [27]. Antileukotriene modifiers such as zileuton and montelukast can block bronchospastic responses during oral ASA challenges but often do not inhibit ASA-induced respiratory tract reactions [28,29].

Some medications, however, should be discontinued 24 hours before challenge. They include anticholinergics, antihistamines, cromolyn, and short-acting inhaled β-agonists. Simultaneous use of anticholinergics and short-acting β-agonists may lead to false-positive reactions [30]. After the effect of the medication disappears, the immediate decline in lung function might be misinterpreted as a true reaction. Antihistamines can block upper respiratory tract reactions to ASA, which interferes with the accuracy of clinical assessment [31]. Cromolyn has minor inhibitory effects on the severity of the respiratory reaction induced by ASA, but pretreatment with cromolyn delays the onset of ASA-induced asthmatic reactions [32].

Scripps Clinic developed and modified an oral ASA challenge protocol (Table 10-2). ASA oral challenges are conducted over 3 days. All patients receive 30 mg of ASA as their first dose. Very few patients react to 30 mg of ASA. Depending on the patient's history, he or she may be advanced by 15- or 30-mg doses at 3-hour intervals for a total of three doses. Therefore, individualization of doses is encouraged. A maximum of three doses is given per day. If 650 mg is administered without reaction and the patient is not taking more than 10 mg of prednisone or a leukotriene-modifier drug, the challenge is determined to have a negative result.

The onset of reactions after ASA ingestion occurs between 15 minutes and 1 hour. Respiratory reactions last 1 to 24 hours after the start of reactions. Respiratory tract signs and symptoms, which commonly occur during positive oral ASA and NSAID challenges, include nasal congestion, anosmia, and headaches. After the reaction begins, it is reversed with appropriate treatment, and subsequent ASA challenges are suspended for that day.

Table 10-2. ASPIRIN ORAL CHALLENGE PROTOCOL AT SCRIPPS CLINIC

Time*	Day 1	Day 2, *mg*	Day 3, *mg*
8 AM	Placebo†	15 to 30‡§	150
11 AM	Placebo	45 to 60	325
2 PM	Placebo	100	650

*FEV₁ (forced expiratory volume in 1 s) every h for 3 h after each dose.
†Placebo day: FEV₁, baseline or first AM value, > 70% predicted.
‡First AM FEV₁, value should be within 5% (up or down) from placebo.
§FEV₁, values should not change (ie, < 15%) during 9-h placebo challenges.

INHALATION CHALLENGE WITH ASPIRIN-LYSINE

Although not available in the United States, inhalation challenge is routinely performed in other parts of the world and deserves mention. Bianco *et al.* [33] introduced inhalation challenge with ASA-lysine in 1977. The onset of respiratory reaction with inhalation challenge is commonly less than 30 minutes, and bronchospasm is easily reversed with an inhaled β-agonist. Therefore, each increasing concentration can be delivered at 30-minute intervals [34]. This appears more convenient and allows the test to be performed in an outpatient setting.

Then why have we not adopted this type of ASA challenge in the United States? First, the test is unavailable here. In addition, Dahlen and Zetterstrom [34] performed a study comparing oral and bronchial inhalation ASA challenges in 22 patients. Both routes accurately detected bronchospastic reactions. Inhalation challenge produced limited and short bronchospastic reactions. Only two of 22 patients experienced only naso-ocular reactions in the oral challenge group, and none in the bronchial challenge group experienced reactions. This is not surprising because there is no direct naso-ocular contact in bronchial challenges. Oral ASA challenges more closely approximate real-life challenges with ASA and NSAIDs.

Another type of ASA challenge is the nasal inhalation challenge with ASA-lysine. ASA-lysine can induce local swelling of the nasal membranes in AERD asthmatic patients. The study is limited, however, by limited sensitivity when compared with oral or inhalation provocation testing. Nevertheless, the test provides a rapid and safe means of confirming the diagnosis when the result is positive [26].

ASPIRIN DESENSITIZATION

The first ASA desensitization for an episode of anaphylaxis was reported in 1922 by Widal *et al.* [35]. Desensitization is used in its broadest sense because IgE-mediated mechanisms have not been established for ASA respiratory sensitivity. Historically, desensitization has been viewed as repeated exposure to injected antigens, leading to the reduction of IgE-mediated reactions.

In 1977, Bianco *et al.* [33] induced "tolerance" to inhaled ASA-lysine after repeated inhalations in ASA-sensitive asthmatic patients. In 1980, Stevenson *et al.* [36] reported two ASA-sensitive asthmatic patients who became refractory to ASA after single-blind oral challenges with ASA. Both patients, after desensitization, experienced improvement in respiratory disease while taking daily doses of ASA.

A state of tolerance can be induced and maintained by aspirin desensitization. This process includes administration of small incremental doses of ASA over 2 to 3 days until 400 to 650 mg of ASA are tolerated. Thereafter, ASA can be administered daily to maintain desensitization, between doses of 80 mg and 325 mg. After desensitization, the desensitized state persists for 2 to 5 days [37]. During this refractory period, NSAIDs may be taken with relative safety. Stevenson *et al.* [38] compared clinical outcomes after 1 to 6 years of daily ASA treatment. They found that patients who remain on maintenance therapy at doses of 325 to 650 mg twice a day usually respond with improvement of respiratory symptoms.

From a practical standpoint, patients with a history of arthritis or rheumatic diseases or those who require antiplatelet therapy may be desensitized to ASA and then take daily ASA indefinitely. The patient can be switched to any cross-reacting NSAID as long as ASA or the NSAID is continued daily.

NSAIDS, which preferentially inhibit COX-1 in vitro, cross-react with ASA on first exposure to the new NSAID. The NSAIDs that inhibit COX-1 with the least concentration require the smallest doses of NSAIDs in cross-reacting with ASA [39]. Furthermore, cross-desensitization between ASA and any of the NSAIDs that inhibit COX-1 occurs routinely.

CROSS-REACTIVE MEDICATIONS

Acetaminophen is a weak inhibitor of COX-1; therefore, it poses a challenge in determining element of cross-reactivity. Acetaminophen partially cross-reacts with ASA in patients with AERD, but only when high doses are administered. Delaney [40] challenged ASA-sensitive asthmatic patients with 1000 mg of acetaminophen and found that 28% of patients developed respiratory reactions. Similarly, in a large study, Settipane and Stevenson [41] challenged 50 ASA-sensitive asthmatic patients with 1000 mg and then 1500 mg of acetaminophen. They found that 34% of the subjects developed respiratory reactions. However, 650 mg of acetaminophen appears safe in ASA-sensitive asthmatic patients and can be recommended for analgesia and antipyresis.

Chemicals, dyes, and additives, such as azo and nonazo dyes, sulfites, and hydrocortisone succinate, have been reported to crossreact with ASA. However, their compounds have not been shown to inhibit COX-1. Azo dyes, frequently found in coloring for food, drinks, drugs, and cosmetics, have been reported to induce bronchospasm. However, more recent studies [40–42] have shown that azo intolerance is rare among ASA-sensitive asthmatic patients. Reports of severe bronchospasm within minutes of receiving hydrocortisone intravenously led to a study by Feigenbaum *et al.* [43], who found that only one of 44 ASA-sensitive asthmatic patients reacted to both hydrocortisone succinate and methylprednisone succinate. Readministration of hydrocortisone succinate after ASA desensitization continued to induce a respiratory reaction in this patient. This suggests a coincidental IgE-mediated reaction rather than cross-reactivity with ASA.

The recent development of highly selective COX-2 inhibitors, such as rofecoxib and celecoxib, has reduced many of the adverse side effects commonly seen with COX-1 inhibitors. Theoretically, these drugs should not cross-react with ASA or those COX-1 NSAIDs. In a recent double-blind placebo controlled study by Stevenson and Simon [44•] at the Scripps Clinic, of 60 (now 100 by personal communication) patients with demonstrated aspirin sensitivity, none had reacted to rofecoxib at therapeutic doses. A recent study by the same group found similar results with celecoxib.

TREATMENT

Education of the patient with ASA-induced disease is very important. Avoidance of ASA and all cross-reacting NSAIDs prevents respiratory and urticarial cross-reacting events in previously sensitized patients. However, avoidance of only the specific inciting NSAID or ASA is important in preventing a recurrence of acute urticarial reactions, anaphylaxis, aseptic meningitis, and hypersensitivity pneumonitis. In patients with single NSAID-induced urticaria, some blended reactions, anaphylaxis, hypersensitivity pneumonitis, and aseptic meningitis, it is not necessary to avoid dissimilar NSAIDs. Patients who are cross-reactive should receive a list of drugs that are contraindicated and the reaction potentials of the drugs.

Patients with ASA-sensitive asthma can take acetaminophen for analgesic or antipyretic properties. However, a cross-reaction was reported after ingestion of 1000 to 1500 mg of acetaminophen in patients with ASA-sensitive asthma [45]. Patients can also take drugs with no activity or weak activity such as sodium salicylate, salicylamide, choline magnesium trisalicylate, benzydamine, chloroquine, azapropazone, or dextropropoxyphene [11•]. Selective COX-2 inhibitors are safe for patients with ASA-sensitive asthma because COX-1 will continue to produce PGE_2. AERD is ongoing inflammation of both the upper and lower respiratory tract. Therefore, a major goal in controlling ASA disease is to reduce this inflammation. Prevention of nasal polyp formation, sinusitis, and worsening asthma are important goals. Many patients require bursts of oral corticosteroids.

If leukotrienes are responsible for most of the respiratory reactions seen in ASA-sensitive asthma, then theoretically preventing synthesis of leukotrienes may modify these reactions. Recently, the antileukotriene drugs have been introduced as treatment of ASA-sensitive asthma. These drugs act by inhibiting synthesis of leukotrienes by blocking 5-lipoxygenase or by blocking the cysLT receptors. Several early studies have shown that pretreatment with leukotriene modifiers attenuates nasal

and bronchial reactions in ASA-sensitive asthmatic patients. However, these studies used minimal provoking doses of ASA. More recent studies [28,29] using escalating doses of ASA showed that about 50% of subjects experienced breakthrough asthmatic responses. This may indicate that leukotriene modifiers are incomplete in their blockade or alternative mediators may be involved in ASA-induced respiratory reactions. For the most part, treating with a 5-lipoxygenase inhibitor provides only partial control of symptoms. However, a recent Swedish-Polish study [46] of 40 patients with ASA-sensitive asthma found that treatment with zileuton provided acute and chronic improvement of pulmonary function measurements. This is thought to be caused by its bronchodilating effects. In patients treated with leukotriene receptor antagonists, such as montelukast, variable responses may be seen. In a study by Kuna *et al.* [47], montelukast was given to 80 patients with ASA-sensitive asthma who were not controlled with inhaled or oral steroids. After 4 weeks, patients had improvement in pulmonary function as measured by FEV_1 (forced expiratory volume in 1 second), less nocturnal asthma symptoms, more asthma-free days, and improvement in quality of life. However, overall, the effects of treating ASA-sensitive asthmatic patients are moderate at best and no different than seen in non–ASA-sensitive asthmatic patients.

There is an alternative to treating patients with ASA-sensitive asthma. Through desensitization, ASA tolerance can be induced and maintained. Selection of patients for ASA desensitization therapy should include all AERD patients, except those whose disease is controlled with inhaled corticosteroids and leukotriene-modifier drugs. Also, ideal candidates are patients with recurrent or chronic sinusitis and nasal polyps. In some cases, "triple therapy," including 5-lipoxygenase inhibitor, cysLT-receptor antagonist, and desensitization, are required.

CONCLUSIONS

The past two decades have provided many advances into understanding the pathogenesis of ASA-exacerbated respiratory disease. The discovery of the many important mediating properties of the leukotriene modifiers has allowed further research into finding appropriate treatment opportunities. It is evident that much more research is needed and expected in this area. ASA sensitivity remains a complex, heterogeneous disease with many clinical manifestations. Proper classification of reactions to ASA and NSAIDs will enable more accurate understanding of the literature. Without in vitro tests to determine patients at risk, making a definitive diagnosis becomes an even more tedious process.

REFERENCES AND RECOMMENDED READING

Papers of particular interest, published recently, have been highlighted as:
- • *Of importance*
- •• *Of major importance*

1.• Stevenson D, Simon RA, Zuraw B: Sensitivity to aspirin and non-steroidal anti-inflammatory drugs. In *Allergy: Principles and Practice*. Edited by Middleton E Jr, Ellis EF, Yunginer JW, *et al*. St. Louis: Mosby, 2002.
This must-read chapter nicely summarizes the pathogenesis and treatment options for a complicated disease.

2. Samter M, Beers RF Jr: Intolerance to aspirin. Clinical studies and consideration of its pathogenesis. *Ann Intern Med* 1968, 68(5):975–983.

3. Vane JR: Inhibition of prostaglandin synthesis as a mechanism of action for aspirin-like drugs. *Nature* 1971, 231:232–235.

4. Moneret-Vautrin DA, Hsieh V, Wayoff M, *et al*.: Nonallergic rhinitis with eosinophilia syndrome a precursor of the triad: nasal polyposis, intrinsic asthma, and intolerance to aspirin. *Ann Allergy* 1990, 64:513–518.

5. Sladek K, Dworski R, Soja J, *et al*.: Eicosanoids in broncho-alveolar lavage fluid of aspirin-intolerant patients with asthma after aspirin challenge. *Am J Respir Care Med* 1994, 149:940–946.

6. Yamashita T, Tsuyi H, Maeda N, *et al*.: Etiology of nasal polyps associated with aspirin-sensitive asthmatic subjects. *Rhinology* 1989, 8:15–24.

7. Samuelsson B, Hammarstroem S, Murphy RC, *et al*.: Leukotrienes and slow reacting substance of anaphylaxis. *Allergy* 1980, 35:375–381.

8. Christie PE, Tagari P, Ford-Hutchinson AW, *et al*.: Urinary leukotriene E4 concentrations increase after aspirin challenge in aspirin-sensitive asthmatic subjects. *Am Rev Respir Dis* 1991, 143:1025–1029.

9. Smith DM, Hawksworth RJ, Thien FC, *et al*.: Urinary leukotriene E4 in bronchial asthma. *Eur Respir J* 1992, 5:693–699.

10. Szczeklik A: The cyclooxygenase theory of aspirin-induced asthma. *Eur Respir J* 1990, 3:588–593.

11.• Szczeklik A, Stevenson DD: Aspirin-induced asthma: advances in pathogenesis and management. *J Allergy Clin Immunol* 1999, 104:5–13.
This is a wonderful summary of recent advances in determining the pathogenesis and treatment of aspirin exacerbated respiratory disease.

12. Juergens UR, Christiansen SC, Stevenson DD, *et al*.: Arachidonic acid metabolism in monocytes of aspirin-sensitive patients before and after oral aspirin challenge. *J Allergy Clin Immunol* 1992, 90:636–645.

13. Arm JP, O'Hickey SP, Spur BW, *et al*.: Airway responsiveness to histamine and leukotriene E4 in subjects with aspirin-induced asthma. *Am Rev Respir Dis* 1989, 140:148–153.

14. Sestini P, Armetti L, Gambaro G, *et al*.: Inhaled PEG2 prevents aspirin-induced bronchoconstriction and urinary LTE4 excretion in aspirin-sensitive asthma. *Am J Respir Crit Care Med* 1996, 153:572–575.

15. Ferreri NR, Howland WC, Stevenson DD, *et al*.: Release of leukotrienes, prostaglandins, and histamine into nasal secretions of aspirin-sensitive asthmatics during reactions to aspirin. *Am Rev Respir Dis* 1988, 137:847–854.

16. Juergens UR, Christiansen SC, Stevenson DD, *et al*.: Inhibition of monocyte leukotriene B4 production following aspirin desensitization. *J Allergy Clin Immunol* 1995, 96:148–156.

17.• Stevenson D, Sanchez-Borges M: Classification of allergic and pseudoallergic reactions to drugs that inhibit cyclooxygenase enzymes. *Ann Allergy* 2001, 87:177–180.
This article provides interesting clinical scenarios and walks the reader through the classification of each one.

18. Weber JCP, Eissigman WK: Pulmonary alveolitis and NSAIDs: fact or fiction. *Br J Rheumatol* 1986, 25:5–6.

19. Nader DA, Schillaci RF: Pulmonary infiltrates with eosinophilia due to naproxene. *Chest* 1983, 83:280–282.

20. Buscaglia AJ, Cowden FE: Pulmonary infiltrates associated with naproxene. *JAMA* 1984, 1:65–66.

21. Goodwin SD, Glenny RW: Nonsteroidal anti-inflammatory drug-associated pulmonary infiltrates with eosinophilia: review of the literature and Food and Drug Administration Adverse Drug Reaction reports. *Arch Intern Med* 1992, 152:1521–1524.

22. Londino AV, Wolf GL, Calabro JJ: Naproxen and pneumonitis. *JAMA* 1984, 252:1853–1854.

23. Giraldo B, Blumenthal MN, Spink WW: Aspirin intolerance and asthma: a clinical and immunological study. *Ann Intern Med* 1969, 71:479–496.

24. McDonald JR, Mathison DA, Stevenson DD: Aspirin intolerance in asthma, detection by oral challenge. *J Allergy Clin Immunol* 1972, 50:198–207.

25. Szczeklik A, Nizankowska E, Duplaga M: Natural history of aspirin-induced asthma. AIANE Investigators. European Network on Aspirin-Induced Asthma. *Eur Respir J* 2000, 16:432–436.

26.• Stevenson D: Adverse reactions to nonsteroidal anti-inflammatory drugs. *Immunol Allergy Clin North Am* 1998, 18:773–798.
This chapter is a great reference that reflects Dr. Stevenson's expertise and understanding of ASA and NSAID sensitivity.

27. Pleskow WW, Stevenson DD, Mathison DA, *et al*.: Aspirin-sensitive rhinosinusitis/asthma: spectrum of adverse reactions to aspirin. *J Allergy Clin Immunol* 1983, 71:574–579.

28. Pauls JD, Simon RA, Daffern PJ, *et al*.: Lack of effect of the 5-lipoxygenase inhibitor zileuton in blocking oral aspirin challenges in aspirin-sensitive asthmatics. *Ann Allergy Asthma Immunol* 2000, 85:40–45.

29. Stevenson D, Simon RA, Mathison DA, *et al*.: Montelukast is only partially effective in inhibiting aspirin responses in aspirin sensitive asthmatics. *Ann Allergy Asthma Immunol* 2000, 85:477–482.

30. Stevenson DD: Oral challenges to detect aspirin and sulfite sensitivity in asthma. *N Engl Reg Allergy Pro* 1988, 9:135–142.

31. Szczeklik A, Serwonska M: Inhibition of idiosyncratic reactions to aspirin in asthmatic patients by clemastine. *Thorax* 1979, 34:654.

32. Stevenson DD, Simon RA, Mathison DA: Cromolyn pretreatment delays onset of aspirin (ASA) induced asthmatic reactions. *J Allergy Clin Immunol* 1984, 73:162.

33. Bianco S, Robuschi M, Petrigini G: Aspirin-induced tolerance in aspirin-asthma detected by a new challenge test. *IRCS J Med Sci* 1977, 5:129.

34. Dahlen B, Zetterstrom O: Comparison of bronchial and per oral provocation with aspirin in aspirin-sensitive asthmatics. *Eur Respir J* 1990, 3:527–534.

35. Widal MF, Abrami P, Lermeyez J: Anaphylaxie et idiosyncrasie. *Presse Med* 1922, 30:189.

36. Stevenson DD, Simon RA, Mathison DA: Aspirin-sensitive asthma: tolerance to aspirin after positive oral aspirin challenges. *J Allergy Clin Immunol* 1980, 66:82–85.

37. Pleskow WW, Stevenson DD, Mathison DA, *et al.*: Aspirin desensitization in aspirin-sensitive asthmatic patients: clinical manifestations and characterization of the refractory period. *J Allergy Clin Immunol* 1982, 69:11–19.

38. Stevenson DD, Hankammer MA, Mathison DA: Long term ASA desensitization-treatment of aspirin-sensitive asthmatic patients: clinical outcome studies. *J Allergy Clin Immunol* 1996, 98:751.

39. Szczeklik A, Gryglewski RJ, Czernigwska-Mysik G: Clinical patterns of hypersensitivity to nonsteroidal anti-inflammatory drugs and their pathogenesis. *J Allergy Clin Immunol* 1977, 60:276–284.

40. Delaney JC: The diagnosis of aspirin idiosyncrasy by analgesic challenge. *Clin Allergy* 1976, 6:177–184.

41. Settipane RA, Stevenson DD: Cross-sensitivity with acetaminophen in aspirin-sensitive subjects with asthma. *J Allergy Clin Immunol* 1989, 84:26–33.

42. Stevenson DD: Cross-reactivity between aspirin and other drugs/dietary chemicals: a critical review. In *Progress in Allergy and Clinical Immunology*. Edited by Pichler WJ, Stadler MM, Dahinden CA, *et al.* Lewiston, NY: Hogrefe and Huber; 1989:462–473.

43. Feigenbaum BA, Stevenson DD, Simon RA: Lack of cross-sensitivity to IV hydrocortisone in aspirin-sensitive subjects with asthma. *J Allergy Clin Immunol* 1995, 96:545–548.

44.• Stevenson DD, Simon R: Lack of cross-reactivity between rofecoxib and aspirin in aspirin-sensitive patients with asthma. *J Allergy Clin Immunol* 2001, 108:47–51.
This paper describes the outcome of 60 patients with aspirin sensitivity who underwent challenge with rofecoxib. None developed reactions at therapeutic doses.

45. Settipane RA, Shrank PJ, Simon RA, *et al.*: Prevalence of cross-sensitivity with acetaminophen in aspirin-sensitive asthmatic subjects. *J Allergy Clin Immunol* 1995, 96:480–485.

46. Dahlen B, Nizankowska E, Szczeklik A: Benefits from adding the 5-lipoxygenase inhibitor zileuton to conventional therapy in aspirin-intolerant asthmatics. *Am J Respir Crit Care Med* 1998, 157:1187–1194.

47. Kuna P, Malmstrom K, Dahlen SE, *et al.*: Montelukast (MK-0476) a cysLT1 receptor antagonist improves asthma control in aspirin-intolerant asthmatic patients. *Am J Respir Care Med* 1997, 155(suppl A):975.

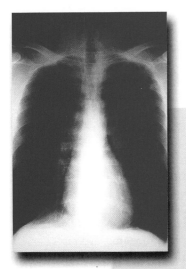

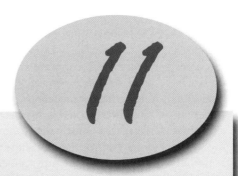

Pregnancy and Asthma

Michael Schatz

Asthma is one of the most common potentially serious medical problems to complicate pregnancy. Recent prevalence data suggest that up to 7% of pregnant women manifest asthma [1]. Managing asthma during pregnancy is unique because the effect of both the illness and the treatment on the developing fetus as well as the patient must be considered. In addition, pregnancy may alter the course of asthma. This chapter discusses the interrelationships between asthma and pregnancy, nonpharmacologic management of gestational asthma, and general and specific aspects of pharmacologic therapy during pregnancy.

INTERRELATIONSHIPS BETWEEN ASTHMA AND PREGNANCY

Effect of Asthma on the Mother and Fetus

Controlled studies that have evaluated outcomes of pregnancy in asthmatic compared with nonasthmatic women have been reviewed recently [2]. These studies suggest that maternal asthma may increase the risk of perinatal mortality, pre-eclampsia, low-birth-weight infants, and preterm births compared with that of nonasthmatic women. These conclusions were confirmed by the largest study to date [3••], which described the outcomes of pregnancy in 36,985 women identified as having asthma in either the Swedish Medical Birth Registry, the Swedish Hospital Discharge Registry, or both (Table 11-1). These outcomes were compared with the total of 1.32 million births that occurred in the Swedish population during the years of the study (1984 to 1995). Prior data and the Swedish study suggest that patients with more severe asthma are at greater risk [2,3••]. In the Swedish study, patients identified as having asthma by both the hospital discharge registry and the medical birth registry, who would presumably be more definite and more severe asthmatic patients, manifested higher risks than all asthmatic patients identified (*see* Table 11-1). The literature also contains case reports of perinatal mortality associated with severe uncontrolled asthma [2]. Finally, in addition to fetal morbidity and mortality, severe asthma during pregnancy may be a cause of maternal mortality.

A definition of the mechanism or mechanisms of maternal asthma's adverse effect on pregnancy will help to develop an optimal intervention strategy. Mechanisms postulated to explain the possible increased perinatal risks have included 1) hypoxia and other physiologic consequences of poorly controlled asthma, 2) medications used to treat asthma, and 3) demographic or pathogenic factors associated with asthma but not actually caused by the disease or its treatment. Data supporting specific mechanisms for the most common specific adverse outcomes have been recently reviewed [2]. The published data do not fully define the mechanism or mechanisms of maternal asthma's potential adverse effects on pregnancy and infants. Available information, however, suggests that poor asthma control, by causing acute or chronic maternal hypoxia, may be the most remedial responsible factor and supports the important generalization that adequate asthma control during pregnancy is important in improving maternal and fetal outcome.

Effect of Pregnancy on Asthma

Asthma severity may worsen, improve, or remain unchanged during pregnancy, and the overall data suggest that these various courses occur with approximately equal frequency [4,5]. The course of asthma may also vary by stage of pregnancy [4,5]. Whereas the first trimester is generally well tolerated in asthmatic patients and is associated with infrequent exacerbations, the second and early third trimesters are associated with increased symptoms and exacerbations. In contrast, asthmatic women generally tend to experience fewer symptoms and less frequent asthma exacerbations during weeks 37 to 40 of pregnancy than during any prior 4-week gestational period. Finally, asthma generally remains quiescent during labor and delivery itself, at least in prospectively managed patients.

The variable effect of pregnancy on the course of asthma appears to be more than just random fluctuation in the natural history of the disease, because the changes in asthma course that women attribute to pregnancy generally revert toward the prepregnancy course in the 3 months postpartum [4,5]. It is also of interest that the course of asthma is often consistent in an individual woman during successive pregnancies [4,5].

The mechanisms responsible for the altered asthma course during pregnancy are unknown and represent a fertile area for additional research. Many biochemical and physiologic changes during pregnancy could potentially ameliorate or exacerbate gestational asthma [4,5]. However, it is not clear which, if any, of these factors are actually important in determining asthma course during pregnancy.

Two observations may be mechanistically and clinically important regarding the course of asthma during pregnancy. First, whereas more severe asthma tends to worsen during pregnancy, less severe asthma tends to remain unchanged or improve. For example, in a recent study, patients with persistent asthma or those taking regular medications were more likely to experience asthma exacerbations during pregnancy than patients with intermittent asthma did [6]. Secondly, there is a significant concordance between rhinitis course and asthma course during pregnancy [7]. This suggests that the same mechanisms may influence both levels of the airway during pregnancy; gestational rhinitis course may predict asthma course during pregnancy; and, possibly, rhinitis management during pregnancy may improve asthma.

Physician reluctance to treat may also affect asthma severity during pregnancy. A recent surveillance study [8•] identified 51 pregnant women and 500 nonpregnant women presenting to the emergency department with acute asthma. Although asthma severity appeared to be similar in the two groups based on peak flow rates, pregnant women were significantly less likely to be treated with systemic steroids in the emergency department (44% vs 66%) and significantly less likely to be discharged on oral steroids (38% vs 64%). Presumably related to this undertreatment, pregnant women were three times more likely than nonpregnant women to report an ongoing exacerbation 2 weeks later ($P = 0.02$).

ASTHMA MANAGEMENT DURING PREGNANCY

Goals of Therapy

The two main goals of asthma management appear appropriate to optimize both maternal and fetal health.

Table 11-1. ODDS RATIOS FOR OUTCOMES OF PREGNANCY IN ASTHMATIC VERSUS ALL WOMEN IN A LARGE POPULATION-BASED STUDY*†

Outcome	All Asthmatic Subjects ($N = 36,985$)	Most Severe Asthma ($N = 1396$)
Perinatatal mortality	1.21 (1.08–1.35) ‡	1.28 (0.76–2.17) ‡
Pre-eclampsia	1.15 (1.08–1.23) ‡	1.42 (1.09–1.86) ‡
Preterm birth (< 37 wk)	1.15 (1.09–1.21) ‡	1.56 (1.27–1.90) ‡
Low-birth-weight (< 2500 g)	1.21 (1.14–1.29) ‡	1.98 (1.52–2.59) ‡
Congenital malformations	1.05 (0.99–1.10)	1.08 (0.83–1.40)

* *Adapted from Kallen et al. [3••].*
†*Numbers in parentheses are 95% CI.*
‡*P < 0.05 asthmatic versus all women.*

Prevention of acute episodes should prevent potentially harmful acute hypoxia. Optimization of chronic maternal pulmonary function should reduce the potential for chronic hypoxia, maternal symptoms, and the likelihood of acute episodes.

Nonpharmacologic Management

The identification of potentially avoidable triggering factors is an important aspect of nonpharmacologic management that may prevent acute episodes, improve clinical well-being, and decrease the need for pharmacologic intervention. It is particularly important for pregnant asthmatic women to discontinue smoking during pregnancy. First, smoking may predispose to increased asthma, complicating bronchitis or sinusitis, and thus contribute to an increased need for medication. Second, the increased perinatal morbidity attributed to smoking may be additive to that conferred by uncontrolled maternal asthma [2].

Historical information or prior skin testing will often suggest mite, mold, dander, or pollen sensitivity for which avoidance may be advised. Routine skin testing in previously untested patients is usually deferred in our clinic until postpartum because skin testing with potent antigens may be associated with systemic reactions. In vitro tests for specific IgE may be obtained if confirmation of historically relevant allergens is necessary during pregnancy.

Spontaneous abortions associated with systemic reactions after allergen immunotherapy have been reported. In addition, anaphylaxis caused by other agents has been associated with maternal and fetal mortality and morbidity [9]. Aside from systemic reactions, allergy immunotherapy appears safe during pregnancy. Based on this information, it is recommended that allergen immunotherapy be continued carefully during pregnancy in patients already receiving it who appear to be deriving benefit, who are not prone to systemic reactions, and who are receiving a maintenance or at least a substantial dosage [9]. Dose reduction is recommended to further decrease the risk of a systemic reaction; similarly, it is also usually appropriate to discontinue immunotherapy in patients who would require further increases to achieve therapeutic doses. Benefit–risk considerations do not favor beginning immunotherapy during pregnancy for most patients because of 1) the undefined propensity for systemic reactions, 2) the increased likelihood of systemic reactions during initiation of immunotherapy, 3) the latency of immunotherapy effect, and 4) the frequent difficulty in predicting which asthmatic patients will benefit from immunotherapy [9].

Asthma may add to the stress of normal pregnancy, and, conversely, this stress may aggravate asthma. It is important that anxiety in pregnant patients regarding their asthma and its interrelationships with pregnancy be reduced by giving patients the opportunity to express their concerns and by educating them regarding their illness and its interactions with pregnancy. Educational material

for pregnant asthmatic patients has been published [10]. Such education should also improve patient adherence.

Careful follow-up by physicians experienced in managing asthma is an essential aspect of optimal gestational asthma management. Pregnant asthmatic women requiring regular medication should be evaluated at least monthly. In addition to symptomatic and auscultatory assessment, objective measures of respiratory status (optimally spirometry, minimally peak expiratory flow rate [PEF]) should be obtained on every clinic visit. In addition, patients with more severe or labile asthma should be considered for home PEF monitoring. All pregnant patients should have facilitated access to their physician for increased symptoms. It is also important that effective communication exists among the physician managing the asthma, the patient, and the obstetrician.

Pharmacologic Management

GENERAL CONSIDERATIONS

Medications used during pregnancy may have several adverse effects on the fetus or the pregnancy: 1) abortion, 2) fetal death, 3) congenital malformation (especially first trimester exposure), 4) effect on fetal growth, 5) effect on function of developing organs (*eg*, the central nervous system), 6) effect on maternal or uteroplacental vasculature or uterine smooth muscle, and 7) effect of transplacentally administered drugs in the newborn. Although few drugs have been proven harmful, and fewer than 1% of congenital malformations can be attributed to drugs [11], statistical and ethical considerations make it unlikely that any drug will ever be "proven safe." Although unnecessary use of medication during pregnancy should be avoided, the potential risks of untreated disease often make pharmacologic intervention for gestational asthma necessary.

The choice of a specific medication for use during pregnancy is based on a number of considerations.

HUMAN DATA

Human data exist in the form of case reports, cohort studies, and case-control studies [12,13]. Case reports, in which an exposure and an outcome are presented, should not be used to infer cause and effect. Cohort studies prospectively evaluate exposed and nonexposed populations to determine outcome, and case-control studies retrospectively evaluate affected and unaffected subjects for whether or not they were exposed. Negative cohort studies are reassuring but rarely include sufficient numbers of exposed individuals to rule out a small (but important) increase in adverse pregnancy outcome, especially when dealing with outcomes such as specific malformations, the most common of which may only occur in three per 1000 births [12]. Positive cohort or case-control studies do not of themselves prove causation and generally must be considered to suggest hypotheses requiring independent confirmation [11]. Nonetheless, when effective alternatives are available, it seems advisable to avoid drugs that were negatively implicated in cohort or case-control studies.

ANIMAL DATA

Although animals differ from humans in a number of ways, animal teratology experiments can be useful in evaluating human drug risks. Animal studies are designed to maximize the response of the system to potential toxic effects of the test agent by using large doses [11]. It is believed that a testing scheme using appropriate doses in at least two species, one of which is not a rodent, is sufficient to raise suspicion of human developmental risk. There are, in fact, no known human developmental toxicants that would not have been identified in this manner [11]. Therefore, if an agent is appropriately tested in animals and found not to be a developmental toxicant, its potential for human developmental toxicity is low. Positive data in animal studies are not as useful because it is often not possible to know whether species differences, the clinically irrelevant high doses used, or maternal toxicity was responsible for the adverse effects on the offspring [11].

FOOD AND DRUG ADMINISTRATION CATEGORIES

In 1979, the United States Food and Drug Administration (FDA) established five categories to describe a drug's potential for causing adverse effects during pregnancy (Table 11-2) and mandated that newly approved drugs introduced after November 1, 1980 be classified into one of these categories in the package insert. The categories are based on the results of animal studies, "adequate and controlled" human data, and consideration of whether the benefit of the drug's use during pregnancy outweighs the risk. No asthma or allergy medication labeled to date meets the requirements for category A. Most category B drugs are labeled as such

because of reassuring animal studies, without adequate and controlled human data. One may wish to choose class B versus C drugs among equally effective alternatives because of the reassuring animal studies. The FDA recently elevated the classification of budesonide to a category B drug based on reassuring data from the population-based Swedish Medical Birth Registry [14••].

OTHER CONSIDERATIONS

A topical medication is preferable to a systemic one because of reduced likelihood of fetal penetration. An older medication with a "track record" may be preferable to a newer one. Finally, absolute and relative efficacy must also be considered in the choice of a medication for use during pregnancy.

Specific Medications

Cohort studies have been reassuring regarding a lack of adverse effects on human pregnancy outcomes of metaproterenol, albuterol, theophylline, cromolyn, beclomethasone, and budesonide [13]. In contrast, data regarding the use of oral corticosteroids during pregnancy have not been totally reassuring. Park-Wyllie *et al.* [15] recently published a meta-analysis of 1) the cohort studies evaluating the relationship between first trimester maternal oral corticosteroid use and total congenital malformations, and 2) the case-control studies evaluating the relationship between first trimester maternal oral corticosteroid use and oral clefts (cleft lip with or without cleft palate). No definite increased risk of total malformations was identified from the six cohort studies (summary odds ratio, 1.45; 95% CI, 0.80–2.60). However, meta-analysis of the four case-control studies revealed a significantly increased risk of oral clefts in infants of corticosteroid-treated mothers (summary odds ratio, 3.35; 95% CI, 1.97–5.69).

Table 11-2. US FOOD AND DRUG ADMINISTRATION PREGNANCY CATEGORIES*

Category	Animal Studies	Human Data	Benefit May Outweigh Risk
A	Negative[†]	Studies[‡] negative	Yes
B	Negative	Studies not done	Yes
B	Positive[§]	Studies negative	Yes
C	Positive	Studies not done	Yes
C	Not done	Studies not done	Yes
D	Positive or negative	Studies or reports positive	Yes
X[¶]	Positive	Studies or reports positive	No

Adapted from Schatz et al. [24].
[†]*No teratogenicity demonstrated.*
[‡]*"Adequate and well-controlled" studies in pregnant women.*
[§]*Teratogenicity demonstrated.*
[¶]*Drug is contraindicated in pregnancy.*

Other adverse outcomes have also been attributed to oral corticosteroids, including an increased risk of pre-eclampsia, preterm birth, and lower birth weight [13]. In many of these studies, it is difficult to exclude an adverse effect of the underlying disease itself. Moreover, authors of most of these studies have pointed out that these potential gestational risks of oral corticosteroids must be balanced against the risks to the mother or the infant with inadequately treated disease. In the case of asthma, as described previously, the risks of severe uncontrolled asthma (which may include maternal or fetal mortality) would usually constitute the greater risk, suggesting that oral corticosteroids must still be used when indicated for the management of severe gestational asthma.

No human data exist for a number of newer medications that are currently used for asthma. These include drugs with reassuring animal studies (*eg*, ipratropium, nedocromil, zafirlukast, and montelukast) and those with nonreassuring animal studies (*eg*, salmeterol, formoterol, and zileuton). Recommendations for the use of these newer medications, based on the animal studies, route of administration, and efficacy considerations, are provided in Table 11-3.

Treatment Protocols

In 1993, the National Asthma Education Program Working Group on Asthma and Pregnancy published consensus recommendations for the management of gestational asthma [9]. More recently, these recommendations were updated by a joint ad hoc committee of the American College of Allergy, Asthma and Immunology and the American College of Obstetricians and Gynecologists [16••].

CHRONIC ASTHMA

The consensus recommendations for the management of chronic asthma during pregnancy are shown in Table 11-3. Although no recommendations regarding a specific inhaled β-agonist were made in either of the reports, the data reviewed previously suggest that metaproterenol or albuterol would be good choices. Based on the published human data, beclomethasone or budesonide were recommended if inhaled corticosteroids were being initiated during pregnancy, but the consensus statement suggested that other inhaled corticosteroids could be continued if the patient's asthma was well controlled on one of these medications before pregnancy. However, because budesonide is now the only inhaled corticosteroid with a category B classification, it may be appropriate to use budesonide for all pregnant patients who require inhaled corticosteroids unless there is reason to think that an alternate inhaled corticosteroid would provide better asthma control for an individual patient. Finally, avoidance of zileuton was recommended, but montelukast or zafirlukast could be considered for patients with recalcitrant asthma who have shown a uniquely favorable response before pregnancy.

ACUTE ASTHMA

The management of patients with acute asthma during pregnancy has been recently reviewed [17], and the recommended pharmacologic management of acute gestational asthma is summarized in Table 11-4. In addition to pharmacologic therapy, supplemental oxygen (initially 3 to 4 L/min by nasal cannula) should be administered, adjusting forced inspiratory oxygen (FiO_2) to

---

Table 11-3. ACAAI-ACOG RECOMMENDATIONS FOR THE PHARMACOLOGIC STEP THERAPY OF CHRONIC ASTHMA DURING PREGNANCY*

Category	Step Therapy
Mild intermittent	Inhaled β$_2$-agonists as needed (for all categories) [†]
Mild persistent	Inhaled cromolyn
	Continue inhaled nedocromil in patients who have shown a good response before pregnancy
	Substitute inhaled corticosteroids[‡] if above not adequate
Moderate persistent	Inhaled corticosteroids[‡]
	Continue inhaled salmeterol in patients who have shown a very good response before pregnancy
	Add oral theophylline or inhaled salmeterol (or both) for patients inadequately controlled by medium-dose inhaled corticosteroids
Severe persistent	Above plus oral corticosteroids (burst for active symptoms, alternate-day or daily if necessary)

*Based on the recommendations of the National Asthma Education Program Report of the Working Group on Asthma During Pregnancy [9], updated to incorporate newer information [16••].
[†]Most published human data using albuterol, metaproterenol, or terbutaline.
[‡]Beclomethasone or budesonide if inhaled corticosteroids are being initiated during pregnancy; continuation of other inhaled corticosteroid if patient is well controlled by it before pregnancy; consider budesonide if patient requires high-dose inhaled corticosteroids for adequate control.
ACAAI—American College of Allergy, Asthma and Immunology; ACOG—American College of Obstetricians and Gynecologists.

maintain a partial pressure of oxygen (PO_2) at 70 or above and/or O_2 saturation by pulse oximetry less than 95%. In addition, intravenous (IV) fluids (containing glucose if the patient is not hyperglycemic) should be administered, initially at a rate of at least 100 mL/h.

Three doses of inhaled β-agonists spaced every 20 to 30 minutes can be given safely as initial therapy to patients without coexistent cardiovascular disease. Thereafter, the frequency of administration varies according to the severity of the patient's symptoms and occurrence of adverse side effects. It would also seem reasonable to administer one dose (500 μg in 2.5 mL) of nebulized ipratropium to patients who have not significantly improved after the first dose of albuterol, because recent data show that its bronchodilatory effect is additive to that of inhaled β-agonists in the management of acute asthma [17].

Parenteral corticosteroids should be administered along with initial therapy to patients taking regular corticosteroids. In addition, IV corticosteroids should be used in patients with severe airflow obstruction (PEFR < 200 L/min or FEV_1 [forced expiratory volume in 1 second] < 40% predicted) that persists after 1 hour of intensive β-agonist therapy [9]. Although there are insufficient data to determine the optimal dose of parenteral corticosteroids to be used in patients with acute asthma, 1 mg/kg methylprednisolone every 6 to 8 hours has been recommended [9].

Intravenous aminophylline is not generally recommended in the emergency department management of patients with acute gestational asthma because it has been demonstrated that aminophylline provides no additional benefit to optimal inhaled β-agonist therapy in the first 4 hours of treatment [9]. Moreover, when used in combination with intensive inhaled β-agonist therapy,

IV aminophylline causes increased adverse side effects without providing additional bronchodilation [9].

Patients who adequately respond to emergency department therapy (PEFR or FEV_1 > 60% to 70% predicted) may usually be discharged from the emergency department. All patients who require more than a single inhaled β-agonist treatment should be discharged on a course of oral corticosteroids as well as on inhaled corticosteroids. Recommended doses of oral corticosteroids upon emergency department discharge are 30 to 60 mg/d of prednisone for 7 to 14 days [17]. Appropriate patient education regarding the discharge treatment plan, especially concerning inhaler and spacer technique, as well as clear instructions for follow-up care are essential to preventing relapses.

Patients who do not adequately respond as above require hospitalization. When a pregnant woman with asthma is hospitalized, both medical and obstetrical supervision is required. Patients in frank or impending respiratory failure (PCO_2 > 35 mm Hg) should be hospitalized in an intensive care unit. In the hospital, oxygen, inhaled β-agonists and IV corticosteroids should be continued. Inhaled β-agonists should be administered continuously every 4 hours, depending on the severity and response. Nebulized ipratropium every 4 to 8 hours may be considered. Because recent studies suggest that IV magnesium sulfate (1.0 to 2.0 g) may be beneficial in acute severe asthma as an adjunct to inhaled β-agonists and IV corticosteroids, magnesium sulfate could also be considered, especially in patients with coexistent hypertension or preterm uterine contractions [17]. In addition, IV aminophylline may be considered. When IV aminophylline is used, pharmacokinetic studies during pregnancy suggest that the loading dose recommendation for theophylline requires no modification during

---

Table 11-4. PHARMACOLOGIC MANAGEMENT OF ACUTE ASTHMA DURING PREGNANCY

β$_2$-agonist bronchodilator (see text)
  Up to 3 doses in first 60–90 min
  Every 1–2 h thereafter until adequate response
Nebulized ipratropium
IV methylprednisolone (with initial therapy in patients on regular corticosteroids and for those with poor response during the first hour of treatment)
  1 mg/kg every 6–8 h
  Taper as patient improves
Consider IV aminophylline (generally only if patient requires hospitalization). If it is to be used:
  6 mg/kg loading dose
  0.5 mg/kg/h initial maintenance dose
  Adjust rate to keep theophylline level between 8 and 12 μg/mL
Consider SC terbutaline 0.25 mg or magnesium sulfate if patient not responding to the above therapy

IV—intravenous; SC—subcutaneous.

pregnancy (5 mg/kg over 20 to 30 minutes), but the initial maintenance dose should be lower (0.5 mg/kg/h) [17]. Studies have also suggested that protein binding of theophylline decreases during pregnancy such that there is an approximately 15% increase in free drug for any total drug concentration. This suggests that a lower therapeutic range (8 to 12 µg/mL) than is usually recommended is appropriate during pregnancy [9].

Antibiotics should be used for hospitalized patients with purulent sputum containing polymorphonuclear leukocytes or if pneumonia is documented on chest radiography. In addition, a high index of suspicion for sinusitis must be maintained, and sinus radiographs should be considered in hospitalized asthmatic patients who have substantial nasal congestion or postnasal drainage, even in the absence of purulent discharge. IV cefuroxime is recommended initially for hospitalized pregnant asthmatic patients with suspected bacterial respiratory infections [17]. Erythromycin should be included as part of initial therapy if *Mycoplasma pneumoniae*, *Chlamydia pneumoniae*, or *Legionella* spp infection is suspected. After the first 24 to 72 hours, oral therapy with amoxicillin-clavulanate or cefuroxime may be substituted for IV cephalosporin therapy in most hospitalized asthmatic patients with pneumonia or sinusitis.

Respiratory failure during pregnancy is beyond the scope of this chapter and is reviewed elsewhere [17,18]. One recent report described a helium-oxygen mixture being successfully used in a patient with asthma-induced respiratory failure during pregnancy [19].

OBSTETRIC CONSIDERATIONS IN PREGNANT ASTHMATIC PATIENTS

Detailed obstetric management of pregnant women with asthma is described elsewhere [20,21]. A number of medications potentially used for obstetric indications should be avoided in patients with asthma because they have been shown to trigger bronchospasm. These include β-blockers, 15 methylprostaglandin $F_{2\alpha}$, transcervical or intra-amniotic prostaglandin E_2, methylergonovine or ergonovine, and NSAIDs (in aspirin-sensitive asthmatics). Use of intravaginal or intracervical prostaglandin E_2 gel for cervical ripening before labor induction or prostaglandin E_2 suppositories for therapeutic abortion or labor induction with a dead fetus have not been reported to cause bronchospasm in asthmatic patients [21]. Magnesium sulfate and calcium channel blockers, which have been shown to possess bronchodilator properties, should also be well tolerated in patients with asthma.

Obstetric management of women with controlled asthma during labor and delivery is identical to management in nonasthmatic women, including the preference for regional versus general anesthesia. When general anesthesia is required for cesarean section, the following medications are recommended in asthmatic women because of their bronchodilating properties: 1) pre-anesthetic use of atropine and glycopyrrolate, 2) induction of anesthesia with ketamine, and 3) low concentrations of halogenated anesthetic agents [9].

Although only 10% of prospectively managed asthmatic women experience symptoms of asthma during labor or delivery [4], prophylactic medications should be continued. Patients who experience asthma symptoms during labor should be treated as described in Table 11-4. For patients taking regular corticosteroids or who have received frequent courses during pregnancy, supplemental corticosteroids for the stress of labor and delivery are recommended: 100 mg of hydrocortisone IV at admission followed by 100 mg IV every 8 hours for 24 hours or until the absence of complications is established [9].

CONCLUSIONS

Managing asthma during pregnancy can be as satisfying as it is challenging. In our litigation-oriented society, however, the medical-legal implications of treating pregnant women with asthma must be considered [22,23]. A number of steps have been recommended to reduce medicolegal jeopardy in managing gestational asthma [24].

1. Discuss with the patient that, although relatively few medications of any kind have been "proven harmful" during pregnancy, no asthma or allergy medication can be considered to be "proven absolutely safe."

2. Discuss with the patient the potential direct and indirect consequences for the mother and for the baby of inadequately controlled asthma.

3. Discuss with the patient the concept that there are medications that appear safe enough that their use is preferable to the uncontrolled illness that would result if they were not used.

4. Discuss the alternative medication choices available for the patient's particular situation and the rationale for choosing among those alternatives.

5. A written informed consent document is not recommended. However, clearly document in the chart that the above discussion has taken place; that the benefits, risks, and alternatives of the specific pharmacologic approach have been discussed with the patient; and that her informed consent to that approach has been obtained.

REFERENCES AND RECOMMENDED READING

Papers of particular interest, published recently, have been highlighted as:
* • Of importance
* •• Of major importance

1. Alexander S, Dodds L, Armson BA: Perinatal outcomes in women with asthma during pregnancy. *Obstet Gynecol* 1998, 92:435–440.

2. Schatz M, Dombrowski M: Outcomes of pregnancy in asthmatic women. *Immunol Allergy Clin North Am* 2000, 20:715–727.

3.••Kallen B, Rydhstroem H, Aberg A: Asthma during pregnancy: a population based study. *Eur J Epidemiol* 2000, 16:167–171.
This is the largest study reported to date comparing outcomes of pregnancy in asthmatic versus nonasthmatic women. The data suggest that maternal asthma increases the risk of perinatal mortality, preterm births, pre-eclampsia, and low-birth-weight infants.

4. Schatz M: Interrelationships between asthma and pregnancy: a literature review. *J Allergy Clin Immunol* 1999, 103(suppl):330–336.

5. Gluck JC, Gluck PA: The effect of pregnancy on the course of asthma. *Immunol Allergy Clin North Am* 2000, 20:729–743.

6. Schatz M, Dombrowski M, Wise R, *et al.*: Asthma morbidity during pregnancy can be predicted by severity classification. 2002 (In press).

7. Kircher S, Schatz M, Long L: Variables affecting asthma course during pregnancy. *Ann Allergy Asthma Immunol* 2002 (In press).

8.• Cydulka RK, Emerman CL, Schreiber D, *et al.*: Acute asthma among pregnant women presenting to the emergency department. *Am J Respir Crit Care Med* 1999, 160:887–892.
This study compared the course and management of pregnant patients presenting with acute asthma with that of nonpregnant women. It documents undertreatment with steroids and poorer clinical outcomes in the pregnant patients.

9. *National Asthma Education Program: Management of asthma during pregnancy: report of the Working Group on Asthma and Pregnancy.* Bethesda, MD: National Institutes of Health, NIH Pub. No. 93-3279; 1993.

10. Lipkowitz MA, Schatz M, Cook TJ, *et al.*: Advice from your allergist: when allergies and asthma complicate pregnancy. *Ann Allergy Asthma Immunol* 1998, 81:30–34.

11. Scialli A, Lone A: Pregnancy effects of specific medications used to treat asthma and immunological diseases. In *Asthma and Immunological Diseases in Pregnancy and Early Infancy.* Edited by Schatz M, Zeiger RS, Claman HN. New York: Marcel Dekker; 1998:157–227.

12. Petitti DB: Perinatal epidemiology: studying the effects of illness and medications during pregnancy. *Immunol Allergy Clin North Am* 2000, 20:673–685.

13. Schatz M: The efficacy and safety of asthma medications during pregnancy. *Semin Perinatol* 2001, 25:145–152.

14.••Kallen B, Rydhstroem H, Abeg A: Congenital malformations after the use of inhaled budesonide in early pregnancy. *Obstet Gynecol* 1999, 93:392–395.
This large population-based study showed that the risk of congenital malformations in 2014 infants whose mothers received budesonide during early pregnancy was not significantly greater than that in the general Swedish population of infants evaluated over the same time period.

15. Park-Wyllie L, Mazzotta P, Pastuszak A, *et al.*: Birth defects after maternal exposure to corticosteroids: prospective cohort study and meta-analysis of epidemiological studies. *Teratology* 2000, 62:385–392.

16.••The use of newer asthma and allergy medications during pregnancy [position statement]. *Ann Allergy Asthma Immunol* 2000, 84:475–480.
A consensus statement by a joint subcommittee of the American College of Allergy Asthma and Immunology and the American College of Obstetricians and Gynecologists presenting recommendations for the pharmacologic management of asthma during pregnancy.

17. Schatz M, Wise RA: Acute asthma in pregnancy. In *Acute Asthma: Assessment and Management.* Edited by Hall JB, Corbridge J, Rodrigo G, *et al.* New York: McGraw-Hill; 2000.

18. Catanzarite V, Cousins L: Respiratory failure in pregnancy. *Immunol Allergy Clin North Am* 2000, 20:775–806.

19. George R, Berkenbosch JW, Fraser RF, Tobias JD: Mechanical ventilation during pregnancy using a helium-oxygen mixture in a patient with respiratory failure due to status asthmaticus. *J Perinatol* 2001, 21:395–398.

20. Cousins L: Fetal oxygenation, assessment of fetal well-being, and obstetric management of the pregnant patient with asthma. *J Allergy Clin Immunol* 1999, 103(suppl):343–349.

21. Dombrowski MP: The obstetrical management of pregnant asthmatics. In *Asthma and Immunological Diseases in Pregnancy and Early Infancy.* Edited by Schatz M, Zeiger RS, Claman HN. New York: Marcel Dekker; 1998:487–497.

22. Aaronson DW: Medical-legal aspects of prescribing during pregnancy. *Immunol Allergy Clin North Am* 2000, 20:699–714.

23. Fern FH, Orlando CP, Hobart JA: Medical/legal aspects of prescribing during pregnancy. In *Asthma and Immunological Diseases in Pregnancy and Early Infancy.* Edited by Schatz M, Zeiger RS, Claman HN. New York: Marcel Dekker; 1998:229–260.

24. Schatz M, Hoffman CP, Zeiger RS, *et al.*: The course and management of asthma and allergic diseases during pregnancy. In *Allergy: Principles and Practice.* Edited by Middleton E, Reed CE, Ellis EF, *et al.* St. Louis: Mosby; 1998:938–952.

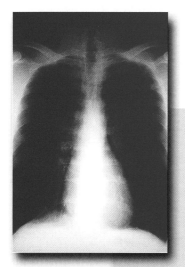

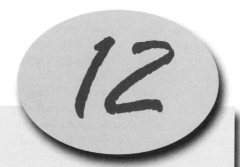

Treatment of Asthma in Children

Athena Economides and Martha V. White

Asthma is the most common chronic illness in children, affecting 6.9% of children younger than 18 years of age, or 5 million children in the United States [1]. It is the leading cause of school absenteeism, and leads to missed workdays in 36% of parents of school-age asthmatic patients [2]. Americans spend over 10 billion dollars each year on asthma, and as many as 50% of asthma patients spend more than 18% of their family income on asthma therapy [3]. Despite improvements in our understanding of asthma and in delivery systems for asthma medications, the incidence of asthma and of deaths due to asthma is rising. Asthma deaths have doubled for children 14 years of age and younger from 1979 to 1995, with the 5- to 14-year-old group driving this rise in mortality [4]. Asthma must be regarded as a potentially life-threatening disorder, even in mild cases; a recent population-based study in Victoria, British Columbia showed that the majority of asthma deaths occurred in patients who could not be classified as high risk [5]. Seventy-eight percent of parents of asthmatic patients report that asthma has a negative impact on their family; indeed, even in mild cases the disruption of family dynamics, school attendance, and social interactions can be significant [3].

Our understanding of the pathology and, therefore, the treatment of asthma has improved dramatically since the 1980s [3,6••,7,8••]. There is, primarily, involvement of small bronchi and bronchioles, sparing the alveoli, with extensive denudation of airway epithelium, sub-basement membrane fibrosis, collagen deposition, mucus hypersecretion because of goblet cell hyperplasia, and smooth muscle hyperplasia with increased contractility. There is, also, inflammatory cell infiltration of the lamina propria by CD4+ lymphocytes of the Th2 phenotype, activated mast cells, eosinophils, and neutrophils. The eosinophil is the most specific of all the infiltrating cells, and is seen rather exclusively in asthma and not in other inflammatory diseases of the airway. Wheezing is attributed to airway lumen plugs of mucus, edema fluid, eosinophils, Charcot-Leyden crystals, and Curschmann's spirals.

Typical asthma attacks consist of an early, short-lived bronchoconstrictive response to an asthma trigger and a later onset, longer reaction, called late-phase reaction (LPR). The bulk of evidence suggests that the airway inflammation observed in asthma is caused by mast cell–initiated LPR. This phase lasts hours to days, is characterized by wheezing that is poorly responsive to bronchodilators, and can render a patient's airways hyperreactive to additional asthma triggers for prolonged periods. Such airway hyperreactivity (AHR) also increases during the allergy season and during rhinovirus infections.

Airway hyperresponsiveness and LPR are closely linked to asthma severity and death. For example, the degree of AHR to nonspecific stimuli, *eg*, histamine, methacholine, pollution, and tobacco smoke, correlates closely with asthma severity. Excessive use of symptomatic medications rather than pathology-reversing treatments and restricted access to long-term follow-up care have also been associated with asthma deaths. Thus, specialists now agree that the primary focus of asthma management should be early diagnosis to reduce and prevent AHR and LPR. Indeed, guidelines for the management of asthma, published through the National Institutes of Health and other world agencies, stress the importance of anti-inflammatory medications [6••]. Although there are differences between adult and pediatric asthma, the principal goals of asthma therapy in children are not different from those in adults (*see* Table 12-1).

DIAGNOSIS

Asthma is a disease characterized by episodic wheezing, cough, or chest tightness responsive to defined asthma management protocols, for which other causes have been eliminated. Although it is true that not all that wheezing is asthma, asthma is common, and the other causes of wheezing are rare. Asthma can present as recurrent dry cough or wheeze occurring at night and/or associated with exercise, viral infections, or smoke exposure. It should be pointed out that wheezing might not always be present.

The diagnosis of asthma in a child is not always as easily made as in the adult patient [6••], who can perform the spirometer maneuver, the gold standard for asthma diagnosis, easily and reliably. In children, a careful history and physical examination are the most useful diagnostic aids, especially in young children who are unable to perform spirometry. Key questions in the history can help determine frequency of symptoms, *eg*, wheezing, shortness of breath (with or without exercise), chest tightness felt below the sternum, or cough (throat versus chest, with or without exercise), as well as quantity and quality of sputum. Questions about daytime wheezing episodes, nocturnal awakenings, morning versus evening symptoms, days missed from school per year, emergency room visits, and/or hospitalizations all help determine the severity of disease. The majority of pediatric asthma is strongly associated with atopy, but asthma attacks are frequently triggered by natural exposures. It is particularly important to determine the atopic risk, and to identify triggers such as cold air, exercise, animal or food exposure, irritating chemicals, and laughter, or the association of symptoms with school or home.

Assuming that the child can adequately perform spirometry, he or she may have asthma despite normal measures of FEV_1 (forced expiratory volume in 1 second), a problem that may be related to the lack of reliable standards for pediatric pulmonary function. Thus, in most normal children, the percent predicted value for FVC (forced vital capacity), FEV_1, and FEF_{25-75} (forced expiratory flow at 25% to 75% of forced vital capacity) are similar, with FEF_{25-75} (percent predicted) often exceeding the other two. In asthma, the FEV_1 (percent predicted) is reduced compared with FVC, with FEF_{25-75} more severely affected. Thus, an FEF_{25-75} with a percent of predicted value proportionally lower than that of the FVC and FEV_1 percent of predicted values should raise the index of suspicion of asthma, even if all values are in the normal range. When the FEV_1 percent of predicted value is proportionally lower than that of the FVC, with the FEF_{25-75} more severely affected, asthma is even more likely. In these children, a 12% improvement in FEV_1 and/or a 20% increase in FEF_{25-75} after inhalation of albuterol will confirm the diagnosis.

Several alternative techniques for confirming the asthma diagnosis in children can be used when spirometry is normal. A post-bronchodilator increase of 12% in the FEV_1 or 20% in FEF_{25-75} or the performance of an exercise challenge is diagnostic for asthma. Bronchial constriction usually occurs about 10 minutes after a simple exercise challenge, in which the child runs in place or up and down the stairs until he or she feels too tired to continue. Peak flow meter measurements during asthma attacks and after bronchodilator use are especially helpful in diagnosing the young child who cannot do full spirometry. Although peak flow meter measurements are routinely recommended for all asthmatic patients, they do not reflect small airway disease, which takes the longest to resolve, and cannot take the place of complete pulmonary function testing.

For children too young to cooperate, a therapeutic trial with asthma therapy may be useful. If a more definite diagnosis is required, the methacholine or histamine challenge is considered the gold standard. An antigen challenge can also be diagnostic of antigen-induced asthma, but it carries the risk of inducing a late-phase reaction. Such challenges are time consuming, require precision, and are best left to physicians trained in these techniques.

Table 12-1. GOALS OF ASTHMA TREATMENT

Prevent chronic and troublesome symptoms

Maintain (near) normal pulmonary function

Maintain or normalize daily activity levels

Prevent recurrence of the disease, and need for emergency treatments or hospitalization

Provide optimal control with lowest effective dose of medication and minimal side effects

Meet child and family's expectations of asthma control

Despite inherent difficulties in diagnosing the very young, a particular urgency for the early diagnosis of asthma is borne out of recent studies. While it is estimated that 80% of asthma patients experience onset by 5 years of age [9] it is also widely recognized that asthma is grossly underdiagnosed in children under 6 years of age. The Tucson Children's Respiratory Study [10•] prospectively studied wheezing patterns in children 6 years of age and younger and showed that there are transient, persistent, and late wheezers, based on the ages when wheezing occurs. However, in the case of the persistent wheezer, significant loss of pulmonary function occurs after 1 year of age, but before 6 years of age [10•]. Furthermore, longitudinal data from Melbourne, Australia, where children between 7 and 10 years of age were followed periodically up to 35 years of age, suggests that the development of persistent deficits in lung function appears by the first 7 to 10 years of life, and few patients develop new-onset airway hyperreactivity during adolescence [11,12•].

TREATMENT

The therapeutic management options for asthma can be divided into two groups: anti-inflammatory interventions that heal and prevent airway inflammation that leads to airway hyperreactivity (controllers), and bronchodilators that relax smooth muscle, thus relieving the acute symptoms of asthma (rescuers). Controllers work slowly and do not produce immediate relief of symptoms. Thus, patient compliance with these products is poor unless their role in asthma management and their expected benefits are clearly outlined for the patient [13]. Controllers include allergen avoidance and immunotherapy, inhaled or nebulized corticosteroids, mast cell stabilizers such as cromolyn and nedocromil, leukotriene modifiers, long-acting bronchodilators, and even oral corticosteroids. Symptomatic treatments are short-acting bronchodilators, anticholinergics, and theophylline.

Management Strategies

Optimal management of asthma requires the cooperation of a knowledgeable patient or parent who has been taught to recognize triggers and early signs of asthma to help abort the late signs. In addition, the appropriate device for the age and ability of the child must be carefully chosen for both monitoring asthma control (peak flow meters) and administrating the medications (spacer devices). A daily peak flow graph, filled out three times a day, helps assess the severity of disease and recognize asthma symptoms and triggers. In this case, the peak flow meter becomes an inexpensive, easy to use, and accurate "asthma thermometer." Thus, once an individual's personal best peak flow is established, an asthma management plan can be devised based on ranges of peak flow readings relative to the personal best.

Impending asthma attacks can be detected before they become severe. It follows that peak flow meters allow self-management because they provide objective measurements of lung function that can guide medication decisions, which can accommodate the variability of airflow obstruction so characteristic of asthma.

The devices currently available to deliver inhaled medications include jet nebulizers, ultrasonic nebulizers, metered-dose inhalers (MDI), and dry-powder inhalers (DPI). Most of these were created with the adult patient in mind, and none of them fulfills all the requirements for an ideal inhaler. Lung dose, convenience, safety, efficacy, reliability, and environmental issues should be weighed against the requirements, abilities, and needs of the patient [14••]. Spacer devices are available to facilitate proper MDI technique, especially in the younger child, and should always be employed with steroid MDIs. They trap most large particles, providing excellent aerosol delivery to the lungs, and may contain a whistle that blows when the inhalation is too rapid.

Just as there is no single inhaler that is successful, there is no single asthma management strategy that is successful for all patients; cooperative management is based on patient education regarding asthma pathophysiology and mechanisms of action of available medications, as well as on avoidance of triggers and appropriate use of monitoring devices and medications. Parents and older children should be taught to monitor peak flow readings, listen to chest sounds, and watch out for retractions or flaring. In addition, they should be taught to track more subtle signs of decreasing asthma control, *eg*, tracking the use of bronchodilators (if used as required) and nighttime awakenings due to asthma, as well as observing for windedness with exercise and a dry, hacking cough with exercise or laughter.

The patient should also be provided with a written asthma management plan, including prescriptions for maintenance medications and details about expected medication effects and common side effects ("well plan"). The asthma management plan should detail additional medications that are to be taken when peak flow readings begin to drop or when known triggers, such as an upper respiratory infection, are encountered ("sick plan"). The school nurse should also be provided with a written medication plan for handling flares. Instructions about when to contact the physician should be clear.

Graded asthma management plans must be individualized, but Tables 12-2 and 12-3 can be used as guidelines. These guidelines have been adopted by the National Institutes of Health and apply to most patients [6••,8••,13,15]. The frequency of bronchodilator use should be monitored as an accurate indicator of symptom control, as well as an index of success of prophylactic therapy. To gauge the success of therapy, it is necessary to determine the maximal lung functions achievable by the patient, often after a therapeutic trial of pharmacotherapy.

AVOIDANCE OF TRIGGERS AND IMMUNOTHERAPY

Most cases of pediatric asthma are strongly correlated with allergies; therefore all children with asthma should undergo skin or serum allergy testing. The development of allergies and the severity of existing allergies depend upon genetic predisposition and the level of exposure to a given allergen. For example, recent monozygotic twin data suggest a hereditary contribution of 60% for serum IgE levels, whereas the remaining 40% contribution was attributed to unshared environmental factors [16]. Exposure to high levels of house dust mites or cockroaches during infancy increases the atopic child's risk of developing asthma fourfold in some studies. In addition, the CAMP (Childhood Asthma Management Program) study [17•] suggested a strong correlation between increased sensitivity to methacholine and skin test reactivity to tree, weed, cat, dog, *Alternaria*, and indoor molds. Optimization of asthma therapy becomes, therefore, difficult without rigorous avoidance of allergic triggers (*see* Chapter 20, *Allergen Avoidance*).

If allergen exposure cannot be completely eliminated, immunotherapy can be helpful in asthmatic patients with known allergic triggers and significantly positive confirmatory skin tests. Carefully performed trials of allergens used to treat well-defined allergic asthmatic patients (*eg*, birch pollen-induced asthma) have documented that immunotherapy reduces symptoms and prevents the increases in airway reactivity normally seen during the allergy season [3,6••]. In addition, data from a recent European study suggest that immunotherapy given for 3 years to children with allergic rhinitis can prevent the development of asthma in these school-age children [18•]. Thus, immunotherapy is currently the only treatment that has been shown to prevent asthma, or to induce a long-term remission of asthma, and is indicated either when the patient does not respond to avoidance and pharmacotherapy or when avoidance may not be possible. It can be used as an inhaled corticosteroid-sparing agent in asthmatic patients. If no improvement occurs after 2 years and the child has not developed new allergies that might explain the persistent symptoms, the immunotherapy should be stopped.

Nonallergic triggers also need to be dealt with. Passive smoke inhalation is unequivocally deleterious to the pulmonary functions of healthy and asthmatic children and should not be permitted in the home of asthmatic children. In some studies, atopic mothers who smoked were four times as likely to have an asthmatic child as were nonsmoking atopic mothers. Upper airway-related infections, such as otitis and sinusitis, are significant triggers of asthma and should be sought and treated aggressively. All asthmatic patients with frequent or difficult asthma flares, especially those requiring hospitalization, should be evaluated for sinusitis. Chronic sinusitis can be indolent and generally requires 3 to 6 weeks of therapy with appropriate antibiotics.

Table 12-2. TREATMENT OF ASTHMA IN INFANTS AND TODDLERS

Degree of Asthma	Therapy
Intermittent	
Mild, brief symptoms < 2×/wk, nocturnal symptoms 2×/mo, normal PFT	Nebulized or oral β_2-agonist as needed
Persistent	
Mild to moderate	
Symptoms > 2×/wk, exacerbations may last days, occasional ER visit, FEV_1 60%–80%	Daily leukotriene modifier or nebulized cromolyn sodium plus nebulized β_2-agonist as needed
	Replace cromolyn sodium with nebulized corticosteroids + leukotriene modifiers
	Add short-term oral corticosteroids
	Wean as tolerated, beginning with oral corticosteroids
Severe	
Continuous symptoms, restricted activity, frequent nocturnal symptoms, FEV_1 < 60%, occasional hospitalizations/ER visits	Daily nebulized corticosteroids plus nebulized β_2-agonist, as needed
	Add leukotriene modifiers
	Add LABA, followed by theophylline or ipratropium
	Add short-term oral corticosteroids, daily or every other day
	Wean as tolerated, beginning with oral corticosteroids

ER—emergency room; FEV_1— forced expiratory volume in 1 second; LABA—long-acting β_2-agonist; PFT—pulmonary function test.

ANTI-INFLAMMATORY AND RESCUE MEDICATIONS
Inhaled Corticosteroids

Inhaled corticosteroids (ICSs) are potent topical anti-inflammatory medications and are considered the backbone of any long-term controller treatment plan. However, sustained ICS use at very high doses can cause linear growth rate suppression in children, glaucoma, cataracts, increased bone mineral loss, and adrenal suppression. This is why the Food and Drug Administration (FDA) called in 1998 for ICS use at the lowest effective dose. Subsequent studies of several ICS substances show that the controversial issue of growth velocity deficits with long-term ICS use seems unsubstantiated with newer inhaled steroid molecules such as fluticasone and budesonide [19••,20•]. The CAMP study was designed primarily to evaluate whether continuous long-term treatment with either budesonide or nedocromil could safely improve lung growth (measured as post-albuterol FEV_1) in mild to moderate asthmatic children 5 to 13 years of age as compared with placebo. Surprisingly, however, a significant improvement in lung function did not occur, in agreement with a growing body of evidence that asthmatic changes in lung function occurring before 6 years of age tend to persist. An alternative explanation is that the mean FEV_1 in the group of children in the CAMP study was 95% of predicted, and there may have been little room for improvement in those children.

An equal body of literature has shown that ICSs are not equal or interchangeable. Beclomethasone has been used extensively in children, but provides unacceptably high systemic exposure and is therefore no longer considered appropriate for pediatric use. Triamcinolone offers the advantage of a built-in spacer, whereas flunisolide may be prohibitive in some children because of the unpleasant taste. The two most popular ICSs for the moment are fluticasone, available in a variety of different strengths, and budesonide, which is also available as the first ICS approved for use in a nebulizer.

There are several recommendations for safe ICS use. First, gargling, rinsing the mouth, or brushing the teeth after each use minimizes thrush. Second, using a spacer (equipped with a child's facemask in young patients) or DPI increases delivery to the lung rather than the gut. Third, use whatever amount is required to maximize peak flow, then step down to the lowest dose that will maintain maximal lung function. Fourth, try to stay below 2000 µg budesonide, triamcinolone, or flunisolide, or 880 µg of fluticasone per day. For mild persistent asthma use 100 to 600 µg per day (44–200 µg/d fluticasone); for moderate persistent asthma, use 600 to 1200 µg per day (220–500 µg/d fluticasone); and for severe persistent asthma, use 1000 to 2000 µg per day (660–1000 µg/d fluticasone). Fifth, children requiring moderate to high doses of ICS should be

---

Table 12-3. TREATMENT OF ASTHMA IN CHILDREN AGED 4 YEARS TO ADOLESCENCE

Degree of Asthma	Therapy
Intermittent	
Mild, brief symptoms < 2×/wk, nocturnal symptoms 2×/mo, normal PFT	Inhaled β₂-agonist as needed
Persistent	
Mild to moderate	
Symptoms > 2×/wk, exacerbations may last days, occasional ER visit, FEV_1 60%–80%	Daily ICS, leukotriene modifiers, or inhaled cromolyn sodium plus inhaled β₂-agonist as needed
	Replace leukotriene modifier or cromolyn sodium with ICS plus LABA and/or leukotriene modifier
	Substitute inhaled for nebulized β₂-agonists and add short-term oral corticosteroids for exacerbations
	Wean as tolerated, beginning with oral corticosteroids
Severe	
Continuous symptoms, restricted activity, frequent nocturnal symptoms, FEV_1 < 60%, occasional hospitalizations/ER visits	Daily inhaled corticosteroids plus LABA or leukotriene modifiers, plus β₂-agonist as needed
	Add LABA and/or leukotriene antagonist or ipratropium or theophylline
	Substitute inhaled with nebulized β₂-agonists and add short-term oral corticosteroids for exacerbations
	Add short-term oral corticosteroids, daily or every other day
	Wean as tolerated, beginning with oral corticosteroids

ER—emergency room; FEV_1— forced expiratory volume in 1 second; ICS—inhaled corticosteroid; LABA—long-acting β₂-agonist; PFT—pulmonary function test.

given long-acting β-agonists and/or leukotriene modifiers in combination with the ICS in an attempt to lower the ICS dose, because moderate- to high-dose ICS use may be associated with systemic side effects. Last, use ICSs at a maximum of twice daily dosage to minimize side effects and encourage compliance.

Mast Cell Stabilizers

Cromolyn or nedocromil are probably the safest drugs for asthma treatment, but unfortunately, they are not very effective. A lethal dose is unobtainable in animal models, and adverse effects are not seen below several grams per kg per day of inhaled cromolyn sodium. Although the exact mechanism of action is not fully understood, these medications prevent early- and late-phase allergic reactions. Mast cell stabilizers protect against bronchospasm by preventing release of mast cell mediators. Both cromolyn and nedocromil may be useful for cough-variant asthma patients, or prophylactically for exercise or allergen exposure when used 10 to 20 minutes in advance. They might be used after a patient has been well controlled with an ICS, as part of a step-down plan. Contrary to a popular belief, it is not recommended that patients stop these medications during an asthma attack. The disadvantage of mast cell stabilizers is the dosing frequency, which encourages noncompliance. It can take 4 to 6 weeks of 3 to 4 times daily use to achieve efficacy, and it is recommended that patients try larger doses if a standard dose (2 puffs at a time) fails. Long build-up times are not required for prophylactic use prior to allergen exposure (possibly the best and most practical use for mast cell stabilizers) or exercise, however, because single doses are effective. Nedocromil may taste so bad that patients will not use it; therefore, it is recommended that patients try nedocromil in the office before receiving a prescription. In small children, cromolyn should be given via a nebulizer because of its superior drug delivery.

Leukotriene-modifying Drugs

Leukotriene blockers are effective bronchodilators that also inhibit airway hyperreactivity. There are currently two classes of blockers: leukotriene-synthesis inhibitors (zileuton [Zyflo; Abbott Laboratories, Abbott Park, IL]) and leukotriene-receptor antagonists (zafirlukast [Accolate; AstraZeneca, Wilmington, DE] and montelukast [Singulair; Merck, West Point, PA]). Leukotriene-receptor antagonists have pediatric dosage formulations and are approved by the Food and Drug Administration (FDA) for use in children. They are well tolerated and have the capacity to allow reduction in ICS dosing. About 30% to 50% of patients will improve with each product, some dramatically. Zileuton is probably the most potent but also has the greatest number of potential side effects; 3% of patients will experience a three- to fivefold rise in liver enzymes. It is not FDA-approved for use in children.

Coumadin levels need adjustment with zafirlukast, and liver enzymes may need to be screened if higher than recommended doses are needed. These precautions, coupled with the drug's twice-daily dosage, have led to underutilization of a potentially very useful medication. Leukotriene-receptor antagonists may also be useful in aspirin-sensitive patients and patients with rhinosinusitis, polyposis, and urticaria.

LONG-ACTING BRONCHODILATORS

Selective long-acting β_2-receptor agonists, relatively specific for airway smooth muscle, offer several advantages for control of chronic symptoms. There are two long-acting bronchodilators medications available: salmeterol (Serevent; GlaxoSmithKline, Research Triangle Park, NC) and formoterol (Foradil; Novartis, East Hanover, NJ). The latter has the advantage of quick initial onset, but both offer bronchodilation for more than 12 hours. Thus, their use is recommended when multiple inhalations per day of a short-acting β-agonist are required despite appropriate therapy, or in nocturnal wheezing that fails other appropriate therapy. They may be considered in the prevention of exercise-induced symptoms, when exercise is prolonged, or for prophylaxis of intermittent exposure to irritants in the environment (*eg*, school). The addition of either of the long-acting bronchodilators to an ICS has been more efficacious than increasing the dose of the ICS; thus, many consider long-acting bronchodilators to be ICS-sparing agents. Either salmeterol or formoterol could be used in combination with an ICS for exacerbations. These products are not appropriate for rapid symptom relief and, therefore, should be left at home and not be carried, in order to avoid confusion with short-acting bronchodilators. Salmeterol is available as an MDI that would need a spacer device and as a DPI, and formoterol is only available as a DPI. In 2001, Advair Diskus (GlaxoSmithKline, Research Triangle Park, NC), a DPI combination of fluticasone and salmeterol, was approved for adult use in the US. Studies have been done in children using the lowest dose, and approval is pending. A similar combination of formoterol and budesonide is also available in Europe.

SHORT-ACTING BRONCHODILATORS

Selective, short-acting β_2-receptor agonists for the airway are the prototype of emergency medication for asthma and should be used only when symptoms require prompt bronchodilation. Although their use results in bronchodilation within minutes if inhaled, they possibly also modulate mediator release from mast cells and basophils. These medications frequently are used for prevention of exercise-induced asthma (EIA), given 10 to 20 minutes before exercise. Short- and long-acting oral preparations exist, lasting 4 to 12 hours, respectively, and are easily administered to infants, but have more side effects. Inhaled forms have fewer side effects and work within 15 minutes. Pirbuterol (Maxair Autohaler; 3M, Northridge,

CA), administered via a breath-actuated MDI, eliminates the need for hand-eye coordination. Levalbuterol, the active L-isomer of albuterol (racemic albuterol contains both L- and S-isomers), is available as a nebulized medication (Xopenex; Sepracor, Marlborough, MA). Levalbuterol is active at lower doses than racemic albuterol, has fewer of the albuterol-related side effects, and therefore is more easily tolerated.

Since the National Institutes of Health guidelines recommend the lowest possible dose and frequency of short-acting bronchodilators, these are the *only* medications for asthma that we strictly monitor to assess the degree of symptoms control. Thus, one canister with about 200 puffs allows enough medication for twice-a-week use over 1 year, or 7 puffs per day over 1 month, and should be more than adequate for any well-controlled patient for a years' use. Use of one or more canisters per month indicates grossly inadequate control and should signal the need for aggressive anti-inflammatory treatment.

THEOPHYLLINE, ANTICHOLINERGICS, AND ANTIHISTAMINES

Three types of medications have some, albeit not significant, use in asthma: phosphodiesterase inhibitors, *eg*, theophylline; anticholinergics, *eg*, ipatropium bromide; and antihistamines. Theophylline can be used in patients who are not adequately controlled symptomatically with β-agonists, and can even be considered as an ICS-sparing agent. However, it has fallen out of favor in recent years because of its tight therapeutic ratio and side-effect profile. Blood levels must be checked yearly (5–15 µg/mL; < 12 µg/mL if pregnant), and care must be given to avoid drug interactions. It remains an attractive option for nocturnal disease, when compliance needs to be monitored very carefully and when an oral, long-acting bronchodilator is preferred.

Anticholinergics have limited use in young asthmatic patients. Ipratropium bromide (Atrovent; Boehringer Ingelheim, Ingelheim, Germany) is the anticholinergic of choice because it has poor absorption and few of the systemic side effects of atropine. It may be beneficial in asthmatic patients with excessive mucus production, *eg*, during acute asthma attacks, although this use is controversial [21]. Ipratropium bromide can prolong the effectiveness of concomitantly administered β-adrenergic agonists and may be useful in cold-, air-, irritant-, and emotionally-induced asthma. Available as both an MDI and a nebulizable solution, ipatropium bromide is not FDA-approved for use in children younger than 12 years of age, and can be used 3 to 4 times per day. Atropine is administered only by nebulization.

Currently, antihistamines are not contraindicated in asthma, because previous concerns about their mucus-drying effects have proven to be irrelevant clinically. Some data suggest that high-dose, non-sedating antihistamines offer statistically significant benefits in asthma. Furthermore, a subset of children receiving antihistamines

in the ETAC (Early Treatment of the Atopic Child) study developed fewer asthma symptoms than the placebo group, suggesting that the role of antihistamines in asthma is still being refined [22]. Certainly, their role in asthma is not as significant as in allergic rhinitis or eczema.

Age Considerations

Relevant asthma triggers and the therapeutic agents available to treat children vary with age. A general rule is to include the day care provider or school nurse in the team of asthma managers, complete with action plans and an extra set of medications.

INFANTS AND TODDLERS

There are two major types of asthmatic infants: those who wheeze only with infections and frequently improve with age (transient wheezers), and those who wheeze continuously and may experience considerable difficulty (persistent wheezers). Overlap exists between the two groups, and it is impossible to predict which infants will enter remission [3]. In the Tucson study [10•], 60% of children younger than 3 years of age who wheezed were actually transient wheezers, and their wheezing resolved by age 6. A formidable 40%, however, were persistent wheezers, characterized by the presence of atopy, bronchial hyperresponsiveness, a parent with asthma, and significant lung deterioration in lung function by age 6 [10•].

Close monitoring of the infant with asthma is a challenge, because typical wheezing may be difficult to detect. Parents should pay particular attention to cough and labored breathing, especially labored exhalation that occurs after hard play, nursing, crying, or at night, especially in association with respiratory infections. A symptom diary of the parent's observations can be an invaluable aid to the physician, because pulmonary function cannot be measured reliably in young children.

Asthma management is also particularly challenging. Environmental control measures can be applied when they are clearly defined. Limiting exposure to viral infections and triggers in general should also limit frequency and severity of attacks. The choices of pharmacotherapy frequently are tailored to the patient's cooperation and the caretaker's ability to ensure delivery. The dosage of pharmacotherapy is frequently adjusted according to symptoms, because the dosage of medications for children younger than 4 to 5 years of age is not always clear [23••].

Response to therapy in infancy is often poor. The preferred routes for medication delivery are either by mouth or by inhalation via a nebulizer with a facemask. Infant masks can also be attached to spacers, allowing use of MDIs. Controversy exists as to the efficacy of nebulized delivery versus MDI via spacer with facemask; however, neither option is ideal. Ultimately, physicians and parents choose the method most likely to produce the desired results and enlist patient cooperation [23••].

Available asthma medications for infants generally are oral β-adrenergic agonists (for mild symptoms as needed); nebulized β-adrenergic agonists that may be diluted in saline, cromolyn, or budesonide; leukotriene modifiers (for more persistent symptoms); inhaled corticosteroids and combination therapies (for severe uncontrolled cases); and oral theophylline (for additional bronchodilation) [6••,8••,13]. The advent of nebulized budesonide in the US, approved for children as young as 1 year of age, revolutionized the treatment of asthma exacerbations in infants, and has provided a real alternative to oral courses of prednisone in the very young. Nebulized budesonide can be considered first-line maintenance therapy for moderate to severe persistent wheezing in an infant or toddler.

THREE- TO SIX-YEAR-OLD CHILDREN

Many 3-year-old and most 4-year-old children can perform peak flow maneuvers, which adds a whole new dimension to the asthma management plan. Most preschoolers can easily use MDIs delivered through spacer devices. Although the nebulizer may still be used, children of this age group can generally inhale their medications quickly and efficiently with spacers equipped with mouthpieces.

In difficult cases, mast cell stabilizers, leukotriene modifiers, and ICSs alone or in combination should be used. Long-acting β-adrenergic agonists, ipratropium bromide, or oral theophylline may be added as additional bronchodilators. Ipratropium bromide may be useful if cholinergic mechanisms are involved (*eg*, emotional upset or cold weather). Prophylactic "controller" medications (leukotriene modifiers or corticosteroids) may need to be increased or instituted at the first sign of an infection in patients susceptible to exacerbations with upper respiratory tract infections [6••,8••,13].

SIX- TO TWELVE-YEAR-OLD CHILDREN

At this age, children should take increasing responsibility for their asthma. It has been demonstrated that regular use of a peak flow meter results in improved perception of airway obstruction and in more accurate early recognition of impending exacerbations. Younger children should be encouraged to guess their peak flow readings and to record the actual values. As children mature, they should be taught the names of their medications and should be encouraged to use their peak flow readings to identify their asthma triggers. Older children can also be given some responsibility (with careful supervision) for keeping their room tidy and dust-free and for taking their own medications. A flow chart on which children can record their symptoms, peak flow readings, and medications taken can help to teach self-management skills.

A frequent problem with medication use in this age group is that administration of medications at school is generally undesirable. Leukotriene modifiers or ICSs should thus be considered instead of cromolyn, because they provide superior control and do not require such frequent dosage. Inhaled β-adrenergic agonists are the bronchodilators of choice, especially if needed for exercise asthma. These agents should always be available for symptom reversal. If bronchodilators are required several times daily, then a long-acting inhaled bronchodilator, *eg*, salmeterol or formoterol, long-acting albuterol tablets (Proventil Repetabs; Schering, Kenilworth, NJ), or theophylline could be prescribed in addition to an anti-inflammatory controller medication such as an ICS. Some specialists prescribe a morning dose of long-acting bronchodilator to be given before school to protect against exercise-induced asthma during the school day [6••,8••,13].

ADOLESCENTS

During adolescence, asthma frequently becomes a battleground between parent and patient, and all too often, poor asthma control ensues. The need for continual patient education cannot be overemphasized. Adolescents must understand that they have control over their disease, and that disruption of their lifestyles and the need for additional medications can be reduced if they monitor themselves closely and follow their asthma management plans. It is preferable, if school policy permits it, to allow adolescents to self-medicate at school.

The agents of choice for reversing inflammation and hyperreactivity are ICSs, because compliance with 4 times daily dosing of cromolyn, which is less effective than ICSs, is often a problem. Leukotriene modifiers are well accepted and easy to take, but are generally less effective than ICSs and more effective than cromolyn. Short-acting inhaled β-adrenergic agonists are likewise overwhelmingly preferred for symptomatic treatment. However, long-acting β-adrenergic agonists, ipratropium bromide, and oral theophylline are also acceptable choices. Advair Diskus is currently preferred over other combinations for controller medications in moderate to severe persistent asthmatic patients. Some adolescent girls experience monthly asthma exacerbations immediately before menses. These episodes can be anticipated and should be treated with increased medications as the peak flows dictate [3].

Emotional Considerations

Parents must be encouraged to expect comparable behavior and, within reason, comparable achievements from their asthmatic and nonasthmatic children. Care must be taken to avoid sibling jealousies over attention given to the asthmatic child. An attitude of achievement and well being can replace an attitude of defeat if the patient and parents are made to realize that they can control asthma. With proper management, most asthmatic children can lead normal lives, engaging in normal activities, as long as they take their regular medications and pre-medicate appropriately [24].

Treatment of Exacerbations

Peak flow readings are useful in the treatment of exacerbations. A fall of 10% to 20% of that predicted should be treated with heightened awareness and a β-adrenergic agonist as needed. More than a 20% drop is often a harbinger of an asthma attack and should be the trigger for instituting the back-up asthma management plan. Treatment of an asthma exacerbation depends on how quickly the pulmonary functions usually fall. Most children deteriorate slowly over several days or weeks, whereas others deteriorate rapidly and require hospitalization within 24 to 48 hours.

MANAGEMENT OF CHILDREN SUBJECT TO SLOW DETERIORATION

Babies with continual symptoms or children with persistent peak flow readings 70% to 80% of that predicted for several days despite 4 times daily bronchodilator use should begin or increase their dose of ICS to reverse the airway hyperreactivity. Addition of a long-acting β-adrenergic agonist and/or leukotriene modifier may also be helpful. When readings drop to 50% to 70%, a short course of oral prednisone is probably needed. The sooner this is instituted, the less medication is required. Prednisone should not be stopped completely until after the peak flows have normalized, and ideally, until the small airways have normalized by pulmonary function testing. Children on maintenance oral prednisone may require higher doses of prednisone during an exacerbation than those not on corticosteroids. When peak flow readings fall below 50% of that predicted, the need for hospitalization is likely, and oral corticosteroids should be instituted immediately.

MANAGEMENT OF CHILDREN SUBJECT TO RAPID DETERIORATION

When children have required hospitalizations within 24 hours of an exacerbation, they should be managed very aggressively [3]. At the first sign of a trigger, ICS use should be instituted or increased, and β-adrenergic agonists should be administered as needed. Addition of a long-acting β-adrenergic agonist and/or leukotriene modifier, if the child is not already taking them, may also be helpful. If peak flow readings drop below 75% of that predicted, oral corticosteroids, nebulized β-adrenergic agonists, and other rescuers should be started immediately. Reliable parents should be permitted to start prednisone on their own at home. When children do not require frequent hospitalization or deteriorate over 24 to 48 hours, a wait and see approach regarding prednisone administration is advised. If peak flow readings fall in the late afternoon, however, oral corticosteroids should be started to avoid deterioration in the middle of the night.

EXACERBATIONS AT SCHOOL

Occasionally, asthma is worse during the week than on the weekend; this pattern can be confirmed with peak flow readings at home and school. If the offending antigen is the class pet, the solution is simple, but often, the problem is more complex and difficult to correct. Frequent administration of cromolyn (every 2 hours) while at school may be useful in these cases, although this dosage is not FDA-approved (*see* Table 12-3).

PATIENT RESOURCES

Several organizations provide plentiful patient resources and support. Allergy & Asthma Network/-Mothers of Asthmatics (Fairfax, VA; telephone 703-385-4403; www.aanma.org) publishes a monthly newsletter filled with practical information and numerous educational and practical resources. They also publish a reference list of asthma resources entitled "Team Work." Local chapters of the American Lung Association sponsor lectures by physicians and other asthma experts, and the Asthma and Allergy Foundation of America sponsors support groups. The Food Allergy & Anaphylaxis Network (Fairfax, VA; telephone 800-929-4040; www.foodallergy.org) publishes helpful information for patients with food allergies, including notices about contamination of commercial foods with possible food allergens. The American Academy of Allergy, Asthma and Immunology (www.aaaai.org) offers a variety of patient information materials on their website.

REFERENCES AND RECOMMENDED READING

Papers of particular interest, published recently, have been highlighted as:
- *Of importance*
- •• *Of major importance*

1. Adams PF, Marano MA: Number of selected reported chronic conditions, by age: U.S. 1994. Current Estimates from the National Health Interview Survey, 1994. *Vital Health Stat* 1995, 10:93–94.

2. Fowler MG, Davenport MG, Garg R: School functioning of US children with asthma. *Pediatrics* 1992, 90:939–944.

3. White MV: Asthma in Children. In *Conn's Current Therapy*. Edited by Rakel RE, Kersey R. Philadelphia; WB Saunders: 1999;764–773.

4. Surveillance for Asthma—US 1960–1995 (CDC Surveillance Summaries). *MMWR* 1998, 47(SS-1):1–26.

5. Robertson CF, Rubinfeld AR, Bowes G: Pediatric asthma deaths in Victoria: the mild are at risk. *Pediatr Pulmonol* 1992, 13:95-100.

6. •• National Heart, Lung and Blood Institute, National Asthma Education and Prevention Program: *Expert Panel Report 2: Guidelines for the Diagnosis and Management of Asthma*. Bethesda, MD: National Institutes of Health, Pub. No. 97-4051; 1997.

7. White MV: Pathophysiology of asthma. In *Current Review of Allergic Diseases*. Edited by Kaliner MA. Philadelphia: Current Medicine; 1999;61–67.

8.•• American Academy of Allergy, Asthma and Immunology: *Pediatric Asthma: Promoting Best Practices.* http://www.aaaai.org/members/resources/initiatives/pediatricasthmaguidelines/default.stm. Accessed September 5, 2002.
The first version of pediatric asthma guidelines, and a must read for those caring for children.

9. Yunginger JW, Reed CE, O'Connell EJ, *et al.*: A community-based study of the epidemiology of asthma. Incidence rates, 1964-1983. *Am Rev Respir Dis* 1992, 146:888-894.

10.• Martinez EF, Wright AL, Taussig LM, *et al.*: Asthma and wheezing in the first six years of life. The Group Health Medical Associates. *N Engl J Med* 1995, 332:133-138.
A landmark study, frequently quoted, attempting to classify subsets of wheezers and risk factors for chronic asthma.

11. Oswald H, Phelan PD, Lanigan A, *et al.*: Childhood asthma and lung function in mid-adult life. *Pediatr Pulmonol* 1997, 23:14-20.

12.• Xuan W, Marks GB, Toelle BG, *et al.*: Risk factors for the onset and remission of atopy, wheeze, and airway hyperresponsiveness. *Thorax* 2002, 57:104-109.
A population-based study following school-aged children with asthma into adulthood, offering evidence for remodeling occurring early in the life of a patient with persistent asthma.

13. Economides A, White MV: The treatment of asthma in children. *Minority Health Today* 2000, 1(4):10-19.

14.•• Bisgaard H: Delivery of inhaled medication to children. *J Asthma* 1997, 34(6):443-467.
An excellent review of delivery devices, pros and cons.

15. Economides A, Kaliner MA: Asthma: diagnosis and management. *Curr Pract Med* 1999, 2(9):1719-1729.

16. Strachan DP, Wong J, Spector TD: Concordance and inter-relationship of atopic diseases and markers of allergic sensitization among adult female twins. *J Allergy Clin Immunol* 2001, 108:901-907.

17.• Nelson HS, Szefler SJ, Jacobs J, *et al.*: *The relationships among environmental allergen sensitization, allergen exposure, pulmonary function and bronchial hyperresponsiveness in CAMP.* J Allergy Clin Immunol 1999, 104:775-785.
A good look at the relationship of asthma and allergens, from the CAMP database.

18.• Moller C, Dreborg S, Ferdousi HA, *et al.*: Pollen immunotherapy reduces the development of asthma in children with seasonal rhinoconjunctivitis (the PAT study). *J Allergy Clin Immunol* 2002, 109:251-256.
A study of the very provocative concept that immunotherapy can be used preventively.

19.•• Long-term effects of budesonide or nedocromil in children with asthma. The Childhood Asthma Management Program Research Group. *N Engl J Med* 2000, 343:1054-1063.
A much awaited study, frequently quoted, both for the reassurance that growth velocity was eventually the same for all study groups, as well as for the surprise that budesonide did not alter the remodeling that had already occurred.

20.• Agertoft L, Petersen S: Effect of long-term treatment with inhaled budesonide on adult height in children with asthma. *N Engl J Med* 2000, 343:1064-1069.
A reassuring study, frequently quoted, that children on budesonide achieve their expected adult height.

21. Goggin N, Macarthus C, Parkin PC: Randomized trial of the addition of ipratropium bromide to albuterol and corticosteroid therapy in children hospitalized because of an acute asthma exacerbation. *Arch Pediatr Adolesc Med* 2001, 155:1329-1334.

22. Allergic factors associated with the development of asthma and the influence of cetirizine in a double-blind, randomised, placebo-controlled trial: first results of ETAC. *Pediatr Allergy Immunol* 1998, 9:116-124.

23.•• Spahn JD, Szefler SJ: Childhood asthma: new insights into management. *J Allergy Clin Immunol* 2002, 109:3-13.
A very thorough recent review of the problems in the management of asthma in children.

24. Szefler SJ: Special issues in managing childhood asthma. *J Resp D* 1998, 19(3A):S35-S41.

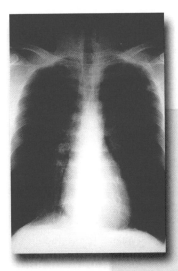

National Heart, Lung, and Blood Institute Guidelines: Classification of Asthma Severity

Homer A. Boushey and Rajeev Venkayya

Historically, the broad consensus that asthma is fundamentally a chronic inflammatory disease of the airways that is characterized by chronic lymphocytic and eosinophilic infiltration of the bronchial mucosa was not achieved until well after the development and introduction of inhaled corticosteroids as a treatment for the condition. But because corticosteroid therapy is regarded as "anti-inflammatory," the reports of inflammatory changes, even in bronchial mucosal biopsy specimens from patients with mild asthma, led to a fundamental shift in the conception of the goals of therapy. By reducing bronchial mucosal inflammation, prolonged use of an inhaled corticosteroid was thought to offer a way of altering the disease on a more fundamental level than accomplished with bronchodilators.

This change in concept was reinforced by well-designed prospective, placebo-controlled, double-blind trials. These have repeatedly shown that regular use of an inhaled corticosteroid reduces the severity and frequency of symptoms, increases measures of airway caliber such as peak expiratory flow (PEF) and the FEV_1 (forced expiratory volume in 1 second), and reduces bronchial reactivity, the frequency of exacerbations, the rate of hospitalization, and even the low but real risk of death from asthma [1–4]. Some studies even suggest that regular use of an inhaled corticosteroid might slow the accelerated rate of loss of pulmonary function associated with asthma [5]. This loss of pulmonary function may be irreversible and can be severe in some patients with asthma, although neither the proportion of patients at risk nor markers for it are now known.

Together, the clinical trials were persuasive that regular use of a "long-term controller" such as an inhaled corticosteroid improved overall asthma control and might affect long-term outcomes. But just as the clinical trials have been too short to prove a beneficial effect on long-term outcomes, they have also been too short to prove the absence of long-term risk, especially of the toxicities associated with chronic use of a corticosteroid.

It seems certain that the risk of these toxicities—especially growth retardation, osteoporosis, and cataracts—is not nil.

Although the magnitude of risk appears to be small, the outcomes feared develop only over years of treatment, so their risk can be truly quantified only by long-term studies. Of these, one 3-year trial showed a small but significant dose-dependent loss in bone density in premenopausal women [6], but a 5-year study of preadolescent children showed only a transient, probably unimportant effect on growth rate [7••]. A short-cut approach to estimating these risks has been to assess the effects of inhaled corticosteroid treatment on cortisol secretion, and several weeks of inhalation of moderate to high doses can indeed affect the levels of cortisol in blood samples obtained hourly overnight [8]. This finding presumably indicates some systemic absorption of the inhaled corticosteroid, but its relationship to corticosteroid toxicities is unknown.

The challenge for proper use of inhaled corticosteroid therapy, or of any long-term controller, is the same as for any drug: to strike the optimal balance between the *benefits* and the *risks* of therapy. To strike this balance, the National Asthma Education and Prevention Program (NAEPP) of the National Heart, Lung, and Blood Institute (NHLBI) proposed in its first set of *Guidelines for the Diagnosis and Management of Asthma* (1992) that the intensity of therapy be matched to the severity of disease, classified as "mild," "moderate," or "severe" [9]. The 1997 update of the guidelines refined this initial categorization by subdividing the mild category into two: "mild intermittent" and "mild persistent" asthma [10•].

RATIONALE FOR CLASSIFICATION BY SEVERITY

The fundamental justification for classifying any disease by severity is prediction of the risks of adverse clinical outcomes. In asthma, gauging disease severity requires assessing different "domains" of function. Assessment of symptoms alone is often misleading because some patients, especially those with long-standing asthma, appear to tolerate airflow obstruction without distress and may minimize their symptoms. These patients are sometimes described as "poor perceivers" [11–13]. Symptoms may also be misleading because many patients with asthma, similar to others with chronic illness, have a high level of denial. Correct estimation of severity during a patient visit thus requires asking direct, specific questions and obtaining an objective measure of pulmonary function.

Severity grading also facilitates the tapering of asthma therapy as the condition improves. Appropriate and timely reduction of therapy is important for the prevention of medication-associated side effects, particularly those that are associated with inhaled corticosteroid use. Although the risk:benefit ratio of inhaled corticosteroid therapy is regarded as quite favorable in asthma, this view is based on the presumption that the patient is being treated with the lowest corticosteroid dose needed to control the disease. Another benefit of appropriate tapering of medications is avoidance of "overmedication" of a patient and the associated increased treatment cost.

Severity grading is also useful for the translation of study findings to clinical practice. By reporting study results in patients grouped according to measurable criteria of disease severity, investigators increase the likelihood that their findings will be applied to the appropriate population in practice.

RATIONALE FOR SELECTING PARAMETERS

The guidelines are based on the premise that asthma severity can be assessed by clinical parameters, including symptom frequency and objective assessments of lung function. Increases in symptom frequency or reductions in FEV_1 or PEF are believed to signify a decline in asthma control and an increase in the risk of important adverse outcomes, such as hospitalizations, emergency department visits, or unscheduled urgent care visits; days lost from work or school; or even death from an asthmatic attack.

In defining the parameters used for grading severity, the National Asthma Expert Panel chose a combination of subjective (symptoms) and objective (pulmonary function) measures. An objective assessment of pulmonary function was thought to be important because both patients and physicians are inaccurate in assessing the degree of pulmonary impairment [14–19]. Moreover, objective measures of lung function ensure some degree of uniformity in classification of disease across different centers.

Symptoms

The frequency of asthma symptoms (*ie*, cough, wheezing, shortness of breath) have long been used to assess asthma severity. Symptom frequency has been shown to correlate with the risk for future morbidity from asthma [17], although "snapshot" assessments are better clues to current asthma status than to long-term disease state [20]. Assessment of asthma severity by symptoms alone, however, is often inaccurate. A significant number of patients underestimate their asthma severity when their assessment is compared with that of the NAEPP guidelines [21]. Moreover, a significant subset of patients have a blunted ability to sense airflow limitation that is demonstrated on objective measurements of pulmonary function [11–13].

Nocturnal Symptoms

Nocturnal symptoms of asthma, especially those that interrupt sleep, have been regarded as important cues of severity since the 1970s, when in-hospital mortality was noted to be greatest in patients with profound falls in PEF in the early hours of the morning (the so-called "morning dipper" pattern) [22]. Subsequent studies [23–25] have shown that asthma deaths do occur most often at night or in the early morning. The importance of nocturnal awakenings from asthma as a sign of severity was emphasized by a survey of asthma deaths in Victoria Province, Australia. Based on retrospective reviews, nearly one third of the patients who died were considered to have had previous evidence of mild disease [26]. The authors were impressed with the frequency with which these patients were recalled to have had nocturnal symptoms that awakened them from sleep. A more recent cross-sectional study [27] of asthmatic children found that nocturnal symptoms correlated with overall symptom severity, high use of reliever medications, days lost from school, poor school performance, and parent absenteeism from work. Nighttime awakenings, however, are often overlooked by patients and providers during office visits. Inquiry about nocturnal symptoms must be explicit, or the symptom may simply be unreported.

Given this information, nocturnal symptoms have a prominent place in the classification of the severity of asthma. It is important to note that incorporation of this historical information often leads to the "upgrading" of a given patient's severity classification, leading some to wonder whether the current grading of nocturnal symptoms is an overly sensitive measure of asthma control [28].

Spirometry

Spirometry, particularly using the FEV_1 unit, is regarded as the gold standard for measurement of lung function in patients with asthma. This is because of its objectivity, reproducibility, and availability [16]. Moreover, it is well documented that symptoms do not always correlate with severity of airflow limitation and that a significant number of asymptomatic persons demonstrate airflow limitation on screening spirometry [14,15,29–31].

The power of FEV_1 measurement in predicting outcomes in asthmatic patients was again first strongly suggested in a study [32] of the most severe form of the disease. Follow-up of patients who had survived an asthma attack requiring intubation and mechanical ventilation showed two patterns among those who died of a second attack: highly variable values for FEV_1 from visit to visit, and progressive worsening from visit to visit [32]. Deaths rarely occurred in those with stable, even if quite low, values. Among patients previously hospitalized for an asthma attack, the FEV_1 (expressed as a percent of the value predicted for the patient's age, height, and ethnicity) was found to predict the risk of rehospitalization [33]. Additionally, a retrospective survey [34•] of nearly 14,000 children seen annually over 15 years showed a strong correlation between the FEV_1 (expressed as percent predicted) and the risk of an attack of wheezing and shortness of breath over the subsequent 12 months. This study also showed that stratification of the degree of airflow obstruction on spirometry correlated with stratification of the risk of attacks. The odds ratio for an attack of wheezing and shortness of breath was greater than 5 among those with an FEV_1 less than 60% predicted and was 1.4 among those with an FEV_1 60% to 79% of predicted.

Because of its ease of measurement, its objectivity, and its strength in predicting clinical outcomes, spirometry features prominently in the guidelines. Spirometry is, however, measured infrequently in patients seen in primary care settings [35].

Peak Flow

Peak expiratory flow measurements are useful for monitoring the course of disease in asthma but are less reliable as isolated measurements. This results from differences in calibration between devices and unreliable reference information for a given subject's age and height. The guidelines allow for the use of PEF measurements (as "percent predicted") to classify severity, but this method is much less reliable than the FEV_1 measurement. In one study [36], the peak flow measurement placed the patient in the same severity class as the FEV_1 only 50% of the time.

The diurnal variability in PEF has been shown to correlate with bronchial reactivity; thus "percent variability" is included as another measure of the severity of disease. When calculating variability in PEF, the morning measurements should be performed within 15 minutes of awakening, before the use of bronchodilators, and again at approximately 2:00 PM after using bronchodilators [37]. It should be noted that the NHLBI guidelines recommend the measurement of the afternoon PEF *after* bronchodilator use, but the European Respiratory Guidelines recommend measurement *before* bronchodilator administration [10,38].

CLASSIFICATION SYSTEM

The NAEPP originally chose to classify asthma severity in three categories: mild, moderate, and severe, as estimated by three "domains" of function. These "domains" include the frequency and severity of symptoms and the frequency of use of an inhaled β-agonist to relieve them, nocturnal awakenings from asthma, and airflow obstruction as measured by spirometry or PEF. The decision in 1997 to divide the "mild" category into "mild intermittent" and "mild persistent" was driven by data suggesting that even mild but persistent asthma may result in accelerated loss of pulmonary function that can be prevented by early introduction of regular maintenance therapy with an inhaled corticosteroid [39,40]. Accordingly, the 1997 revision to the asthma guidelines classify severity as mild intermittent, mild persistent, moderate persistent, and severe persistent. The parameters used are described in Table 13-1. The measurement that falls in the highest severity class dictates the overall disease severity classification.

VALIDATION

Since its publication in 1997, the severity classification outlined by the NAEPP has been evaluated in several studies.

Correlation with Morbidity and Cost of Care

Several studies have demonstrated that asthma severity, as assessed by clinical criteria, correlates with emergency department visits and hospitalization [17,33,41,42]. As might be predicted by these data, the cost of asthma care also correlates with severity [43,44].

Correlation with Airway Inflammation

Airway inflammation has been shown to be increased in patients with fatal asthma compared with subjects with mild to moderate asthma [45]. Although it has not been studied in the context of the NHLBI guidelines, available data suggest that the degree of airway inflammation appears to be roughly correlated with asthma severity, as measured by symptom frequency and pulmonary function.

Intracategory Inconsistencies

Since publication of the guidelines, some investigators have fairly pointed out that the indices of severity reflect a consensus among a broadly representative panel of experts but were not derived from an evidence-based approach. They have also pointed out that symptom frequency in a given severity class often does not correlate with the corresponding measurement of pulmonary function. For instance, it has been shown that the frequency of nocturnal symptoms often places a patient in a higher severity class than that determined by daytime symptoms and pulmonary function [28,46]. Similarly, PEF measurements often do not correlate with the frequency of daytime symptoms [47]. Although a lack of correlation between measures could be viewed as a shortcoming of the guidelines, it might also be considered a strength. If one assumes that each measure carries a different sensitivity for severity of illness, this approach maximizes the likelihood that a patient will be categorized at proper level of severity. Indeed, some studies, such as those that have examined the relationship between the classification of disease severity and costs of care, have found that the composite classification correlates more closely than classification in any single domain. Finally, although classification at a higher level of severity may result in the initial implementation of more aggressive medical therapy, such a practice is unlikely to lead to harm if the therapy is tapered as the clinical indicators improve.

CONCLUSIONS

Publication of the NHLBI guidelines has prompted numerous bodies to incorporate the recommendations into their management guidelines. Several studies have validated the correlation between asthma severity and clinical outcomes, but little is known about the appropriateness of the pairing of individual measures (*ie*, daytime symptom frequency, nocturnal symptoms,

Table 13-1. CLASSIFICATION OF ASTHMA SEVERITY (CLINICAL FEATURES BEFORE TREATMENT)*†

	Symptoms	Nocturnal Symptoms	Lung Function
Step 4 Severe persistent	Continual symptoms / Limited physical activity / Frequent exacerbations	Frequent	FEV_1 or PEF ≤ 60% predicted / PEF variability > 30%
Step 3 Moderate persistent	Daily symptoms / Daily use of inhaled short-acting β_2-agonist / Exacerbations affect activity	> 1 time a week	FEV_1 or PEF > 60%–< 80% predicted / PEF variability > 30
Step 2 Mild persistent	Exacerbations ≥ 2 times a week; may last days / Symptoms > 2 times a week but < 1 time a day / Exacerbations may affect activity	> 2 times a month	FEV_1 or PEF ≥ 80% predicted / PEF variability 20%–30%
Step 1 Mild intermittent	Symptoms ≤ 2 times a week / Asymptomatic and normal PEF between exacerbations / Exacerbations brief (from a few hours to a few days); intensity may vary	≤ 2 times a month	FEV_1 or PEF ≥ 80% predicted / PEF variability < 20%

*The presence of one of the features of severity is sufficient to place a patient in that category. An individual should be assigned to the most severe grade in which any feature occurs. The characteristics noted in this table are general and may overlap because asthma is highly variable. Furthermore, an individual's classification may change over time.
†Patients at any level of severity can have mild, moderate, or severe exacerbations. Some patients with intermittent asthma experience severe and life-threatening exacerbations separated by long periods of normal lung function and no symptoms.
Adapted from [10•].
FEV_1—forced expiratory volume in 1 s; PEF—peak expiratory flow.

spirometry) within categories. Although these guidelines indisputably offer a useful means to standardize management across institutions and to characterize study populations, studies examining the relationships between different markers of asthma severity and important outcomes over time will lead to the selection of more robust, discriminating indices of severity.

The single index of severity that correlates best with the risk of adverse outcomes over time is an objective measurement of pulmonary function, particularly the FEV_1. Given the subjective nature of symptom reporting and interpretation and the existence of a subgroup of asthmatic patients who seem to have an impaired ability to perceive airflow obstruction, it seems prudent to use objective measures of pulmonary function whenever possible. Spirometry has been shown to be an extremely reliable and reproducible measure of severity in asthma, is easily performed in an office setting, and often reveals airflow obstruction to be much more severe than predicted from clinical symptomatology [14]. Whereas PEF is useful for monitoring the course of the disease, its use in categorizing severity according to "percent predicted" values and intraday variability is less clear. Therefore, the performance of spirometry at the time of diagnosis and periodically during the course of medical therapy is indicated. It is important to understand that different measures may point to different severity classification. Until further studies are performed, it is appropriate to tailor therapy to highest severity class indicated by any given parameter.

REFERENCES AND RECOMMENDED READING

Papers of particular interest, published recently, have been highlighted as:
•   Of importance
•• Of major importance

1.   Boushey HA.: Effects of inhaled corticosteroids on the consequences of asthma. *J Allergy Clin Immunol* 1998, 102(suppl):5–16.

2.   Kamada AK, Szefler SJ, Martin RJ, *et al.*: Issues in the use of inhaled glucocorticoids: the Asthma Clinical Research Network. *Am J Respir Crit Care Med* 1996, 153:1739–1748.

3.   Suissa S, Ernst P, Benayoun S, *et al.*: Low-dose inhaled corticosteroids and the prevention of death from asthma. *N Engl J Med* 2000, 343:332–336.

4.   Donahue JG, Weiss ST, Livingston JM, *et al.*: Inhaled steroids and the risk of hospitalization for asthma. *JAMA* 1997, 277:887–891.

5.   van Essen-Zandvliet EE, Hughes MD, Waalkens HJ, *et al.*: Effects of 22 months of treatment with inhaled corticosteroids and/or beta-2-agonists on lung function, airway responsiveness, and symptoms in children with asthma: the Dutch Chronic Non-specific Lung Disease Study Group. *Am Rev Respir Dis* 1992, 146:547–554.

6.   Israel E, Banerjee TR, Fitzmaurice GM, *et al.*: Effects of inhaled glucocorticoids on bone density in premenopausal women. *N Engl J Med* 2001, 345:941–947.

7.•• The Childhood Asthma Management Program Research Group: Long-term effects of budesonide or nedocromil in children with asthma. *N Engl J Med* 2000, 343:1054–1063.
The "CAMP" study compared the effects of an inhaled corticosteroid, nedocromil, and placebo over 4 to 6 years in 1041 children. The inhaled corticosteroid group had significantly better asthma control, missed fewer days of school, and needed fewer courses of treatment. The effects on growth were transient, unsustained, and unimportant. The change in postbronchodilator FEV_1 over time, however, was the same in all three groups.

8.   Martin RJ, Szefler SJ, Chinchilli VM, *et al.*: Systemic effect comparisons of six inhaled corticosteroid preparations. *Am J Respir Crit Care Med* 2002, 165:1377–1383.

9.   National Heart, Lung, and Blood Institute, National Asthma Education and Prevention Program: *Expert Panel Report: Guidelines for the Diagnosis and Management of Asthma.* Bethesda, MD: National Institutes of Health; Pub No. 91-3642; 1991.

10.• National Heart, Lung, and Blood Institute, National Asthma Education and Prevention Program: *Expert Panel Report II: Guidelines for the Diagnosis and Management of Asthma.* Bethesda, MD: National Institutes of Health; Pub No. 97-4051; 1997.
The NIH guidelines reflect a broad consensus of experts from many disciplines. Recommendations based on opinion have so far held up well in subsequent studies. These guidelines are being updated in 2002, and are the definitive guide to care.

11. Connolly MJ, Crowley JJ, Charan NB, *et al.*: Reduced subjective awareness of bronchoconstriction provoked by methacholine in elderly asthmatic and normal subjects as measured on a simple awareness scale. *Thorax* 1992, 47:410–413.

12. Kikuchi Y, Okabe S, Tamura G, *et al.*: Chemosensitivity and perception of dyspnea in patients with a history of near-fatal asthma. *N Engl J Med* 1994, 330:1329–1334.

13. Rubinfeld AR, Pain MC: Perception of asthma. *Lancet* 1976, 1:882–884.

14. Bye MR, Kerstein D, Barsh E.: The importance of spirometry in the assessment of childhood asthma. *Am J Dis Child* 1992, 146:977–978.

15. Coultas DB, Mapel D, Gagnon R, *et al.*: The health impact of undiagnosed airflow obstruction in a national sample of United States adults. *Am J Respir Crit Care Med* 2001, 164:372–377.

16. Enright PL, Lebowitz MD, Cockroft DW: Physiologic measures: pulmonary function tests. Asthma outcome. *Am J Respir Crit Care Med* 1994, 149(suppl):9–18; discussion 149(suppl)9–20.

17. Ng TP: Validity of symptom and clinical measures of asthma severity for primary outpatient assessment of adult asthma. *Br J Gen Pract* 2000, 50:7–12.

18. Shim CS, Williams MH Jr: Evaluation of the severity of asthma: patients versus physicians. *Am J Med* 1980, 68:11–13.

19. Shim CS, Williams MH Jr: Relationship of wheezing to the severity of obstruction in asthma. *Arch Intern Med* 1983, 143:890–892.

20. Osborne ML, Vollmer WM, Pedula KL, *et al.*: Lack of correlation of symptoms with specialist-assessed long-term asthma severity. *Chest* 1999, 115:85–91.

21. Nguyen BP, Wilson SR, German DF: Patients' perceptions compared with objective ratings of asthma severity. *Ann Allergy Asthma Immunol* 1996, 77:209–215.

22. Cochrane GM, Clark JH: A survey of asthma mortality in patients between ages 35 and 64 in the Greater London hospitals in 1971. *Thorax* 1975, 30:300–305.

23. Kinnula V, Nurmela T, Liippo K, *et al.*: Fatal asthma in two regions of Finland. *Ann Clin Res* 1988, 20:189–194.

24. Carswell F.: Thirty deaths from asthma. *Arch Dis Child* 1985, 60:25–28.

25. Campbell S, Hood I, Ryan D *et al.*: Death as a result of asthma in Wayne County Medical Examiner cases, 1975–1987. *J Forensic Sci* 1990, 35:356–64.

26. Robertson CF, Rubinfeld AR, Bowes G: Pediatric asthma deaths in Victoria: the mild are at risk. *Pediatr Pulmonol* 1992, 13:95–100.

27. Diette GB, Markson L, Skinner EA *et al.*: Nocturnal asthma in children affects school attendance, school performance, and parents' work attendance. *Arch Pediatr Adolesc Med* 2000, 154:923–928.

28. Colice GL, Burgt JV, Song J, *et al.*: Categorizing asthma severity. *Am J Respir Crit Care Med* 1999, 160:1962–1987.

29. Kendrick AH, Higgs CM, Whitfield MJ, *et al.*: Accuracy of perception of severity of asthma: patients treated in general practice. *Br Med J* 1993, 307:422–424.

30. Teeter JG, Bleecker ER: Relationship between airway obstruction and respiratory symptoms in adult asthmatics. *Chest* 1998, 113:272–277.

31. Russell NJ, Crichton NJ, Emerson PA, *et al.*: Quantitative assessment of the value of spirometry. *Thorax* 1986, 41:360–363.

32. Westerman DE, Benatar SR, Potgieter PD, *et al.*: Identification of the high-risk asthmatic patient: experience with 39 patients undergoing ventilation for status asthmaticus. *Am J Med* 1979, 66:565–572.

33. Li D, German D, Lulla S, *et al.*: Prospective study of hospitalization for asthma: a preliminary risk factor model. *Am J Respir Crit Care Med* 1995, 151:647–655.

34.• Fuhlbrigge AL, Kitch BT, Paltiel AD, *et al.*: FEV(1) is associated with risk of asthma attacks in a pediatric population. *J Allergy Clin Immunol* 2001, 107:61–67.
This large, retrospective cohort study of nearly 14,000 children seen annually over 15 years showed clear correlation between a reduced value of FEV$_1$ and an increased risk of an attack of wheezing and shortness of breath over the next 12 months.

35. Fried RA, Miller RS, Green LA, *et al.*: The use of objective measures of asthma severity in primary care: a report from ASPN. *J Fam Pract* 1995, 41:139–143.

36. Sawyer G, Miles J, Lewis S, *et al.*: Classification of asthma severity: should the international guidelines be changed? *Clin Exp Allergy* 1998, 28:1565–1570.

37. Quackenboss JJ, Lebowitz MD, Krzyzanowski M: The normal range of diurnal changes in peak expiratory flow rates: relationship to symptoms and respiratory disease. *Am Rev Respir Dis* 1991, 143:323–330.

38. Quanjer PH, Lebowitz MD, Gregg I, *et al.*: Peak expiratory flow: conclusions and recommendations of a Working Party of the European Respiratory Society. *Eur Respir J* 1997, 249(suppl):2–8.

39. Haahtela T, Jarvinen M, Kava T, *et al.*: Comparison of a beta 2-agonist, terbutaline, with an inhaled corticosteroid, budesonide, in newly detected asthma. *N Engl J Med* 1991, 325:388–392.

40. Haahtela T, Jarvinen M, Kava T, *et al.*: Effects of reducing or discontinuing inhaled budesonide in patients with mild asthma. *N Engl J Med* 1994, 331:700–705.

41. Liard R, Leynaert B, Zureik M, *et al.*: Using Global Initiative for Asthma guidelines to assess asthma severity in populations. *Eur Respir J* 2000, 16:615–620.

42. Diette GB, Krishnan JA, Dominici F *et al.*: Asthma in older patients: factors associated with hospitalization. *Arch Intern Med* 2002, 162:1123–1132.

43. Godard P, Chanez P, Siraudin L, *et al.*: Costs of asthma are correlated with severity: a 1-yr prospective study. *Eur Respir J* 2002, 19:61–67.

44. Serra-Batlles J, Plaza V, Morejon E, *et al.*: Costs of asthma according to the degree of severity. *Eur Respir J* 1998, 12:1322–1326.

45. Synek M, Beasley R, Frew AJ, *et al.*: Cellular infiltration of the airways in asthma of varying severity. *Am J Respir Crit Care Med* 1996, 154:224–230.

46. Fix A, Sexton M, Langenberg P, *et al.*: The association of nocturnal asthma with asthma severity. *J Asthma* 1997, 34:329–336.

47. Atherton HA, White PT, Hewett G, *et al.*: Relationship of daytime asthma symptom frequency to morning peak expiratory flow. *Eur Respir J* 1996, 9:232–236.

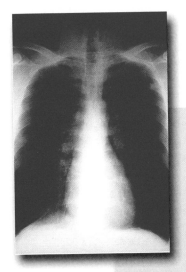

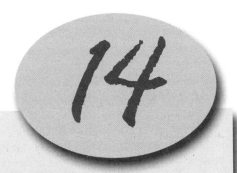

National Heart, Lung, and Blood Institute Guidelines: Treatment of Asthma

Jill Ohar and Eugene R. Bleecker

The goal of treatment of any disease is control. Elements of control include symptoms, pulmonary function, frequency of exacerbations, and disease progression. Asthma symptoms include chest tightness, wheezing, cough, dyspnea on exertion or at rest, nocturnal awakenings due to wheezing, cough, or shortness of breath, and limitation of activities of daily living. Elements of asthma that are associated with frequency of exacerbations are bronchial hyperresponsiveness, excessive peak flow variability, number of asthma-related hospitalizations, emergency room, or unscheduled physician visits, need for rescue short-acting β_2-agonists, and, while relatively rare, asthma-related mortality or intensive care unit admission with intubation. Progression of asthma refers to loss of FEV_1 (forced expiratory volume in 1 second) or anatomic remodeling of the airways in response to chronic or uncontrolled inflammation.

ASSESSMENT OF CONTROL

Symptoms

Symptoms and clinical signs of asthma should be assessed at each health care visit by an appropriate medical history that evaluates asthma control, by physical examination, and, when available, by an assessment of pulmonary function by spirometry (preferred) or peak flow assessment [1]. Patients should be taught to recognize the symptom patterns that characterize loss of asthma control and predict exacerbations. In addition to the symptoms noted above, the Baylor Health Care System's "Rules of Two" provide a simple way to assess control (www.bhcs.com/rules of two). Violation of one of these three rules is an indication of escape of asthma control: an increase in short-acting β_2-agonist use (using these drugs more than twice a week to control acute symptoms); more than two nocturnal awakenings per month; or use of more than two albuterol canisters each year.

Peak Flow

The National Asthma Education and Prevention Program (NAEPP) of the National Heart, Lung, and Blood Institute (NHLBI), in its first set of guidelines, recommended periodic monitoring of lung function by spirometry at the onset of an acute exacerbation and after treatment has stabilized symptoms. Additional spirometric evaluations may be performed on an "as needed" basis as clinical conditions dictate and at least once every 1 to 2 years thereafter. Lung function may also be monitored by peak expiratory flow (PEF). In contrast to spirometry, PEF meters are inexpensive, portable, and ideal for home use. They are designed as tools for monitoring, not diagnosis, because they are more dependent upon patient effort and technique. Furthermore, PEF only measures the initial peak of the forced expiration and is therefore less accurate than spirometry. For reliable PEF meter use, patient instruction with frequent review of technique is mandatory. The NHLBI guidelines advocate long-term daily PEF monitoring to evaluate the efficacy of therapy and to detect early changes in disease status that may require urgent intervention in moderate and severe persistent asthma. In contrast to the NHLBI guidelines, the recently published Agency for Healthcare Research and Quality (AHRQ) Evidenced-based Practice Program: Management of Chronic Asthma report found that the evidence available to date is insufficient to advocate the use of a written asthma management program based on PEF or symptoms compared to medical management alone [2]. Many patients are unable to sense large changes in lung function that may place them at risk for worsening asthma and exacerbations [3]. PEF monitoring may be particularly important in these individuals. Short-term PEF monitoring may be used to assess response to a medical intervention, identify pulmonary function changes induced by environmental exposures, or establish a patient's personal baseline or "best" PEF. Specific monitoring techniques are described in the NHLBI Guidelines for the Diagnosis and Management of Asthma [1].

Patient Perception of Control

One of the pitfalls in the assessment of asthma control is patient perception. Just as there is a subset of asthma patients that fails to sense changes in lung function, some asthma patients believe that their disease is far better controlled than it really is. A recent random digit dialing telephone survey contacted 42,022 households. Among them were 2,509 adult asthmatic patients or parents of asthmatic patients [4]. These respondents were queried as to their level of asthma control based on criteria set forth by the asthma guidelines. The results of this survey revealed a number of important findings about asthma management in the United States. According to the NHLBI guidelines, patients with well-controlled asthma do not require urgent interventional medical care, do not miss school or work because of asthma symptoms, do not awaken at night with asthma symptoms, and do not experience disruption of activities of daily living because of asthma symptoms. The Asthma in America survey found that 9% of respondents had been hospitalized, 23% had at least one emergency room visit, and 29% had an unscheduled outpatient visit for urgent care during the previous year. In the preceding

year, at least one school day was missed by 49% of children, and 25% of adults missed work because of asthma symptoms. Sleep disruption due to asthma was experienced by 30% of respondents at least once a week. Sports and recreational activities were limited in 48% of respondents, and 36% said asthma limited their normal physical activity. Only 22% of asthmatic patients whose symptoms were consistent with severe persistent asthma classified themselves as severe. Furthermore, only 41% of respondents whose symptoms were considered moderate persistent asthma classified themselves as moderate. Clearly, many patients with asthma underestimate the severity of their disease and the effects of asthma on their daily activities and quality of life.

Treatment of Chronic Asthma

Management of asthma is based upon understanding its pathogenesis (Fig. 14-1). Asthma is caused in susceptible individuals by interactions between environmental exposures and genetic factors that cause bronchial inflammation, airway obstruction, and asthma symptoms. Environmental factors important in the initiation and progression of asthma require nonpharmacologic therapy. These include patient education, environmental control, and immunotherapy. Airway inflammation and bronchial hyperresponsiveness that result from the interaction of genetic and environmental factors require long-term anti-inflammatory controller medications. Thus, medications such as inhaled corticosteroids reduce markers of inflammation, whereas acute airway smooth muscle contraction (bronchospasm) requires use of quick relief medication (short-acting β_2-agonists).

The goals of asthma therapy are the prevention of symptoms, maintenance of normal or near-normal lung function, maintenance of normal activity levels, prevention of exacerbations while limiting adverse effects from therapy, and meeting the expectations of patients and their families. This should be achieved in a stepwise approach based on the severity of the patient's disease (Fig. 14-2).

Long-term Controller Therapy in Asthma

Mild intermittent asthma should be treated with short-acting β_2-agonists as needed. Caution should be used in determining the appropriate level of severity of asthma, because patients at all degrees of asthma severity tend to underreport their symptoms. If "as needed" short-acting β_2-agonists are required more frequently than twice a week, the patient should be reclassified as having mild persistent asthma. This level of severity requires treatment with long-term controller therapy. Anti-inflammatory controller therapy with inhaled corticosteroids is the preferred pharmacologic intervention for persistent asthma (mild, moderate, and severe). Other controller medications include leukotriene modifiers, cromolyn or nedocromil, and long-acting bronchodilators [5]. Inhaled corticosteroids are regarded as the most effective long-term controller medications because they reduce asthma symptoms, improve pulmonary function, reduce bronchial responsiveness, decrease the frequency of exacerbations, and appear to reverse airway remodeling [6–18]. These clinical effects are attributable to their broad action on the inflammatory process in the airways that includes a reduction of inflammatory cells (especially eosinophils), decreased production of inflammatory mediators (especially cytokines), and a possible reversal of airway remodeling [6,7,9,11,17–20]. With regular use of inhaled corticosteroids, studies have shown a reduction in symptoms scores, the need for quick-relief medication, the frequency of exacerbations, and asthma-related emergency room visits and hospitalizations [7,8,12,14–16]. The use of inhaled corticosteroids is safe and effective in children [21]. The available evidence sug-

gests that the use of inhaled corticosteroids at recommended doses does not have significant or irreversible effects on vertical growth, bone mineral density, ocular toxicity, and the adrenal/pituitary axis in children [21].

Preliminary reports suggest that inhaled corticosteroids may prevent inflammation-induced airway remodeling [6,9,14,22]. However, the AHRQ report states that evidence is currently insufficient to support the assumption that patients with mild to moderate asthma have a progressive decline in lung function that can be prevented by early initiation of inhaled corticosteroids [2]. It cites the Childhood Asthma Management Study (CAMP) as the primary evidence for that conclusion. In the CAMP study, children with mild to moderate asthma managed without inhaled corticosteroids did not experience a significant decline in lung function over the 4-year

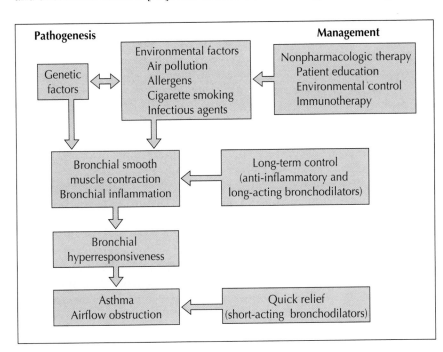

Figure 14-1.
Pathogenesis and management of asthma.

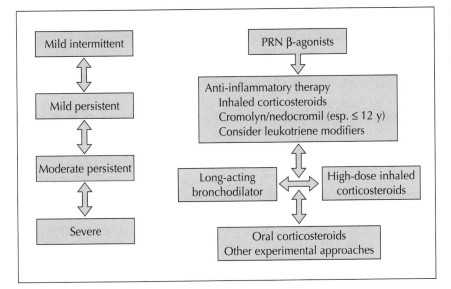

Figure 14-2.
Progression of pharmacologic therapy in asthma. PRN—as needed.

period of follow-up, and asthma patients who stopped using inhaled corticosteroids returned to predose PFT values [23]. However, the study did not assess the long-term effects over decades or the effects of delayed intervention in adult asthma. In accordance with the concept that inhaled corticosteroids may prevent airway remodeling, retrospective cohort studies suggest that delayed use of inhaled corticosteroids may be associated with progressive loss of lung function measured by FEV_1 and PEF, and earlier intervention with inhaled corticosteroids may improve long-term outcomes [8,9,22,24].

Other long-term anti-inflammatory medications are less efficacious than inhaled corticosteroids [25–27]. In general, the leukotriene modifiers, zafirlukast and montelukast, cause an increase in FEV_1 from baseline that is about half the magnitude of change produced by inhaled corticosteroids when compared in direct clinical trials [28,29].

The AHRQ report concluded that no alternate controller medication appears to be superior to inhaled corticosteroids [21]. The CAMP trial found no difference in pulmonary function or asthma symptoms in children treated with nedocromil compared with placebo. However, nedocromil did reduce the frequency of exacerbations compared with placebo [23]. The AHQR report concluded that the evidence was inadequate to determine relative efficacy of inhaled corticosteroids compared with the long-acting bronchodilators with salmeterol, formoterol, or theophylline [2].

Clinical Rationale for Combination Controller Therapy in Asthma

Long-acting β_2-agonists (LABAs) (salmeterol and formoterol) are drugs with a duration of action lasting 12 hours or more, more than twice as long as that obtained with short-acting β_2-agonists. While formoterol has a more rapid onset of action than salmeterol, these agents in general should not be used as rescue therapy to treat acute symptoms. They are most beneficial when added to inhaled corticosteroids. LABAs improve lung function, alleviate symptoms, and reduce the use of rescue treatment when added to inhaled corticosteroids in the treatment of asthma. The AHRQ found that there is a large body of evidence that shows a complimentary effect when inhaled corticosteroids are used in combination with LABAs [21]. Furthermore, the dose of inhaled corticosteroid may be reduced when added to LABAs without losing asthma control. Studies have shown that dual therapy with a low-dose inhaled corticosteroid plus an LABA is more effective than increasing the dose of inhaled corticosteroids. In the first of these studies, Greening *et al.* [30] demonstrated that the combination of low-dose beclomethasone and salmeterol was superior to high-dose beclomethasone in the control of asthma. These results were subsequently confirmed by Woolcock *et al.* [31], who demonstrated that a twofold increase in beclomethasone was inferior to the combination of low-dose beclomethasone in combination with

salmeterol. Condemi *et al.* [32], in a study of 437 patients, showed that low-dose fluticasone (88 µg bid) plus salmeterol was more effective than fluticasone 220 µg twice a day in a 3-month trial. The combination produced a significant improvement in symptom-free days, days without rescue short-acting β_2-agonists, as well as a large increase in morning peak flow (20 L compared with 50 L). Baraniuk *et al.* [33] studied three therapies: fluticasone alone, fluticasone concurrently with salmeterol, or triamcinolone alone in 680 patients in a 12-week trial. The combination of fluticasone 88 µg plus salmeterol was superior to the higher doses of inhaled corticosteroid, with regard to symptom-free days and rescue short-acting β_2-agonist use. Improvement in the FEV_1 with fluticasone plus salmeterol was 600 mL versus 425 mL with higher doses of fluticasone alone and 300 mL with triamcinolone alone. Ind *et al.* [34] showed that salmeterol 50 µg plus fluticasone 250 µg twice a day was superior to fluticasone 250 µg twice a day, as well as fluticasone 500 µg twice a day, with regard to symptom-free days, symptom-free nights, and changes in morning peak flow rate. Similar results were reported by Murray *et al.* [35], van Noord *et al.* [36], and Pearlman *et al.* [37], all favoring the combination of salmeterol plus low-dose inhaled corticosteroids to doubling the dose of inhaled corticosteroids. The European FACET (Formoterol and Corticosteroids Establishing Therapy) study [38] of formoterol plus budesonide showed similar effects. The combination of formoterol with budesonide 200 µg twice a day plus formoterol was associated with similar numbers of severe exacerbations with therapy as for budesonide 800 µg twice a day. Thus, similar effects on asthma control were found with therapeutic combinations that consisted of a lower dose of inhaled corticosteroid and an LABA.

The observed benefits of combination therapy with inhaled corticosteroids in combination with LABAs appear to represent a class effect combining these two controller medications rather than the effect of specific corticosteroids or LABAs. These studies clearly reassure prescribers that combinations of LABAs plus low-dose inhaled corticosteroids are appropriate for Step 3 management of persistent asthma.

Molecular and Cellular Mechanisms for Combination Therapy

Molecular and cellular mechanisms for the complimentary action of LABAs added to inhaled corticosteroids include the following: corticosteroids increase β_2-receptor synthesis, and LABAs may prime the glucocorticoid receptors for activation. Baraniuk *et al.* [39] has reported that corticosteroids increase the number of nasal mucosal β_2-receptors. Eickelberg [40] showed that in the presence of a glucocorticosteroid, the glucocorticoid receptor is translocated from the cytosol into the nucleus of the cell, a step that is necessary for steroid-mediated anti-inflammatory effects. When salmeterol is added, there is more complete translocation of the cytosolic glucocorticoid receptor to the nucleus promoting anti-inflammatory activity. This finding may explain in part the observations from clinical trials that in the presence of LABAs, a lower dose of inhaled corticosteroids may be used to maintain asthma control. In addition, there are other in vitro effects of corticosteroids that appear to have clinical relevance, *eg*, enhanced eosinophil apoptosis. Salmeterol increases the effect of fluticasone on eosinophil apoptosis [41]. Combinations of salmeterol and dexamethasone more effectively inhibit the release of granulocyte-macrophage colony-stimulating factor, interleukin (IL)-2, tumor necrosis factor (TNF), and IL-16 after monocyte activation [42]. The same authors found there was an additive effect of salmeterol and dexamethasone inhibiting T-cell proliferation. Pang and Knox [43] showed that airway smooth muscle cells release eotaxins when stimulated by TNF-α. Eotaxin release by stimulated smooth muscle cells is inhibited by corticosteroids; this effect is further inhibited by combinations of LABAs and corticosteroids. These authors also demonstrated that dexamethasone and salmeterol inhibit TNF-α–stimulated IL-8 release by human airway smooth muscle cells.

The combination of an inhaled corticosteroid and LABAs is available in a single delivery device. In the United States, a combination of fluticasone and salmeterol (Advair; GlaxoSmithKline, Research Triangle Park, NC) has been shown to be as effective as its component agents [44–46]. Symbicort (AstraZeneca, Auckland, NZ), a combination of budesonide and formoterol, is in use in Europe and other countries but is not approved for use in the United States [31,47].

Leukotriene Modifier and Antihistamine Combinations for Asthma Therapy

Other combinations of controller drugs have been shown to provide greater efficacy than either component alone, but these combinations demonstrate inferior efficacy to an LABA–inhaled corticosteroid combination. Corticosteroids do not inhibit in vivo leukotriene synthesis in asthmatic patients, and the combination of an inhaled corticosteroid coupled with a leukotriene modifier therefore is of potential benefit. Studies examining the effect of combining leukotriene-modifying drugs with inhaled corticosteroids have revealed an additive clinical effect. When zileuton is added to existing corticosteroid therapy and compared with the addition of placebo, the improvement in FEV_1 from baseline was 12.7% compared with 6.8% [48]. In another study, FEV_1 improved 9% from baseline in response to zafirlukast added to inhaled corticosteroids compared with 4% for placebo added to inhaled corticosteroids [49]. When pranlukast was given to patients treated with high-dose beclomethasone and the dose of beclomethasone was reduced by half, FEV_1 was unchanged. Patients treated with beclomethasone and placebo experienced a 330 ± 200

mL decline in FEV_1 with reduction of high-dose beclomethasone [50].

Other studies have evaluated efficacy of leukotriene modifiers in combination with corticosteroids compared with the LABA-inhaled corticosteroids combination. Busse *et al.* [27] evaluated the efficacy of zafirlukast compared with salmeterol in patients with moderate to severe asthma concurrently treated with inhaled corticosteroids. Peak flow increased over baseline by 15% in the zafirlukast-treated group and 30% in the salmeterol-treated group. A limitation of this trial was that only 80% to 83% of the enrolled subjects were concurrently treated with inhaled corticosteroids. Fish *et al.* [26] studied the addition of salmeterol to montelukast in patients currently receiving inhaled corticosteroids. This study showed greater improvement with the LABA for the following parameters: symptom-free days, puffs per day of the short-acting β_2-agonist, and change from baseline peak flow. Similarly, Laviolette *et al.* [51] studied montelukast as add-on therapy and as a substitute for inhaled corticosteroids. When patients were weaned off beclomethasone, there was a slight decline in the FEV_1 ($\approx$ 4%). When montelukast was added to beclomethasone, there was an increase in FEV_1 of about 7%. Dempsey *et al.* [52] evaluated the relative efficacies of montelukast combined with salmeterol compared with salmeterol alone in a placebo-controlled, cross-over study. Treatment groups included 12 patients treated with montelukast 10 mg daily, salmeterol 50 µg twice a day, montelukast 10 mg plus salmeterol 50 µg twice a day, and montelukast 10 mg plus salmeterol 100 µg twice a day. FEV_1 and FEF_{25-75} (forced expiratory flow at 25%–75% of forced vital capacity) were greater in patients treated with both combination therapies compared with placebo and montelukast [52]. To confirm these preliminary results, a large-scale trial involving 125 centers in Europe, Latin America, Africa, Asia, and the Mideast is currently in progress to evaluate the relative efficacies of salmeterol plus fluticasone versus montelukast plus fluticasone. Therefore, the combination of a leukotriene-receptor antagonist plus a low dose of inhaled corticosteroids is also effective, but does not improve FEV_1 or reduce asthma symptoms as much as the combination of salmeterol and inhaled corticosteroids. Additional comparisons of different LABAs as asthma therapies are underway [53]. Studies evaluating the effects of combinations of inhaled corticosteroids, LABAs, and a leukotriene modifier in patients with more severe asthma will be important.

Leukotrienes and histamine are both released from mast cells in response to allergen challenge. This combination would have the theoretical benefit of inhibition of both the early and late phase of allergen-induced airway obstruction. Furthermore, the combination of an antihistamine and a leukotriene modifier could potentially ameliorate symptoms of seasonal allergic rhinitis, a known trigger of asthma. The combination of antihistamines and leukotriene-modifying agents have been shown to block allergen-induced bronchospasm in animal models and in vitro [54]. Three clinical trials have evaluated the efficacy of these combinations. Roquet *et al.* [55] demonstrated a 75% reduction of early airway obstruction in response to antigen challenge with zafirlukast in combination with loratadine. Zafirlukast effected a 62% reduction and loratadine a 25% reduction in early airway obstruction. The inhibition of allergen-induced obstruction by the combination of zafirlukast and loratadine quantified by area under the FEV_1 curve was deemed therapeutically synergistic by the authors. In a preliminary report, Reicin *et al.* [56] demonstrated superiority of montelukast in combination with loratadine compared with loratadine alone when FEV_1 was used as a study endpoint. Combination therapy in asthmatic patients resulted in a 14% improvement in FEV_1, whereas montelukast alone effected a 10% improvement in FEV_1. In patients with seasonal allergic rhinitis, the combination of montelukast and loratadine resulted in a significant reduction in nasal symptom score compared with therapy with montelukast, loratadine, and placebo [57].

Stepwise Management of Asthma

In general, a stepwise approach is advocated by the NHLBI guidelines (Table 14-1). This approach implies increasing the level of therapy initially or during exacerbations to gain control and potentially reducing therapy in a stepwise fashion when control is achieved. Step 1 (mild intermittent asthma) does not require daily maintenance medication. Short-acting β_2-agonists as needed are adequate for this group. Preferred therapy for Step 2 (mild persistent asthma) is low-dose inhaled corticosteroids. The updated NHLBI guidelines recommend combined therapy (low- to medium-dose inhaled corticosteroids with LABAs) for Step 3 (moderate persistent) asthma [21]. High-dose inhaled corticosteroids in combination with LABAs is recommended for Step 4 (severe persistent asthma).

ESCAPE FROM CONTROL

As discussed, escape from control is defined by numerous criteria. These include nocturnal symptoms, the need for urgent care visits, increased need for rescue short-acting β_2-agonists, a reduction in PEF of 20% or more from personal best, or a reduction in quality of life such as missed school or work, reduction in usual home, school, and work, recreational, or social activities. When optimal control is not achieved or sustained, patient adherence to medications and the delivery device technique should be assessed. Review of pharmacy records from large national practice plans reveals that patients refill on

---

Table 14-1. STEPWISE MANAGEMENT OF ASTHMA*

	Symptoms	Lung Function	Medication
Step 4 Severe persistent	Continual daytime symptoms	FEV_1 or PEF ≥ 60% predicted	LABA in combination with high-dose ICS
	Frequent nocturnal symptoms	PEF variability > 30%	Consider addition of LTM
			Systemic corticosteroids as needed (taper to lowest dose)
Step 3 Moderate persistent	Daily/nocturnal symptoms > 1 time a week	FEV_1 or PEF > 60%– < 80% predicted	LABA in combination with low- to moderate-dose ICS
		PEF variability > 30	
Step 2 Mild persistent	Daytime symptoms > 2 times a week but < 1 time a day	FEV_1 or PEF ≥ 80% predicted	Low-dose ICS
	Nocturnal symptoms > 2 times a month	PEF variability 20%–30%	
Step 1 Mild intermittent	Daytime symptoms < 2 times a week	FEV_1 or PEF ≥ 80% predicted	PRN SABA
	Nocturnal symptoms < 2 times a month	PEF variability < 20%	

For children less than 5 years of age who are unable to a metered-dose inhaler (MDI), corticosteroid syrup (2 mg/kg/d) may be substituted for the long-acting β_2-agonist (LABA)/inhaled corticosteroid (ICS) combination in Steps 3 and 4. Repeated attempts should be made to reduce systemic corticosteroids to the lowest possible dose. Use of an MDI holding chamber with a facemask or nebulized corticosteroid may avoid the need for systemic corticosteroids in young children.
‡Adapted from *National Heart, Lung, and Blood Institute* [1].
FEV_1—forced expiratory volume in 1 second; LABA—long-acting β_2-agonist; LTM—leukotriene modifier; PEF—peak expiratory flow; PRN—as needed; SABA—short-acting β_2-agonist.

average 3 canisters of inhaled corticosteroids annually. Noncompliance with prescribed inhaled corticosteroids has been linked not only to an increase in hospitalization rate but also to asthma-related deaths [15,16]. In population studies, compliance with inhaled corticosteroids as little as 50% of the time is associated with a dramatic drop in death rate from asthma [16]. In a study assessing the efficacy of combined therapy of salmeterol and inhaled corticosteroids, 49% of patients with mild to moderate persistent asthma whose inhaled corticosteroids were withdrawn experienced a loss of asthma control [44]. In a similarly designed trial, 62% of patients with moderate persistent asthma experienced a loss of asthma control after inhaled corticosteroid withdrawal [46]. Once patient compliance is assured during periods of poor asthma control, a temporary increase in the dose of inhaled corticosteroid therapy should be considered to reestablish control. Control of asthma "triggers" should also be addressed and, whenever possible, reduced. These include upper respiratory infections, changes in environment, sinusitis, nasal polyps, gastroesophageal reflux, postnasal drip, and exposure to allergens and irritants. Medications, such as NSAIDs and β-blockers, can also be responsible for worsening asthma. If environmental triggers are persistent, they may precipitate an asthma exacerbation. A common pitfall in the management of asthma exacerbations is to treat the inflammation with systemic corticosteroids and reduce bronchospasm with bronchodilators but not control the environmental triggers, leading to a pattern of recurrent hospital or emergency room admissions and prolonged systemic steroid therapy. Finally, a step up to the next level of therapy may be required to reestablish control.

When to Consult a Specialist

Consultation with an asthma specialist is recommended for asthma patients requiring Step 3 and Step 4 care. Consultation with an asthma specialist should be considered in infants and young children requiring Step 2 care [1]. Other indications for referral to an asthma specialist are life-threatening asthma, atypical signs and symptoms of asthma, immunotherapy, the need for occupational exposure assessment, long-term therapy with systemic steroids, or the inability to achieve control with standard therapy. Risk factors for life-threatening asthma are listed in Table 14-2. These factors are the common characteristics of patients with severe asthma; however, a recent study showed that patients with mild to moderate asthma were as likely to die from an asthma exacerbation as patients with severe asthma [58]. A small fraction of asthma patients with persistent symptoms despite the use of high doses of inhaled or oral corticosteroids who frequently require high use of health care resources are described as having severe asthma [59]. Severe asthma represents a heterogeneous subset of asthma patients who share a risk for adverse outcomes but who can be characterized by several different clinical patterns of disease

expression. In some patients, frequent and severe symptoms occur despite aggressive therapy with anti-inflammatory as well as other control medications. The number of emergency room visits or hospitalizations has been used to assess asthma severity and define disability. However, this may in part reflect limited access or adherence to appropriate asthma care. Other patients with asthma may have fixed and progressive reductions in pulmonary function that do not reverse completely either after intense acute or long-term therapy. These abnormalities in lung function may reflect structural changes in the airways that have been classified as airway remodeling. A very small group of patients without many of the clinical features found in severe asthma have infrequent but life-threatening acute exacerbations, perhaps related to heightened bronchial hyperresponsiveness.

The varied clinical patterns found in severe asthma may reflect genetic differences that regulate bronchial inflammation and its interplay with environmental stimuli, resulting in the characteristic pathophysiologic abnormalities as well as the propensity to airway remodeling. In addition, pharmacogenetic responses may alter expected therapeutic responses and influence asthma severity. It is important to define and characterize patients with severe asthma. Specific disease patterns may emerge during a comprehensive evaluation that will facilitate management of these difficult patients.

THERAPY OF EXACERBATIONS

Clearly, a continuum exists between "escape from control" and asthma exacerbation. This is why it is important to teach patients how to monitor symptoms

Table 14-2. RISK FACTORS FOR LIFE-THREATENING ASTHMA

History of past sudden severe exacerbations

Exacerbations requiring intensive care unit admission

Two or more hospitalizations in the preceding year

Three or more emergency room visits in the preceding year

Emergency care or hospitalization within the past month

Use of two or more rescue short-acting β₂-agonist canisters in the preceding month

Current or recent need for systemic steroids

Inability to perceive fluctuations in peak expiratory flow

Comorbid conditions

Psychiatric or psychosocial problems

Low socioeconomic status

Urban residence

and recognize early signs of deterioration. Signs and symptoms of an acute exacerbation include cough, breathlessness, chest tightness, wheeze, and a declining PEF. While a fall below 80% of a patient's personal best is consistent with escape from control, a PEF 50% or less than one's personal best is consistent with a severe exacerbation. PEF between 50% and 80% of personal best represents a yellow or caution zone, where very close

communication between the patient and health care provider should take place. Knowledge of the patient's past history should aid in determining the level of pharmacologic intervention. Monitoring with a peak flow meter is an important method for assessing asthma severity and dictating specific therapy. Some exacerbations can be managed at home. Initial therapy should be up to three treatments of 2 to 4 puffs by metered-dose

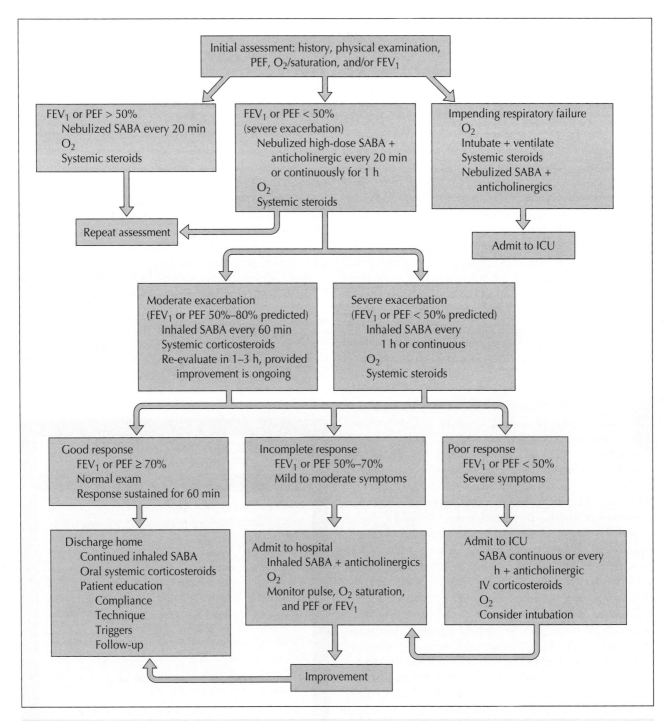

Figure 14-3.

Emergency room management of asthma exacerbation. FEV_1—forced expiratory volume in 1 second;

ICU—intensive care unit; PEF—peak expiratory flow; SABA—short-acting β_2-agonist.

inhaler of a short-acting β_2-agonist at no less than 20-minute intervals [1]. Objective responses to medical therapy will dictate further treatment options, including treatment with oral corticosteroids or transport to the health care provider's office or emergency room (Fig. 14-3). The NHLBI guidelines classify severity of exacerbations by symptoms and functional assessment (Table 14-3). Treatment goals for exacerbations of

Table 14-3. CLASSIFYING SEVERITY OF ASTHMA EXACERBATIONS

Symptoms	Mild	Moderate	Severe	Respiratory Arrest Imminent
Breathlessness	While walking	While talking (infant: softer, shorter cry, difficulty feeding)	While at rest (infant: stops feeding)	
	Can lie down	Prefers sitting	Sits upright	
Talks in	Sentences	Phrases	Words	
Alertness	May be agitated	Usually agitated	Usually agitated	Drowsy or confused
Signs				
Respiratory rate	Increased	Increased	Often > 30/min	

Guide to rates of breathing in awake children

Age	Normal rate
< 2 mo	< 60/min
2–12 mo	< 50/min
1–5 y	< 40/min
6–8 y	

Symptoms	Mild	Moderate	Severe	Respiratory Arrest Imminent
Use of accessory muscles; supra-sternal retractions	Usually not	Commonly	Usually	Paradoxical thoraco-abdominal movement
Wheeze	Moderate, often only end expiratory	Loud; throughout exhalation	Usually loud; inhalation and exhalation	Absence of wheeze
Pulse/minute	< 100	100–120	> 120	Bradycardia

Guide to normal pulse rates in children

Age	Normal rate
2–12 mo	< 160/min
1–2 y	< 120/min
2–8 y	< 110/min

Symptoms	Mild	Moderate	Severe	Respiratory Arrest Imminent
Pulsus paradoxus	About < 10 mm Hg	May be present 10–25 mm Hg	Often present >25 mm Hg (adult), 20–40 mm Hg (child)	Absence suggests muscle fatigue

Functional Assessment

	Mild	Moderate	Severe	
PEF % Predicted % Personal best	> 80%	≈ 50%–80% or response lasts < 2 h	< 50% predicted or personal best	
P_aO_2 (on air) and/or	Normal (test not usually necessary)	> 60 mm Hg (test not usually necessary)	< 60 mm Hg: possible cyanosis	
PCO_2	< 42 mm Hg (test not usually necessary)	< 42 mm Hg (test not usually necessary)	≥ 42 mm Hg: possible respiratory failure	
SaO_2 (on air) at sea level	> 95% (test not usually necessary)	91%–95%	< 91%	

Hypercapnia (hypoventilation) develops more readily in young children than in adults and adolescents

Note: The presence of several parameters, but not necessarily all, indicates the general classification of the exacerbation. Many of these parameters have not been systematically studied, so they serve only as general guides.

Adapted from *National Heart, Lung, and Blood Institute* [21].
PEF—peak expiratory flow.

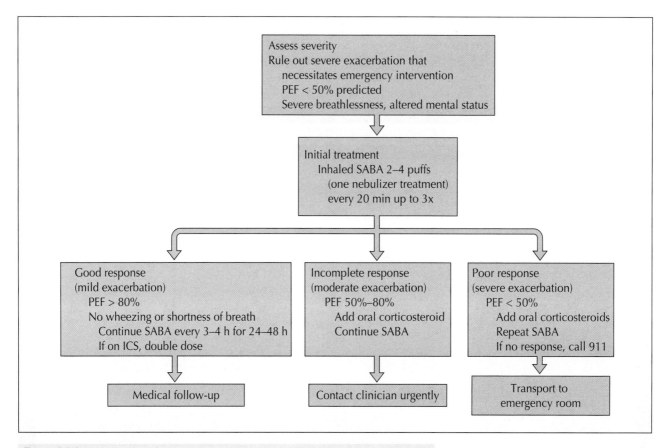

Figure 14-4.
Home management of asthma exacerbation. ICS—inhaled corticosteroid;
PEF—peak expiratory flow; SABA—short-acting β₂-agonist.

asthma include correction of hypoxemia, reversal of airflow obstruction, and comprehensive efforts to reduce recurrence rates. Oxygen is recommended for most patients during an asthma exacerbation. Inhaled short-acting β₂-agonists are recommended for all patients. These can be administered every 20 to 30 minutes. In the case of severe airway obstruction, use of nebulized short-acting β₂-agonists may be necessary. Continuous administration of nebulized short-acting β₂-agonists may be more effective than intermittent therapy [1]. Although less effective in chronic stable asthma, anticholinergics may be a useful and safe form of adjunct therapy during an acute asthma exacerbation [60]. Systemic corticosteroids are recommended for most patients. In addition to the NHLBI algorithm for emergency room and hospital-based care (Fig. 14-4), factors responsible for the exacerbation should be assessed. PEF should be monitored every 15 to 20 minutes during the initial phase of therapy and then at least daily throughout the hospital stay. Wide fluctuations in PEF are suggestive of severe or even life-threatening deterioration. Therapies that are less effective and not recommended to treat an acute exacerbation of asthma include theophylline, primarily because of

its adverse effects profile. Aggressive hydration is not recommended for adults and older children. Mucolytics are irritants that may provoke symptoms during asthma exacerbation, such as cough and bronchospasm, and should not be used. Chest physical therapy and anti-biotics have not been shown to have a role in the therapy of acute exacerbations of asthma unless a specific bacterial cause for the exacerbation can be identified [1]. For a more detailed understanding of the management of asthma, the reader is referred to the 1997 [1] and 2002 NHLBI Guidelines [21].

Asthma guidelines are an important means to standardize diagnosis, assess severity, and determine therapeutic approaches to patients with asthma. A recent survey showed that both primary care physicians and specialists may not be familiar with all of the components of the NHLBI asthma guidelines [61]. Thus, efforts should continue to review these algorithms and to educate all asthma health care providers.

ACKNOWLEDGMENT

The writing of this article was supported by the National Institutes of Health grant number R01 HL69167.

REFERENCES AND RECOMMENDED READING

1. National Heart, Lung, and Blood Institute, National Asthma Education and Prevention Program: *Expert Panel Report 2: Guidelines for the Diagnosis and Management of Asthma.* Bethesda, MD: National Institutes of Health; Pub No. 97-4051; 1997.

2. Agency for Healthcare Research and Quality Evidence Report/Technology Assessment. Management of chronic asthma. http://www.ahcpr.gov/clinic/epcsums/asthmasum.htm. Accessed September 10, 2002.

3. Teeter JG, Bleecker ER: Relationship between airway obstruction and respiratory symptoms in adult asthmatics. *Chest* 1998, 113(2):272–278.

4. Asthma in America. Executive summary. http://www.asthmain-america.com/execsum_over.htm. Accessed September 10, 2002.

5. Salvi SS, Krishna MT, Sampson AP, Holgate ST: The anti-inflammatory effects of leukotriene-modifying drugs and their use in asthma. *Chest* 2001, 119(5):1533–1546.

6. Laitinen LA, Laitinen A, Haahtela T: A comparative study of the effects of an inhaled corticosteroid, budesonide, and a beta$_2$-agonist, terbutaline, on airway inflammation in newly diagnosed asthma: a randomized, double-blind parallel-group controlled trial. *J Allergy Clin Immunol* 1992, 90:32–42.

7. Djukanovic R, Wilson TW, Britten KM, *et al.*: Effect of an inhaled corticosteroid on airway inflammation and symptoms of asthma. *Am Rev Respir Dis* 1992; 145:669–674.

8. Haahtela T, Jarvinen M, Kava T, *et al.*: Comparison of a beta$_2$-agonist, terbutaline, with an inhaled corticosteroid, budesonide, in newly detected asthma. *N Engl J Med* 1991, 325:388–392.

9. Olivieri D, Chetta A, Donno MD, *et al.*: Effect of short-term treatment with low-dose inhaled fluticasone propionate on airway inflammation and remodeling in mild asthma: a placebo-controlled study. *Am J Respir Crit Care Med* 1997, 155:1864–1871.

10. Kerstjens HAM, Brand PLP, Hughes MD, *et al.*: A comparison of bronchodilator therapy with or without inhaled corticosteroid therapy for obstructive airways disease. *N Engl J Med* 1992, 327(20):1413–1419.

11. Barnes PJ: Inhaled glucocorticoids for asthma. *N Engl J Med* 1995, 332:868–875.

12. van Essen-Zandvliet EE, Hughes MD, Waalkens, HJ, *et al.*: Effects of 22 months of treatment with inhaled corticosteroids and/or beta$_2$-agonists on lung function, airway responsiveness, and symptoms in children with asthma. *Am Rev Respir Dis* 1992, 146:547–554.

13. Sont JK, Willems LN, Bel EH, *et al.*: Clinical control and histopathologic outcome of asthma when using airway hyper-responsiveness as an additional guide to long-term treatment. The AMPUL Study Group. *Am J Respir Crit Care Med* 1999, 159:1043–1051.

14. Haahtela T, Jarvinen M, Kava T, *et al.*: Effects of reducing or discontinuing inhaled budesonide in patients with mild asthma. *N Engl J Med* 1994, 331:700–705.

15. Donahue JG, Weiss ST, Livingston JM, *et al.*: Inhaled steroids and the risk of hospitalization for asthma. *JAMA* 1997, 277:887–891.

16. Suissa S, Ernst P, Benayoun S, *et al.*: Low-dose inhaled corticosteroids, and the prevention of death from asthma. *N Engl J Med* 2000, 343:332–336.

17. Jeffery PK, Godfrey RW, Adelroth E, *et al.*: Effects of treatment on airway inflammation and thickening of basement membrane reticular collagen in asthma. *Am Rev Respir Dis* 1992, 145:890–899.

18. Booth H, Richmond I, Ward C, *et al.*: Effect of high dose inhaled fluticasone propionate on airway inflammation in asthma. *Am J Respir Crit Care Med* 1995, 152:45–52.

19. Busse WW, Sedgwick JB, Jarjour NN, Calhoun WJ: Eosinophils and basophils in allergic airway inflammation. *J Allergy Clin Immunol* 1994, 94:1250–1254.

20. Kamada AK, Szefler SJ, Martin RJ, *et al.*: Issues in the use of inhaled glucocorticoids. *Am J Respir Crit Care Med* 1996, 153:1739–1748.

21. Seiroos O, Pientinalho A, Lofroos A, Riska H: Effect of early vs. late intervention with inhaled corticosteroids in asthma. *Chest* 1995, 108:1228–1234.

22. National Heart, Lung, and Blood Institute, National Asthma Education and Prevention Program: *Guidelines for the Diagnosis and Management of Asthma-Update on Selected Topics 2002.* http://www.nhlbi.nih.gov/guidelines/asthma/index.htm. Accessed September 30, 2002.

23. Szefler S, Weiss S, Tonascia J, *et al.*: Long-term effects of budesonide or nedocromil in children with asthma. *N Engl J Med* 2000, 343:1054–1063.

24. Panhuysen CIM, Vonk JM, Koeter GH, *et al.*: Adult patients may outgrow their asthma. A 25-year follow-up study. *Am J Respir Crit Care Med* 1997, 155:1267–1272.

25. Nelson HS, Busse WW, Kerwin E, *et al.*: Fluticasone propionate/salmeterol combination provides more effective asthma control than low-dose inhaled corticosteroid plus montelukast. *J Allergy Clin Immunol* 2000, 106:1088–1095.

26. Fish J, Boone R, Emmett A, *et al.*: Salmeterol added to inhaled corticosteroids (ICS) provides greater asthma control compared to montelukast. *Am J Respir Crit Care Med* 2000, 161:A:203.

27. Busse W, Nelson H, Wolfe J, *et al.*: Comparison of inhaled salmeterol and oral zafirlukast in patients with asthma. *J Allergy Clin Immunol* 1999, 103: 1075–1080.

28. Bleecker ER, Welch MJ, Weinstein SF, *et al.*: Low-dose inhaled fluticasone propionate versus oral zafirlukast in the treatment of persistent asthma. *J Allergy Clin Immunol* 2000, 105:1123–1129.

29. Malmstrom K, Rodriguez-Gomez G, Guerra J, *et al.*: Oral montelukast, inhaled beclomethasone, and placebo for chronic asthma. *Ann Intern Med* 1999, 130:487–495.

30. Greening AP, Wind P, Northfield M, Shaw G: Added salmeterol versus higher-dose corticosteroid in asthma patients with symptoms on existing inhaled corticosteroid. *Lancet* 1994, 344:219–224.

31. Woolcock A, Lundback B, Ringdal N, Jacques LA: Comparison of addition of salmeterol to inhaled steroids with doubling of the dose of inhaled steroids. *Am J Respir Crit Care Med* 1996; 153:1481–1488.

32. Condemi J, Goldstein S, Kalberg C, *et al.*: The addition of salmeterol to fluticasone propionate versus increasing the dose of fluticasone propionate in patients with persistent asthma. *Ann Allergy Asthma Immunol* 1999, 82:383–389.

33. Baraniuk J, Murray J, Nathan R, *et al.*: Fluticasone alone or in combination with salmeterol vs. triamcinolone in asthma. *Chest* 1999, 116:625–632.

34. Ind P, Dal Negro R, Colman N, *et al.*: Inhaled fluticasone propionate and salmeterol in moderate adult asthma. II. Exacerbations. *Am J Respir Crit Care Med* 1998, 157A:415.

35. Murray J, Church N, Anderson W, *et al.*: Concurrent use of salmeterol with inhaled corticosteroids is more effective than inhaled corticosteroid dose increases. *Allergy Asthma Proc* 1999, 20:173–180.

36. van Noord J, Schreurs A, Mol S, Mulder P: Addition of salmeterol versus doubling the dose of fluticasone propionate in patients with mild to moderate asthma. *Thorax* 1999, 54:207–209.

37. Pearlman D, Stricker W, Weinstein S: Inhaled salmeterol and fluticasone: as study comparing monotherapy and combination therapy in asthma. *Ann Allergy Clin Immunol* 1999, 82:257–265.

38. Pauwels RA, Lofdahl CG, Postma DS, *et al.*: Effect of inhaled formoterol and budesonide on exacerbations of asthma. *N Engl J Med* 1997; 337:1405–1411.

39. Baraniuk J, Ali M, Brody D, *et al.*: Glucocorticoids induce beta$_2$-adrenergic receptor function in human nasal mucosa. *Am J Respir Crit Care Med* 1997, 155:704–710.

40. Eickelberg O, Roth M, Rainer L, *et al.*: Ligand-independent activation of the glucocorticoid receptor by beta$_2$-adrenergic receptor agonists in primary human lung fibroblasts and vascular smooth muscle cells. *J Biol Chem* 1999, 274:1005–1010.

41. Anenden V, Egemba G, Kessel B, *et al.*: Institute of Cardiovascular and Respiratory Pharmaceutical Development. Salmeterol facilitation of fluticasone-induced apoptosis in eosinophils of asthmatics pre- and post-antigen challenge. *Eur Respir J* 1998, 12:157S.

42. Oddera S, Silvestri M, Testi R, Rossi G: Salmeterol enhances the inhibitory activity of dexamethasone on allergen-induced blood mononuclear cell activation. *Respiration* 1998, 65:199–204.

43. Pang L, Knox A: Synergistic inhibition by beta$_2$-agonists and corticosteroids on tumor necrosis factor–α-induced interleukin-8 release from cultured human airway smooth-muscle cells. *Am J Respir Cell Mol Biol* 2000, 23:79–85.

44. Kavuru M, Melamed J, Gross G, *et al.*: Salmeterol and fluticasone propionate combined in a new powder inhalation device for the treatment of asthma: a randomized, double-blind placebo-controlled trail. *J Allergy Clin Immunol* 2000, 105:1108–1116.

45. Aubier M, Pieters W, Schlosser N, Steinmetz K: Salmeterol/fluticasone propionate (50/500 µg) in combination in a Diskus inhaler (Seretide) is effective and safe in the treatment of steroid-dependent asthma. *Respir Med* 1999, 93:876–874.

46. Shapiro G, Lumry W, Wolfe J, *et al.*: Combined salmeterol 50 µg and fluticasone propionate 250 µg in the Diskus device for the treatment of asthma. *Am J Respir Crit Care Med* 2000, 161:527–534.

47. Palmqvist M, Arvidsson P, Beckman O, *et al.*: Onset of bronchodilation of budesonide/formoterol vs. salmeterol/fluticasone in single inhalers. *Pulm Pharmacol Ther* 2001, 14:29–34.

48. Dahlen B, Nizankowska E, Szczelik A, *et al.*: Benefits from adding the 5-lipoxygenase inhibitor zileuton to conventional therapy in aspirin-tolerant asthmatics. *Am J Resp Crit Care Med* 1998, 157:1187–1194.

49. Virchow J, Prasse A, Naya I, *et al.*: Zafirlukast improves asthma control in patients receiving high-dose inhaled corticosteroids. *Amer J Resp Crit Care Med* 2000, 162:578–585.

50. Tamaoki J, Kondo M, Sakaj N, *et al.*: Leukotriene antagonist prevents exacerbation of asthma during reduction of high-dose inhaled corticosteroid. *Am J Respir Crit Care Med* 1997, 155:1235–1240.

51. Laviolette M, Malmstrom K, Lu S, *et al.*: Montelukast added to inhaled beclomethasone in treatment of asthma. *Am J Respir Crit Care Med* 1999, 160:1862–1868.

52. Dempsey O, Andrew M, Wilson M, *et al.*: Additive broncho-protective and bronchodilator effects with single doses of salmeterol and montelukast in asthmatic patients receiving inhaled corticosteroids. *Chest* 2000, 117:950–953.

53. Bjermer L, Bisgaad H, Bousquet J *et al.*: Montelukast or salmeterol combined with an inhaled steroid in adult asthma: design and rationale of a randomized, double-blind comparative study (the IMPAC investigation of montelukast as a partner agent for complementary therapy-trial). *Respiratory Med* 2000, 94:612–621.

54. Dahlen S: Lipid mediator pathways in the lung: leukotrienes as a new target for the treatment of asthma. *Clinical and Experimental Allergy* 1998, 28(5):141–146.

55. Roquet A, Dahlen B, Kumlin M, *et al.*: Combined antagonism of leukotrienes and histamine produced predominant inhibition of allergen-induced early and late phase airway obstruction in asthmatics. *Am J Respir Crit Care Med* 1997, 155:1856–1863.

56. Reicin A, White R, Weinstein S, *et al.*: Montelukast, a leukotriene receptor antagonist, in combination with loratadine, a histamine receptor antagonist, in the treatment of chronic asthma. *Arch Intern Med* 2000, 160:2481–2488.

57. Meltzer E, Malmstrom K, Lu S, *et al.*: Concomitant montelukast and loratadine as treatment for seasonal allergic rhinitis: a randomized, placebo-controlled clinical trial. *J Allergy Clin Immunol* 2000, 105:917–920.

58. Robertson CF, Rubinfeld AR, Bowes G: Pediatric asthma deaths in Victoria: the mild are at risk. *Pediatr Pulmonol* 1992, 13(2):95–100.

59. Busse WW, Banks-Schlegel S, Wenzel SE: Pathophysiology of severe asthma. *J Allergy Clin Immunol* 2000, 106:1033–1042.

60. McFadden Jr E, Elsanadi N, Dixon L, *et al.*: Protocol therapy for acute asthma: therapeutic benefit and cost savings. *Am J Med* 1995, 99:651.

61. Doerschug KC, Peterson MW, Dayton CS, Kline JN: Asthma guidelines: an assessment of physician understanding and practice. *Am J Respir Crit Care Med* 1999, 159:1735–1741.

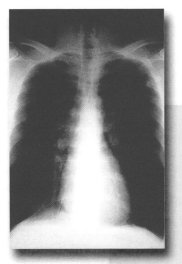

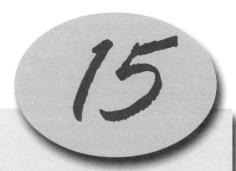

Inhaled Corticosteroids and Their Use in Asthma

Kerry L. Drain and James T. C. Li

Inhaled corticosteroids (ICSs) have revolutionized the treatment of asthma. They are the most potent and effective therapy for persistent asthma and are efficacious in most patients, regardless of age or asthma severity [1••]. ICS use diminishes airway inflammation and hyperresponsiveness, improves lung function, and controls symptoms in asthmatic patients. Clinically, ICS use has been shown to reduce the number of emergency room visits, hospitalizations [2], and deaths [3••]. Histologic studies have found that ICS use may even positively affect the natural course of asthma. However, dose-related adverse effects such as growth suppression and decreased bone mineral density (BMD) may limit ICS use for some patients.

PHARMACOLOGY

Corticosteroids (*ie*, glucocorticoid and mineralocorticoid) are secreted by the adrenal cortex. Whereas hydrocortisone or cortisol is the major glucocorticoid secreted in humans, aldosterone is the major mineralocorticoid. Under normal conditions, the body produces approximately 10 mg of cortisol and 0.125 mg of aldosterone per day. Corticosteroids affect carbohydrates, lipids and proteins, and electrolyte balance. The discovery of the use of corticosteroids for inflammatory diseases such as asthma heralded a new era of disease management. Dosages needed to achieve an anti-inflammatory, immunosuppressive effect may be much greater than that normally produced by the body.

Glucocorticoids share a basic 21-carbon structure arranged within a four-ring complex (Fig. 15-1). Modifications of the basic structure are made to enhance the anti-inflammatory properties while decreasing the mineralocorticoid activity. Corticosteroids are lipophilic, so they are able to pass cellular membranes easily. Minor alterations in chemical structure alter the rate of absorption, the onset of effect, and the duration of action. Certain water-soluble esters of hydrocortisone and its synthetic analogues can be administered intravenously to achieve rapid, high drug concentration within the blood. This is advantageous because after it enters the blood stream, more than 90% of cortisone becomes reversibly bound to proteins within the plasma. Thus, only 10% of the cortisone, the unbound fraction, can enter cells and exert its anti-inflammatory effects. In situations of clinical necessity, supraphysiologic doses are required to increase the availability of free cortisone. Metabolism of these entities occurs in the liver and kidneys, and excretion is via urine and feces.

Mechanism of Action

After they are deposited in the airway, ICSs readily move intracellularly and then bind to the cytosolic glucocorticoid receptor. The receptor complex is activated and translocated into the nucleus, where it acts as a transcription factor binding to specific recognition sequences on the DNA in the promoter region of corticosteroid receptor elements. ICSs can cause activation of suppression or target genes by either increasing or decreasing specific messenger RNA (mRNA) production. Examples of increased transcription in the presence of an ICS include protein lipocortin-1, an inhibitor of phospholipase A2, β_2-adrenergic receptors, interleukin-1 (IL-1) receptor antagonists, and leukocyte inhibitory protein. Inhibited transcription results in decreased production of cytokines such as interleukins, tumor necrosis factor (TNF), and other inflammatory mediators. ICSs inhibit production of inducible nitric oxide synthase, cyclooxygenase (COX), and intracellular adhesion molecule (ICAM). The glucocorticoid receptor complex can interact directly on transcription factors that are activated by cytokine binding to its receptor, thereby inactivating the effects of the cytokine on the cell and preventing further cytokine production [4].

Mechanisms of Action of Inhaled Corticosteroids in Asthma

The pathogenesis of asthma involves many mediators. These include inflammatory cells found in the airways such as eosinophils, lymphocytes, mast cells, macrophages, and neutrophils. ICSs are very effective at suppressing the eosinophilic inflammation in the airways. Corticosteroids affect transcription and expression of anti-inflammatory proteins such as IL-1 receptor antagonists, IL-10, and neutral endopeptidases. Suppression is also achieved by decreased concentrations of inflammatory cytokines IL-4, IL-5, and chemokines involved in eosinophil recruitment, such as eotaxin. ICSs effectively inhibit other inflammatory components in asthma (Fig. 15-2). They inhibit activation and recruitment of cells such as eosinophils, T lymphocytes, macrophages, and dendritic cells. ICSs act on mast cells by reducing their survival at the airway surface, but they do not act in blocking activation. ICSs also act by inhibiting the release of mediators from structural cells of the airway such as fibroblasts and epithelial, smooth muscle, and endothelial cells. These findings have been confirmed by studies of bronchial biopsy specimens taken from asthmatic patients in whom the number of inflammatory cells (*ie*, eosinophils, surface mast cells, and macrophages) and T lymphocytes are significantly decreased [5]. Studies of other parameters of asthmatic inflammation show that cells within bronchoalveolar lavage (BAL) fluid, eosinophil number in induced sputum, amount of local cytokine production, and concentration of exhaled nitric oxide are all affected by ICS use [6].

Airway hyperresponsiveness is affected by chronic ICS use by reducing airway inflammation. In both children and adults, chronic treatment with an ICS has reduced

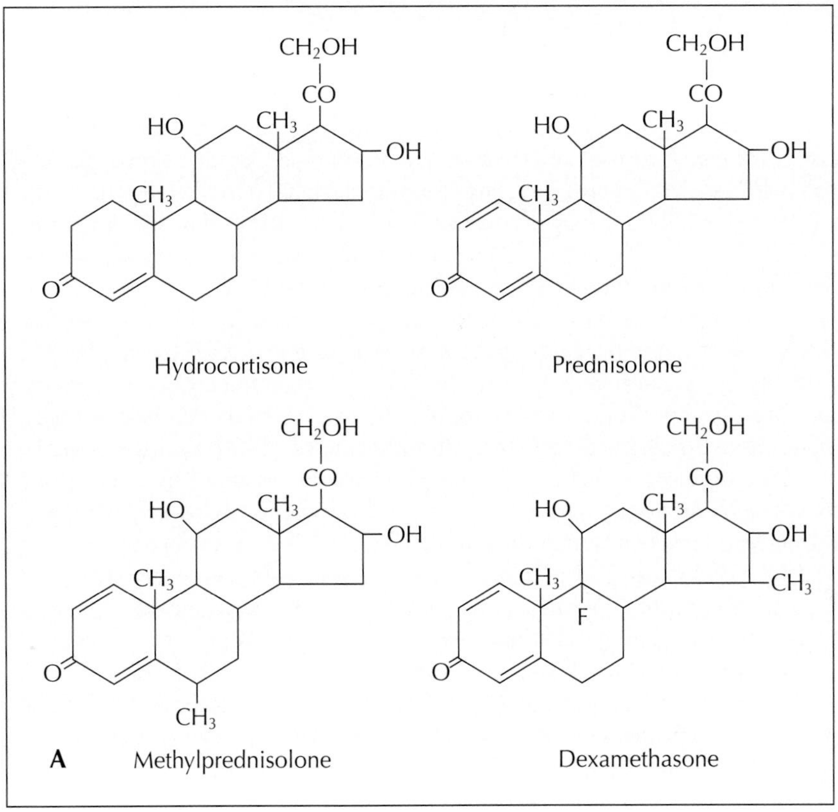

Figure 15-1.
Structure of systemic glucocorticoids. **A,** Hydrocortisone, prednisolone, methylprednisolone, and dexamethasone.
(*Continued on next page*)

responsiveness to histamine, allergen (early and late responses), exercise, and irritants [6]. The reduction in hyperresponsiveness takes place over several weeks and may not be maximal until used consistently for several months. Prolonged administration of ICS can result in decreased responsiveness of the airways to irritants, and may also limit the maximal narrowing in response to these challenges [7]. ICSs have been found to decrease vascularity and collagen deposition that occur with airway remodeling [8].

Efficacy of Inhaled Corticosteroids in Asthma

Inhaled corticosteroids are the first-line agents for patients with persistent asthma. They fulfill the criteria of a good controller medication in that they prevent and control symptoms, reduce the frequency and severity of exacerbations, reverse airflow obstruction, and may prevent the progression of asthma and the development of a fixed obstruction.

Clinical experience with ICSs has accumulated over the past 30 years. The first trials were in patients with

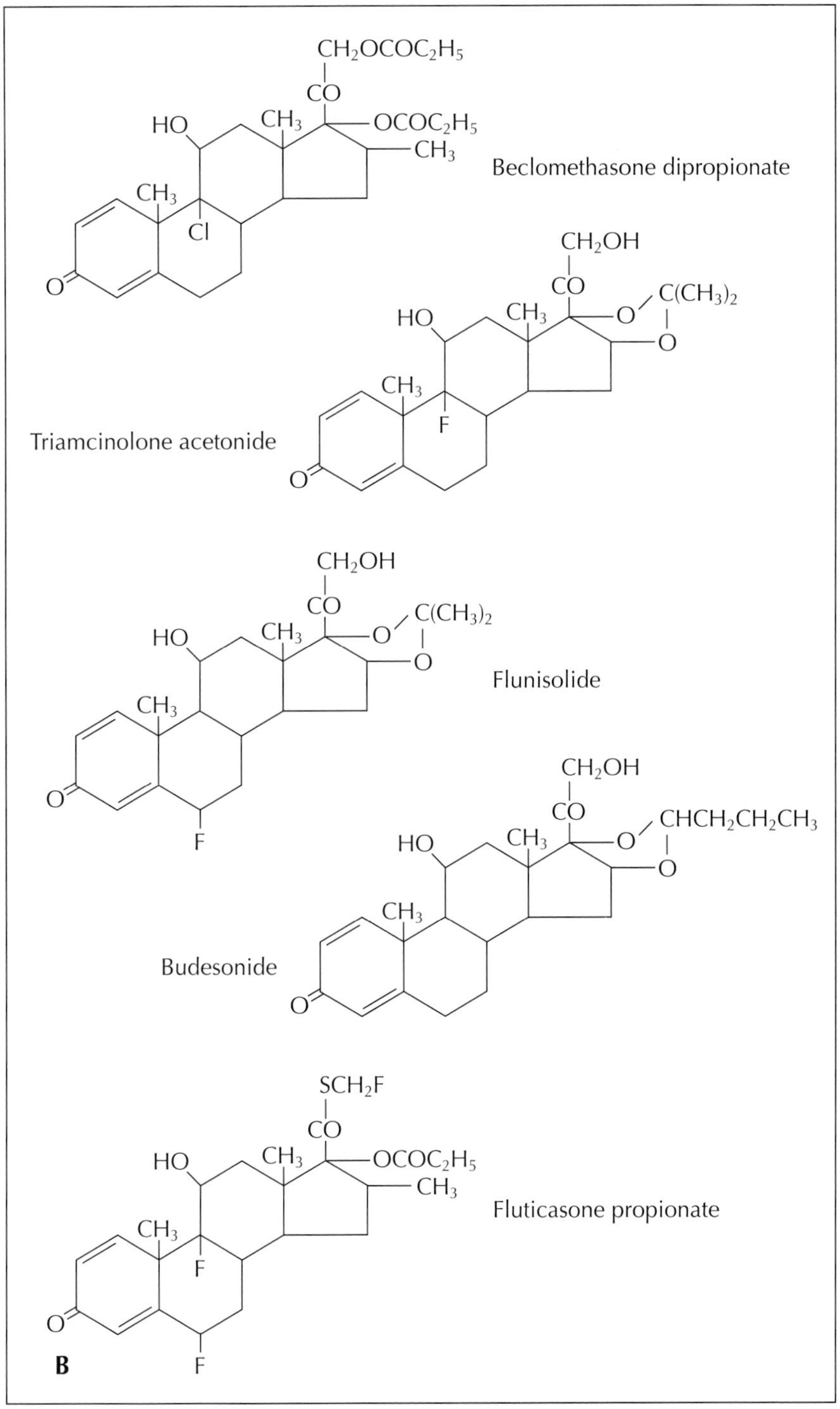

Figure 15-1.
(*Continued from previous page*)
B, Beclomethasone dipropionate, triamcinolone acetonide, flunisolide, budesonide, and fluticasone propionate. (*Adapted from* Miesfeld and Bloom [4].)

moderate and severe asthma. Experience in more mild asthmatic patients has increased over the past 15 years. One of the first studies of ICS use in mild disease was conducted using budesonide 600 μg twice daily versus the short-acting β$_2$-agonist terbutaline in newly diagnosed asthmatic patients. Compared with inhaled terbutaline, patients using inhaled budesonide experienced fewer symptoms, improved lung function, and improved hyper-responsiveness to methacholine [9]. The effectiveness of ICSs has been demonstrated in patients with varying severity of persistent asthma for inhaled beclomethasone, budesonide, flunisolide, triamcinolone, and fluticasone.

Inhaled corticosteroids can reduce the frequency of asthma exacerbations. ICSs reduce the frequency of hospitalization for asthma and the risk of life-threatening attacks. In a study of 11,195 children 3 to 15 years of age recruited from three distinct geographic regions, there was a significant protective effect with the use of inhaled anti-inflammatory agents (either ICS or cromolyn) and the risk of emergency department visits, hospitalizations, or both [2]. In 2002, Eisner *et al.* [10••] demonstrated that the use of ICS was associated with a risk reduction of intensive care unit admission among adults hospitalized with asthma. Interestingly, the same study found the opposite effect for increased use of inhaled β$_2$-agonist.

Suissa *et al.* [3••] showed a dose-response relationship between ICS and death from asthma. Their cohort included 30,569 patients within the Saskatchewan Health database using anti-asthma therapy over a 17-year period. Subjects who died of asthma were compared with control subjects. On the basis of continuous dose-response analysis, the rate of death from asthma was decreased by 21%

with each additional canister of ICS used in the previous year. They also found the rate of death from asthma during the first 3 months after discontinuation of an ICS was higher than the rate among patients who continued to use their medication (Fig. 15-3).

Early intervention with an ICS may reduce or prevent permanent airway obstruction. In one study [11], patients who received an ICS earlier in their course maintained significantly better spirometric results compared with those in whom ICS use was delayed by 2 years while treated with β$_2$-agonist therapy alone. Both groups showed ICS benefit, but there was less improvement in lung function and hyperresponsiveness in the delayed treatment cohort. In a clinical observation study [12], adult patients with asthma who received an ICS earlier in their disease showed significant improvement in peak expiratory flow (PEF) compared with asthmatic patients in whom therapy was delayed. The patients were then categorized by time of initiation of therapy with an ICS compared with initial asthma diagnosis. There was an inverse relationship between improvement in PEF associated with ICS use and the duration of asthma. This relationship was present across all disease durations (6 months to 10 years).

The use of ICS in severe asthmatic patients has reduced the need for maintenance oral corticosteroid. A study by Wenzel *et al.* [13] looked at the use of high-dose fluticasone (880 μg twice daily) in patients with severe, refractory asthma. In conjunction with a referral to an asthma specialty clinic, the use of high-dose fluticasone led to statistically significant improvement in pulmonary function, oral steroid requirement, and health care resources use.

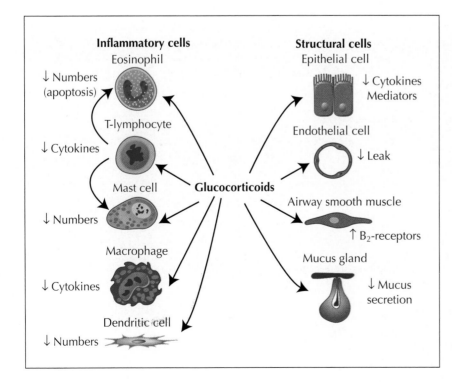

Figure 15-2.
Effects of inhaled corticosteroids. (*Adapted from* Barnes [6].)

Comparisons with Other Medications

The clinical efficacy of ICSs has been studied extensively in comparative trials. Studies comparing ICSs and cromolyn, nedocromil, theophylline, short- and long-acting β_2-agonists, and leukotriene modifiers show improved outcomes in patients using an ICS.

One study included 1041 asthmatic children 5 to 12 years of age treated with either budesonide 200 μg twice daily versus nedocromil 8 mg twice daily [14••]. All subjects were studied for 4 to 6 years. Budesonide was superior to nedocromil and placebo for decreasing airway hyperresponsiveness and improving asthma control, but neither agent was better than placebo when FEV_1 (forced expiratory volume in 1 second) after bronchodilator was compared. Price *et al.* [15] compared low-dose fluticasone (50 μg twice daily) and cromolyn (20 μg daily) in 225 children 4 to 12 years of age during an 8-week period, and found fluticasone to be superior to cromolyn in symptom control and increasing PEF.

Two studies directly compared ICSs with theophylline [16,17]. Galant *et al.* [16] compared two dosages of fluticasone and theophylline capsules in 353 adults and adolescents. In this 12-week study, the fluticasone groups had significantly better FEV_1 and PEF than the theophylline group. Reed *et al.* [17] looked at 747 patients for 1 year using either beclomethasone 84 μg daily or sustained release theophylline twice daily. Beclomethasone was more effective in decreasing symptoms, bronchodilator use, and hyperresponsiveness. Both drugs improved pulmonary function, but theophylline had a high rate of adverse effects.

Inhaled corticosteroids have been compared with short-acting β_2-agonist medications. ICSs were shown to be superior in decreasing airway hyperresponsiveness and increasing lung function. ICSs were also found to be superior to short-acting β-agonists in preventing asthma exacerbations, hospitalizations, and death. In a study of long-acting β_2-agonists [18], patients whose asthma was well controlled by low-dose triamcinolone were switched to salmeterol monotherapy. Those treated with salmeterol alone experienced more exacerbations, treatment failure, and increased indices of airways inflammation.

Leukotriene modifiers block the production of cysteinyl leukotrienes (LTC4, -D4, -E4), which are derived from arachidonic acid as part of the inflammatory response. Malmstron *et al.* [19] studied 895 adults with chronic asthma (FEV_1 50% to 85% predicted) treated with either montelukast (10 mg/d) or beclomethasone (200 μg twice a day). Subjects treated with beclomethasone had larger improvement in FEV_1 and symptom scores [19]. Direct comparisons between low-dose ICSs and leukotriene modifiers universally demonstrate ICSs superior improvement in lung function, symptom control, and reduction in exacerbations [20,21]. When asthmatic patients well controlled on a low-dose ICS were switched to a leukotriene modifier, there was deterioration of lung function and an increased rate of exacerbations [22].

Combination of Inhaled Corticosteroids and Other Medications

Numerous studies have found that the addition of the long-acting β_2-agonist to ICSs was superior to simply increasing the ICS dose. A meta-analysis [23•] of nine trials involving a total of 3685 patients in parallel groups compared the response to an increased dose of ICS with the addition of a long-acting agent, salmeterol, with existing ICS. The combination resulted in improved lung function, decreased daytime and nighttime symptoms, and decreased rescue medication use. The combination group also had fewer exacerbations or, if present, the exacerbations were less severe. These findings have led to the development of combination products delivered within one device.

A recent study looked at theophylline withdrawal in asthmatic patients well controlled on a combination of theophylline and inhaled beclomethasone [24]. After the patients were off theophylline for 1 week, two thirds of the patients had rapid declines in FEV_1, suggesting an additive effect of combined theophylline and beclometha-

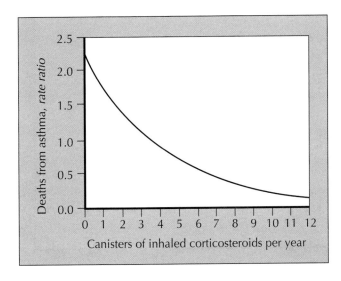

Figure 15-3.

Impact of low-dose inhaled corticosteroids on asthma mortality. (*Adapted from* Suissa *et al.* [3••].)

sone. Another study [25] demonstrated that low-dose theophylline in addition to low-dose ICS had the same effect on relief or clinical symptoms and airway hyper-responsiveness as higher doses of ICS did.

Laviolette *et al.* [26] studied 642 patients 15 years of age and older with incomplete asthma control on beclomethasone (FEV$_1$ 50% to 85% predicted) treated with the combination of montelukast 10 mg/d and beclomethasone 200 µg twice daily, beclomethasone at the same dose, or montelukast alone. After the 16-week treatment period, asthma control was worsened by removing beclomethasone. Some clinical benefit was seen with the addition of montelukast to the ICS.

SAFETY AND SPECIAL CONSIDERATIONS OF INHALED CORTICOSTEROIDS IN ASTHMA TREATMENT

Inhaled corticosteroids at recommended dosages have a proven record of safety and tolerability [1••]. Local effects of ICSs include oral candidiasis and dysphonia. Reported

systemic effects include suppression of the hypothalamic-pituitary-adrenal (HPA) axis, bone demineralization, growth effects in children, and cataracts.

Bioavailability

Inhaled corticosteroids are safer than oral corticosteroids in patients with asthma because they are delivered directly to the affected site (the lung). Despite this direct action, a portion of each dose enters the systemic circulation via the lungs or the gastrointestinal (GI) tract. After they are available systemically and activated, ICSs can exert unintended effects. Glucocorticoid receptors are expressed on many cell types besides those directly related to asthma. Systemically absorbed corticosteroids can affect metabolism, endocrine function, and other systems. Asthma is a chronic disease, so it must be treated over sustained periods of time, which can increase the risk of adverse effects from repeated activation of nonpulmonary sites.

Intrinsic glucocorticoid activity, the amount of systemic bioavailability, and the rate of elimination of the medication from the body all affect the risk of systemic adverse effects of ICSs. The intrinsic glucocorti-

Table 15-1. RECOMMENDED DOSES OF INHALED CORTICOSTEROIDS FOR ADULTS WITH ASTHMA

Drug	Dose		
	Low	Medium	High
Beclomethasone	168–504 µg	504–840 µg	> 840 µg
42 µg/puff	4–12 puffs	12–20 puffs	> 20 puffs
84 µg/puff	2–6 puffs	6–10 puffs	> 10 puffs
Beclomethasone-HFA	40–160 µg	160–320 µg	> 320 µg
40 µg/puff	1–4 puffs	4–8 puffs	> 8 puffs
80 µg/puff	1–2 puffs	2–4 puffs	> 4 puffs
Budesonide	200–400 µg	400–600 µg	> 600 µg
DPI: 200 µg/dose	1–2 inhalations	2–3 inhalations	> 3 inhalations
Flunisolide	500–1000 µg	1000–2000 µg	> 2000 µg
250 µg/puff	2–4 puffs	4–8 puffs	> 8 puffs
Fluticasone	88–264 µg	264–660 µg	> 660 µg
MDI: 44 µg/puff	2–6 puffs	—	—
MDI: 110 µg/puff	2 puffs	2–6 puffs	> 6 puffs
MDI: 220 µg/puff	—	—	> 3 puffs
DPI: 50 µg/inhalation	2–6 inhalations	—	—
DPI: 100 µg/inhalation	—	3–6 inhalations	> 6 inhalations
DPI: 250 µg/inhalation	—	—	> 2 inhalations
Triamcinolone	400–1000 µg	1000–2000 µg	> 2000 µg
100 µg/puff	4–10 puffs	10–20 puffs	> 20 puffs
Fluticasone/salmeterol	100–200 µg	250–500 µg	500–1000 µg
DPI: 100 µg/50 µg	1–2 inhalations	—	—
DPI: 250 µg/50 µg	—	1–2 inhalations	—
DPI: 500 µg/50 µg	—	—	1–2 inhalations

DPI—dry-powder inhaler; HFA—hydrofluoroalkane-134a; MDI—metered dose inhaler.

coid activity is determined by the agent's affinity for the glucocorticoid receptor (GR). Fluticasone has a very high affinity for the human GR. Its affinity is three times that of budesonide and 10 times that of triamcinolone and flunisolide [27]. Generally, the higher the affinity of an ICS to the GR, the more potent it is in both anti-inflammatory action and potential for local and systemic effects. However, with higher affinity, the dose of ICS can be decreased without loss of effect. The current recommended dosages for ICS reflect this strength of GR binding (Tables 15-1 and 15-2). Thus, fluticasone (a more avidly binding ICS) has a lower recommended dose than lower-affinity ICSs such as triamcinolone and flunisolide [1••,28]. It is thought that fluticasone is twice as potent as budesonide, which, in turn, is of equal potency to beclomethasone. Triamcinolone and flunisolide are six to nine times less potent than fluticasone [29].

Absorption from the lung and gastrointestinal tract accounts for systemic corticosteroid availability. Whereas ICS, absorbed from the lung gains direct access to the systemic circulation, ICSs absorbed from the gastrointestinal tract must pass through the liver. Corticosteroid that escapes this first-pass metabolism becomes bioavailable (Fig. 15-4). Most ICSs have high rates of first-pass metabolism. Fluticasone undergoes almost complete metabolism in the liver so that lung absorption is its primary route of systemic availability [27]. The first-pass metabolism of budesonide is approximately 90% and is 60% to 70% for beclomethasone [30]. For drugs with less liver metabolism, the swallowed fraction contributes to the systemic bioavailability. This bioactivity makes it important to consider the manner in which the medication is deposited to the lung and the GI tract.

Metered dose inhalers (MDIs) are among the earliest hand-held devices to deliver medication directly into the airway. Using propellants to aerosolize medication, MDIs are an accurate and precise method of dose delivery. Spacers or holding chambers have been shown to enhance the efficacy and safety of MDIs. The spacing devices reduce the need for hand–lung coordination and decrease the

Table 15-2. RECOMMENDED DOSES OF INHALED CORTICOSTEROIDS FOR CHILDREN WITH ASTHMA

Drug	Dose		
	Low	Medium	High
Beclomethasone	84–336 µg	336–672 µg	> 672 µg
42 µg/puff	2–8 puffs	8–16 puffs	> 16 puffs
84 µg/puff	1–4 puffs	4–8 puffs	> 8 puffs
Beclomethasone-HFA	40–160 µg	160–320 µg	> 320 µg
40 µg/puff	1–4 puffs	4–8 puffs	> 8 puffs
80 µg/puff	1–2 puffs	2–4 puffs	> 4 puffs
Budesonide	100–200 µg	200–400 µg	> 400 µg
DPI: 200 µg/dose	—	1–2 inhalations	> 2 inhalations
Susp 250 µg/dose	—	1–2 nebs	> 2 nebs
Susp 500 µg/dose	—	—	> 1 neb
Flunisolide	500–750 µg	1000–1250 µg	> 1250 µg
250 µg/puff	2–3 puffs	4–5 puffs	> 5 puffs
Fluticasone	88–176 µg	176–440 µg	> 440 µg
MDI: 44 µg/puff	2–4 puffs	—	
MDI: 110 µg/puff	—	2–4 puffs	> 4 puffs
MDI: 220 µg/puff	—	—	> 2 puffs
DPI: 50 µg/inhalation	2–4 inhalations	—	—
DPI: 100 µg/inhalation	—	2–4 inhalations	> 4 inhalations
DPI: 250 µg/inhalation	—	—	> 2 inhalations
Triamcinolone	400–800 µg	800–1200 µg	> 1200 µg
100 µg/puff	4–8 puffs	8–12 puffs	> 12 puffs
Fluticasone/salmeterol	100–200 µg	250–500 µg	> 500 µg
DPI: 100 µg/50 µg	1–2 inhalations	—	—
DPI: 250 µg/50 µg	—	1–2 inhalations	—
DPI: 500 µg/50 µg	—	—	> 1 inhalations

DPI—dry-powder inhaler; HFA—hydrofluoroalkane-134a; MDI—metered dose inhaler; neb—nebulized; susp—suspension.

amount of ICS oropharyngeal deposition [31••]. The use of a spacer or holding chamber can decrease the systemic effects of ICS [32]. In emergency departments, albuterol given by MDIs are as effective as nebulized medications [33]. MDIs can be used in those 5 years of age and older with spacers or holding devices and can be used in those younger than 5 years of age using an age-appropriate spacing device. MDIs have been redesigned recently to adhere to the principles outlined by the Montreal Protocol on Substances that Deplete the Ozone Layer [34]. The chlorofluorocarbon (CFC)-containing propellants are being phased out and replaced by either hydrofluoroalkane-134a (HFA)-containing propellants, which have no effect on ozone, or by dry-powder inhalers (DPIs), which do not require a propellant. Using HFA propellant, beclomethasone is delivered in an extra-fine aerosol (1.1 μm diameter particle size) that greatly increases its lung deposition. In a study [35] that compared radiolabeled CFC-beclomethasone (BDP) with HFA-BDP, lung deposition was 16% ± 9% with CFC-BDP and 53% ± 10% with HFA-BDP. Oropharyngeal deposition was 60% ± 13% and 25% ± 8%, respectively.

Some DPIs deliver a greater fraction of drug to the lower airway compared with MDIs. Some DPIs can deliver only a single dose, but others have multiple doses stored within the device in individual packages or as a solid reservoir [31••].

Dry-powder inhalers differ in their resistances to flow. High-resistance devices such as those that use a reservoir system are more flow dependent than those with lower resistances. The optimal flow for a high-resistance device is 60 L/min. In a study of high resistance DPIs, a range of 28 to 63 L/min flow showed no difference between total emitted doses [36]. In contrast, Prime *et al.* [37] found fine particle fraction produced by DPIs was sensitive to inspiratory flow. This variation was less prominent in lower resistance devices. At 5 years of age, a child should be able to consistently create airflow required for breath activation.

Nebulizers are used to deliver aerosols through either a mouthpiece or a mask. Nebulizers do not require skillful manipulations to deliver medication and are appropriate for young people or those who are unable to use other devices. Budesonide solution for nebulization is available for the treatment of patients with asthma. Studies suggest that the systemic effect of nebulized budesonide is no greater than that of budesonide delivered by DPI or MDI [38].

The elimination half-life of ICS is 7.8 hours for fluticasone, 2.3 hours for budesonide, 1.5 hours for triamcinolone, and 1.6 hours for flunisolide [32]. The risk of systemic effect is thought to mimic persistent levels rather than transient, high peak levels. Lipophilicity of an ICS influences systemic bioavailability. Pulmonary absorption is enhanced by increased lipophilicity. Fluticasone is three times more lipophilic than beclomethasone and more than 1000 times that of triamcinolone or flunisolide. Uptake, binding, retention, and excretion characteristics of lipophilic ICS create an attenuated release from the lipid compartment of the pulmonary tissue, contributing not only to the potency of the medication but also to the risk of systemic effects [39••].

SYSTEMIC EFFECTS

Effects on the Hypothalamic-Pituitary-Adrenal Axis

Serum cortisol levels mirror the effect of exogenous glucocorticoid on the hypothalamic-pituitary-adrenal

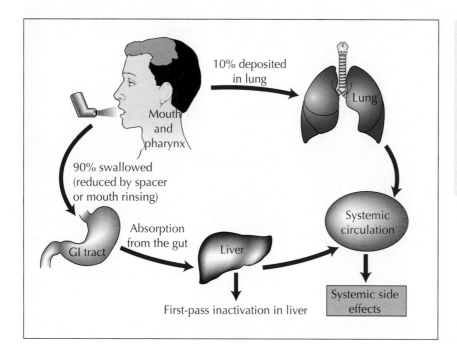

Figure 15-4.
The distribution of inhaled corticosteroid. A corticosteroid absorbed from the lung gains immediate access to systemic circulation, whereas only the portion absorbed from the gut that escapes first-pass metabolism in the gastrointestinal tract and liver becomes bioavailable. (*Adapted from* Barnes [5].)

(HPA) axis. The most reliable measure of HPA axis is the response to stimulation by corticotropin. Peak cortisol levels after stimulation reflects the HPA dynamic and adrenal reserve. An abnormally low response to corticotropin stimulation indicates significant HPA axis suppression. Stimulation can be done with low or high doses of corticotropin. The lower-dose stimulation tests are thought to detect lesser degrees of suppression, but the association with relevant adrenal insufficiency is still unclear [39••].

The clinical significance of ICS-induced HPA axis suppression is unclear. Documented cases of adrenal insufficiency are rare [32]. Low doses of ICS are not associated with significant suppression of the HPA axis in children [40]. In adults with mild to moderate persistent asthma, cortisol suppression was only noted at the highest dosages (1600 µg/d), a dose twice the highest suggested dose [41]. In a study [42] of 700 patients with chronic severe asthma treated with high-dose fluticasone or budesonide, serum cortisol levels were normal during treatment. In a group of study subjects with mild asthma (ages 7 to 9 years), 400 µg of beclomethasone had no effect on overnight cortisol production after 7 months of treatment [40].

A 28-day study of adult asthmatic patients compared fluticasone 440 µg/d with triamcinolone 800 µg/d. After corticotropin stimulation test, whereas the cortisol levels of those treated with fluticasone were comparable with placebo, those treated with triamcinolone had significantly suppressed cortisol as compared with placebo [43].

Thus, short-term ICS use at standard dosages may not significantly suppress the HPA axis. Even long-term use of ICS may not adversely affect the HPA axis. A 2-year study [44] in adults taking fluticasone 500 µg/d found no association between dose and effect on the HPA axis.

Bone Mineralization

Osteocalcin is a protein produced by bone-forming osteoblasts. Serum levels are a sensitive indicator of bone turnover [45]. High-dose corticosteroids have been found to diminish serum osteocalcin levels. Prolonged oral corticosteroid therapy has been shown to cause osteoporosis [46], and studies suggest that ICS use may decrease BMD. A population-based study [47] of patients with asthma demonstrated a negative correlation between cumulative ICS use and BMD in those who took ICS regularly for a median of 6 years. Several other long-term studies [39••] of ICS up to 1000 µg/d have shown no effect on BMD.

Prospective studies indicate that ICS use may affect levels of osteocalcin. In a study [48] of beclomethasone 500 µg twice daily, the mean plasma levels of osteocalcin decreased significantly after 1 week of therapy. In contrast, a 2-year study of adults with mild asthma using fluticasone 500 µg twice daily had no significant effect on osteocalcin levels or BMD [44]. Although plasma osteocalcin may reflect bone turnover, actual measurement of bone mineral content may be more clinically relevant.

Growth Effects

Studies in children with asthma have shown variable results regarding ICS and growth. Some studies [49] have found significant growth suppression, but others have detected little or no change in growth. Any statements regarding growth are complicated by the difference of growth between individuals, the timing of ICS initiation and puberty, the length of individual study, and the fact that patients with poorly controlled asthma have growth issues independent of ICS use.

A study of children with mild asthma treated with beclomethasone 400 µg/d showed a 1-cm growth suppression over 7 months without demonstrable effect on the HPA axis [40]. In contrast, a study of prepubescent adolescents taking 100 to 200 µg/d of fluticasone for 1 year showed no significant difference in growth velocity [50]. Another study [51••] compared children treated with fluticasone 100 µg/d and cromolyn and found no difference in growth velocity after 1 year. A controlled, nonrandomized, long-term growth study by Agertoft and Pedersen [52] showed no significant effect of ICS on adult height. The prospective study followed more than 200 children with asthma treated with a mean dose of 400 µg/d of budesonide for 9.2 years. As control subjects, the study included children with asthma who never received ICS and healthy siblings of the budesonide-treated subjects. Growth rates were reduced during the first year of budesonide treatment, but these changes were not associated with significant changes in adult height. There was no dose-response relationship between daily dose or duration of treatment and the difference between measured and target adult height. The one factor that did influence final adult height was the child's height before budesonide therapy. Transient suppression of growth was again confirmed by a large-scale trial of children 5 to 12 years of age who received nedocromil or budesonide. The reduction of growth (approximately 1 cm) was noted at 1 year in the ICS-treated group [14••]. Therefore, for most children, any growth velocity inhibition that may be associated with ICS use at standard therapeutic doses may be significant only for 1 year and may not have a significant impact on final adult height.

Ocular Effects

An association between oral corticosteroid use and the formation of posterior subcapsular cataracts has been documented. A study of adult asthma patients taking long-term oral corticosteroids and ICS found a 27% prevalence of cataracts in this group [53]. This association has not been found in those treated with ICS alone. In a study of young patients (median age, 13.8 years) taking inhaled budesonide or beclomethasone at a dose of 750 µg/d for 5 years, no cataracts were found [54]. Therefore, the risk of cataracts in patients taking ICS is thought to be negligible.

Local Effects

Candida spp colonization and dysphonia are common adverse effects of patients using ICS. *Candida* organisms can be cultured in about 50% of ICS-treated patients, but clinical thrush is noted in 0% to 34% [1••]. In a large study of 639 children treated with either budesonide or beclomethasone for at least 1 month, hoarseness occurred in 14.1%, and dysphonia was noted in 11.1% [55]. Oral candidiasis occurred in 10.7%. Using a spacer or holding chamber with an MDI or rinsing the mouth with water after DPI reduces colonization of *Candida* organisms and clinical thrush [56]. Dysphonia is reported in 5% to 50% of patients using an ICS, and its incidence is dose-related [57].

Preventing Adverse Effects

The risk of systemic effects is generally low with ICS. Using a spacer or holding chamber with MDIs decreases

---

Table 15-3A. GOALS OF ASTHMA TREATMENT

Prevent chronic and troublesome symptoms (*eg*, coughing or breathlessness in the night, in the early morning, or after exertion)

Maintain (near) "normal" pulmonary function

Maintain normal activity levels (including exercise and other physical activity)

Prevent recurrent exacerbations of asthma and minimize the need for emergency department visits or hospitalizations

Provide optimal pharmacotherapy with minimal or no adverse effects

Meet patients' and families' expectations of and satisfaction with asthma care

---

Table 15-3B. STEPWISE APPROACH FOR MANAGING ASTHMA IN ADULTS AND CHILDREN OLDER THAN 5 YEARS OF AGE

Clinical Features Before Treatment*	Symptoms[†]	Nighttime Symptoms	Lung Function
Step 4 (severe persistent)	Continual symptoms	Frequent	FEV_1 or PEF ≤ 60% predicted
	Limited physical activity		
	Frequent exacerbations		PEF variability > 30%
Step 3 (moderate persistent)	Daily symptoms	> 1 time a week	FEV_1 or PEF > 60%– < 80% predicted
	Daily use of inhaled short-acting β$_2$-agonist		PEF variability > 30%
	Exacerbations affect activity		
	Exacerbations ≥ 2 times a week; may last days		
Step 2 (mild persistent)	Symptoms > 2 times a week but < 1 time a day	> 2 times a month	FEV_1 or PEF ≥ 80% predicted
	Exacerbations may affect activity		PEF variability 20%–30%
Step 1 (mild intermittent)	Symptoms ≤ 2 times a week	≤ 2 times a month	FEV_1 or PEF ≥ 80% predicted
	Asymptomatic and normal PEF between exacerbations		PEF variability < 20%
	Exacerbations brief (from a few hours to a few days); intensity may vary		

*The presence of one of the features of severity is sufficient to place a patient in that category. An individual should be assigned to the most severe grade in which any feature occurs. The characteristics noted in this figure are general and may overlap because asthma is highly variable. Furthermore, an individual's classification may change over time.

[†]Patients at any level of severity can have mild, moderate, or severe exacerbations. Some patients with intermittent asthma experience severe and life-threatening exacerbations separated by long periods of normal lung function and no symptoms.

FEV_1—forced expiratory volume in 1 second; PEF—peak expiratory flow.

oropharyngeal deposition. Rinsing the mouth after DPI administration has a similar effect.

Reducing the dose of ICS to the lowest effective dose may limit unwanted effects. An adjuvant to this approach may be the addition of a second asthma medication. Numerous studies have found this to be preferable to increasing ICS dose, and in most the dose of ICS can be tapered. The recent release of a fluticasone/salmeterol combination inhaler, which comes in three different strengths, has made this an attractive option. The combination of fluticasone and salmeterol has been found to be superior to increasing ICS dose [58] or the addition of leukotriene modifier or theophylline to current ICS dose.

GOALS AND CLASSIFICATION OF ASTHMA

Table 15-3 depicts the goals of asthma treatment and the classification of asthma based on symptoms and lung function. Tables 15-4 and 15-5 outline a stepwise approach for management of asthma in adults and children older than 5 years of age. Table 15-6 describes the treatment of infants and children younger than 5 years of age with acute and chronic symptoms.

Mild Intermittent Asthma

By definition, patients with mild intermittent asthma experience symptoms two or fewer times per week with nocturnal symptoms occurring two or fewer times per month, and these patients show normal lung function. ICS therapy is not indicated for all patients with mild intermittent asthma. Short-acting β_2-agonist is the primary treatment, but long-term control therapy may be indicated if symptoms are troublesome. Low-dose ICSs may be appropriate for some patients with mild intermittent asthma.

Mild Persistent Asthma

Studies suggest (but do not prove) that the earlier one starts an ICS, the better the resultant lung function [8,9]. Patients with mild persistent asthma should use an anti-inflammatory medication along with a short-acting β_2-agonist for symptom relief. Studies suggest that an ICS is the agent of choice in patients with mild persistent asthma because ICSs decrease inflammatory mediators, improve smooth muscle dysfunction, and prevent airway wall remodeling. The addition of budesonide in a nebulizable form makes ICS use appropriate for children younger than 5 years of age.

In patients who are uncomfortable with an ICS or unable to comply with the dosing regimens, leukotriene modifiers, cromolyn, nedocromil, or theophylline may be appropriate. However, head-to-head studies of these agents compared with ICSs showed that ICSs are better at controlling airways responsiveness, asthma control, and increasing PEF.

Moderate Persistent Asthma

Inhaled corticosteroids have been extensively studied in patients with moderate persistent asthma. For these patients, an ICS should be initiated at the medium dosage range. After good asthma control is reached, the dose of ICS should be tapered to the lowest effective dose. If symptoms and lung function do not improve with ICS at moderate doses, then asthma therapy should be intensified. One strategy is to increase the ICS dose. A second strategy is to add a second asthma medication, such as a long-acting β_2-agonist, leukotriene modifier, or theophylline. It is always important to review medication compliance, inhaler technique, and objective measures of lung function. Recent data [59] suggest that the most effective step up in management would be to add a long-acting β_2-agonist to ICS. This has been found to be more effective than the addition of a leukotriene modifier or theophylline.

Severe Asthma

Higher dosages of ICS may be required for patients with severe asthma. If both oral corticosteroids and ICSs are used, patients are at increased risk of corticosteroid systemic effects. Encouraging adequate intake of calcium and vitamin D is a simple measure for all patients taking high-dose ICSs or oral corticosteroids. Monitoring of growth in children and BMD in adults and an eye examination by an ophthalmologist may be useful. Combined therapy of ICS and long-acting β_2-agonists is appropriate for most patients with severe asthma. Review of medication compliance, inhaler technique, and triggers are important. Many studies support the use of a high-potency ICS, such as fluticasone, especially in patients in whom compliance is crucial to asthma control.

A small number of patients with severe asthma fail to respond even to high dosages of oral corticosteroids. By definition, a patient with steroid-resistant asthma fails to improve FEV_1 or PEF by greater than 15% after treatment with oral prednisolone (30 to 40 mg/d for 2 weeks). This complete resistance is rare, with a prevalence of less than one in 1000 asthmatic patients. For asthma unresponsive to corticosteroids, it may be wise to look for other causes of recalcitrant disease such as vocal cord dysfunction, left ventricular failure, or cystic fibrosis.

CONCLUSIONS

Several important clinical questions remain concerning the use of ICSs in patients with asthma. More information must be gathered to understand the effects of ICSs on the natural course of asthma and airway remodeling. The relative benefits and risks of different ICS agents and delivery devices should be studied further.

Inhaled corticosteroids are still the most effective means of long-term control of patients with asthma. ICSs improve lung function, reduce rescue medication requirement, and decrease hospitalization rate and

Table 15-4. STEPWISE APPROACH FOR MANAGING ASTHMA IN ADULTS AND CHILDREN OLDER THAN 5 YEARS OF AGE: TREATMENT OF MODERATE AND SEVERE ASTHMA*

	Long-term Control	Quick Relief	Education
Step 4 (severe persistent)	Daily medications: **Anti-inflammatory: inhaled corticosteroid (high dose)** **AND** Long-acting bronchodilator: either **long-acting inhaled β$_2$-agonist,** sustained-release theophylline, or long-acting β$_2$-agonist tablets AND Corticosteroid tablets or syrup long term (make repeat attempts to reduce systemic steroids and maintain control with high-dose inhaled steroids)	Short-acting bronchodilator: **inhaled β$_2$-agonists** as needed for symptoms Intensity of treatment will depend on severity of exacerbation Use of short-acting inhaled β$_2$-agonists on a daily basis, or increasing use, indicates the need for additional long-term control therapy	Steps 2 and 3 actions plus: Refer to individual education/counseling
Step 3 (moderate persistent)	Daily medication: Either **Anti-inflammatory: inhaled corticosteroid (medium dose)** OR Inhaled corticosteroid (low-medium dose) and add a long-acting bronchodilator, especially for nighttime symptoms; either **long-acting inhaled β$_2$-agonist,** sustained-release theophylline, or long-acting β$_2$-agonist tablets If needed Anti-inflammatory: **inhaled corticosteroids (medium-high dose)** **AND** **Long-acting bronchodilator,** especially for nighttime symptoms; either **long-acting inhaled β$_2$-agonist,** sustained-release theophylline, or long-acting β2-agonist tablets	Short-acting bronchodilator: **inhaled β$_2$-agonists** as needed for symptoms Intensity of treatment will depend on severity of exacerbation Use of short-acting inhaled β$_2$-agonists on a daily basis, or increasing use, indicates the need for additional long-term-control therapy	Step 1 actions plus: Teach self-monitoring Refer to group education if available Review and update self-management plan

Preferred treatments are highlighted in bold.

Table 15-5. STEPWISE APPROACH FOR MANAGING ASTHMA IN ADULTS AND CHILDREN OLDER THAN 5 YEARS OF AGE: TREATMENT OF MILD ASTHMA*

	Long-term Control	Quick Relief	Education
Step 2 (mild persistent)†	One daily medication: **Anti-inflammatory:** either **inhaled corticosteroid (low doses) or cromolyn or nedocromil** Sustained-release theophylline-to-serum concentration of 5–15 µg/mL is an alternative, but not preferred, therapy Zafirlukast or zileuton may also be considered for patients ≥ 12 years of age, although their position in therapy is not fully established	Short-acting bronchodilator: **inhaled β₂-agonists** as needed for symptoms Intensity of treatment will depend on severity of exacerbation Use of short-acting inhaled β₂-agonists on a daily basis, or increasing use, indicates the need for additional long-term control therapy	Step 1 actions plus: Teach self-monitoring Refer to group education if available Review and update self-management plan
Step 1 (mild intermittent)	No daily medication is needed	Short-acting bronchodilator: **inhaled β₂-agonists** as needed for symptoms Intensity of treatment will depend on severity of exacerbation Use of short-acting inhaled β₂-agonists 2 times/wk may indicate the need to initiate long-term-control therapy	Teach basic facts about asthma Teach inhaler/spacer/holding chamber technique Discuss roles of medications Develop self-management plan Develop action plan for when and how to take rescue actions, especially for patients with a history of severe exacerbations Discuss appropriate environmental control measures to avoid exposure to known allergens and irritants

Step down

Review treatment every 1 to 6 mo; a gradual stepwise reduction in treatment may be possible.

Step up

If control is not maintained, consider step up. First, review patient medication technique, adherence, and environmental control (avoidance of allergens or other factors that contribute to asthma severity).

Preferred treatments are in bold.
†*The following points should be kept in mind:*
The stepwise approach presents general guidelines to assist clinical decision making; it is not intended to be a specific prescription. Asthma is highly variable; clinicians should tailor specific medication plans to the needs and circumstances of individual patients. Gain control as quickly as possible; then decrease treatment to the least medication necessary to maintain control. Gaining control may be accomplished by either starting treatment at the step most appropriate to the initial severity of the condition or starting at a higher level of therapy (eg, a course of systemic corticosteroids or higher dose of inhaled corticosteroids).
A rescue course of systemic corticosteroids may be needed at any time and at any step.
Some patients with intermittent asthma experience severe and life-threatening exacerbations separated by long periods of normal lung function and no symptoms. This may be especially common with exacerbations provoked by respiratory infections. A short course of systemic corticosteroids is recommended. At each step, patients should control their environment to avoid or control factors that make their asthma worse (eg, allergens, irritants); this requires specific diagnosis and education.
Referral to an asthma specialist for consultation or comanagement is recommended if there are difficulties achieving or maintaining control of asthma or if the patient requires step 4 care. Referral may be considered if the patient requires step 3 care.

Table 15-6. STEPWISE APPROACH FOR MANAGING INFANTS AND YOUNG CHILDREN (5 YEARS OF AGE AND YOUNGER) WITH ACUTE OR CHRONIC ASTHMA SYMPTOMS

	Long-term Control	Quick Relief
Step 4 (severe persistent)	Daily anti-inflammatory medicine High-dose inhaled corticosteroid with spacer/holding chamber and face mask If needed, add systemic corticosteroids, 2 mg/kg/d, and reduce to lowest daily or alternate-day dose that stabilizes symptoms	Bronchodilator as needed for symptoms (see step 1) up to 3 times/d
Step 3 (moderate persistent)	Daily anti-inflammatory medication. Either: Medium-dose inhaled corticosteroid with spacer/holding chamber and face mask OR, once control is established: Medium-dose inhaled corticosteroid and nedocromil OR medium-dose inhaled corticosteroid and long-acting bronchodilator (theophylline)	Bronchodilator as needed for symptoms (see step 1) up to 3 times/d
Step 2 (mild persistent)	Daily anti-inflammatory medication. Either: Cromolyn (nebulizer is preferred; or MDI) or nedocromil (MDI only) Infants and young children usually begin with a trial of cromolyn or nedocromil OR low-dose inhaled corticosteroid with spacer/holding chamber and face mask	Bronchodilator as needed for symptoms (see step 1)
Step 1 (mild intermittent)	No daily medication needed	Bronchodilator as needed for symptoms ≤ 2 times/wk Intensity of treatment will depend on severity of exacerbation (see below). Either: Inhaled short-acting β_2-agonist by nebulizer or face mask and a spacer/holding chamber OR oral β_2-agonist for symptoms With viral respiratory infection Bronchodilator q 4–6 h up to 24 h (longer with physician consult) but, in general, repeat no more than once every 6 wk Consider systemic corticosteroid if current exacerbation is severe OR patient has history of previous severe exacerbations

Step down

Review treatment every 1–6 mo. If control is sustained for at least 3 mo, a gradual stepwise reduction in treatment may be possible.

Step up

If control is not achieved, consider step up. However, first review patient medication technique, adherence, and environmental control (avoidance of allergens or other precipitant factors).

The following points should be kept in mind:
The stepwise approach presents guidelines to assist clinical decision making. Asthma is highly variable; clinicians should tailor specific medication plans to the needs and circumstances of individual patients.
Gain control as quickly as possible; then decrease treatment to the least medication necessary to maintain control. Gaining control may be accomplished by either starting treatment at the step most appropriate to the initial severity of their condition or by starting at a higher level of therapy (eg, a course of systemic corticosteroids or higher dose of inhaled corticosteroids).
A rescue course of systemic corticosteroid (prednisolone) may be needed at any time and step.
In general, use of short-acting β_2-agonist on a daily basis indicates the need for additional long-term control therapy.
It is important to remember that there are very few studies on asthma therapy for infants.
Consultation with an asthma specialist is recommended for patients with moderate or severe persistent asthma in this age group.
Consultation should be considered for all patients with mild persistent asthma.

mortality. The risk of systemic effects is low when ICS doses are within recommended ranges. ICSs are recommended for patients with mild, moderate, and severe persistent asthma.

REFERENCES AND RECOMMENDED READING

Papers of particular interest, published recently, have been highlighted as:
* • *Of importance*
* •• *Of major importance*

1.•• National Heart, Lung, and Blood Institute, National Asthma Education and Prevention Program: *Expert Panel Report 2: Guidelines for the Diagnosis and Management of Asthma.* Bethesda, MD: National Institutes of Health, Pub. No. 97-4051; 1997.
This is a wonderful set of guidelines to help approach the treatment of patients with asthma.

2. Adams RJ, Fuhlbrigge A, Finkelstein JA, *et al.*: Impact of inhaled antiinflammatory therapy on hospitalization and emergency department visits for children with asthma. *Pediatrics* 2001, 107:706–711.

3.•• Suissa S, Ernst P, Benayoun S, *et al.*: Low-dose inhaled corticosteroids and the prevention of death from asthma. *N Engl J Med* 2000, 343:332–336.
This landmark paper justifies the use of ICS in asthma.

4. Miesfeld RL, Bloom JW: Glucocorticoid receptor structure and function. In *Inhaled Glucocorticoids in Asthma: Mechanisms and Clinical Actions.* Edited by Schleimer RP, Busse WW, O'Byne PM. New York: Marcel Dekker; 1997:3–28.

5. Barnes PJ: Inhaled glucocorticoids for asthma. *N Engl J Med* 1995, 332:868–875.

6. Barnes PJ: Efficacy of inhaled corticosteroids in asthma. *J Allergy Clin Immunol* 1998, 102:531–538.

7. Barnes PJ: Effect of corticosteroid on airways hyperresponsiveness. *Am J Respir Crit Care Med* 1990, 141(suppl):70–76.

8. Olivieri D, Chetta A, Del Donno M, *et al.*: Effect of short-term treatment of low-dose inhaled fluticasone propionate on airway inflammation and remodeling in mild asthma: a placebo-controlled study. *Am J Respir Crit Care Med* 1997, 155:1864–1871.

9. Haahtela T, Jarvinen M, Tuomo K, *et al.*: Comparison of a beta agonist terbutaline with an inhaled steroid, budesonide, in newly detected asthma. *N Engl J Med* 1991, 325:388–392.

10.•• Eisner MD, Lieu TA, Capra AM, *et al.*: Beta agonist, inhaled corticosteroids and the risk of intensive care unit admission for asthma. *Eur Respir J* 2001, 17:233–240.
This is another great paper that provides a basis for continued ICS use in persistent asthma of varying severity.

11. Haahtela T, Jarvinen M, Kava T, *et al.*: Effects of reducing or discontinuing inhaled budesonide in patients with mild asthma. *N Engl J Med* 1994, 331:700–705.

12. Selroos O, Pretnalcho A, Lofroos AB, *et al.*: Effects of early and late interventions with inhaled corticosteroids in asthma. *Chest* 1995, 108:1228–1234.

13. Wenzel SE, Morgan K, Griffin R *et al.*: Improvement in health care utilization and pulmonary function with fluticasone propionate in patients with steroid-dependent asthma at a national asthma referral center. *J Asthma* 2001, 38:405–412.

14.•• Childhood Asthma Management Program Research Group: Long-term effects of budesonide or nedocromil in children with asthma. *N Engl J Med* 2000, 343:1054–1063.
This article sheds light on the treatment of asthma in children.

15. Price JF, Weller PH: Comparison of fluticasone propionate and sodium cromoglycate for treatment of childhood asthma. *Respir Med* 1995, 89:363–368.

16. Galant SP, Lawrence M, Meltzer EO, *et al.*: Fluticasone propionate compared with theophylline for mild to moderate asthma. *Ann Allergy Asthma Immunol* 1996, 77:112–118.

17. Reed CE, Offord KP, Nelson HS, *et al.*: Aerosol beclomethasone dipropionate spray compared with theophylline as primary treatment for chronic mild to moderate asthma: the American Academy of Allergy, Asthma and Immunology Beclomethasone ipropionate Study Group. *J Allergy Clin Immunol* 1998, 101:14–23. •

18. Lazarus SC, Boushey HA, Fahy JV, *et al.*: Long acting beta2-agonist monotherapy versus continued therapy with inhaled corticosteroids in patients with persistent asthma: a randomized controlled trial. *JAMA* 2001, 285:2583–2593.

19. Malmstrom K, Rodriguez-Gomez, G, Guerra J, *et al.*: Oral montelukast, inhaled beclomethasone and placebo for chronic asthma: a randomized, controlled trial: Montelukast/Beclomethasone Study Group. *Ann Intern Med* 1999, 130:487–495.

20. Bleecker E, Welch MJ, Weinstein SF, *et al.*: Low-dose fluticasone propionate versus zafirlukast in the treatment of persistent asthma. *J Allergy Clin Immunol* 2000, 105:1123–1129.

21. Busse W, Raphael GD, Galant S, *et al.*: Low-dose fluticasone propionate compared with montelukast for first line treatment of persistent asthma: a randomized clinical trial. *J Allergy Clin Immunol* 2001, 107:461–468.

22. Kim KT, Ginchansky EJ, Friedman BF, *et al.*: Fluticasone propionate versus zafirlukast: effect in patients previously receiving inhaled corticosteroid therapy. *Ann Allergy Asthma Immunol* 2000, 85:398–406.

23• Shrewbury S, Pyke S, Britton M: Meta-analysis of increased dose of inhaled steroid or addition of salmeterol in symptomatic asthma (MIASMA). *Br Med J* 2000, 320:1368–1373.
This is a wonderful meta-analysis of the additive therapy, salmeterol.

24. Baba K, Sakakibara A, Yagi T, *et al.*: Effects of theophylline withdrawal in well-controlled asthmatics treated with inhaled corticosteroid. *J Asthma* 2001, 38:615–624.

25. Li J, Mo H, Huang H: Effect of low dose inhaled corticosteroid combined with small dose of oral theophylline on treatment of bronchial asthma. *Chin J Tuberculosis Respir Dis* 2000, 23:336–339.

26. Laviolette M, Malmstrom K, Lu S, *et al.*: Montelukast added to inhaled beclomethasone in treatment of asthma. *Am J Respir Crit Care Med* 1999, 160:1862–1868.

27. Johnson M: Development of fluticasone propionate and comparison with other inhaled corticosteroids. *J Allergy Clin Immunol* 1998, 101(suppl):434–439.

28. Holt S, Suder A, Weatherall M, *et al.*: Dose response relation of inhaled fluticasone propionate in adolescents and adults with asthma: meta-analysis. *Br Med J* 2001, 323:253–256.

29. Kelly HW: Establishing a therapeutic index for the inhaled corticosteroids: part 1, pharmacokinetics/pharmacodynamic comparison of the inhaled corticosteroids. *J Allergy Clin Immunol* 1998, 102(suppl):36–51.

30. Dempsey OJ, Wilson AM, Coutie WJ, *et al.*: Evaluation of the effect of a large volume spacer on the systemic bioactivity of fluticasone propionate metered dose inhaler. *Chest* 1999, 116:935–940.

31.•• Rubin BK, Kelly HW: The impact of drug delivery devices in asthma management. *J Respir Dis* 2002, 23(suppl A):36–43.
An excellent review of devices for asthma medication and their efficacy.

32. Barnes PJ, Pedersen S, Busse WW: Efficacy and safety of inhaled corticosteroids: new developments. *Am J Respir Crit Care Med* 1998, 157(suppl):1–53.

33. Schuh S, Johnson DW, Stephens D, et al.: Comparison of albuterol delivered by a metered dose inhaler with spacer versus nebulizer in children with mild acute asthma. *J Pediatrics* 1999, 135:22–27.

34. Montreal Protocol: The Montreal Protocol on substances that deplete the ozone layer. Final Act (Nairobi: UNEP, 1987). *Federal Register* 1994, 59:56276–56298.

35. Vanden Burgt JA, Busse WW, Martin RJ, et al.: Efficacy and safety overview of a new inhaled corticosteroid, QVAR (hydrofluoroalkane-beclomethsaone extrafine inhalation aerosol), in asthma. *J Allergy Clin Immunol* 2000, 106:1209–1226.

36. Meakin BJ, Ganderton D, Panza I, et al.: The effect of flow rate on drug delivery from the Pulvinal, a high-resistance dry powder inhaler. *J Aerosol Med* 1998, 11:143–152.

37. Prime D, Parkes PA, Petchy L, et al.: Evaluation of the pharmaceutical performance of two dry powder inhalers: comparison of Diskus and Turbuhaler inhalers. *Am J Respir Crit Care Med* 1996, 153(suppl A):62.

38. Szefler SJ: A review of budesonide inhalation suspension in the treatment of pediatric asthma. *Pharmacotherapy* 2001, 21:195–206.

39.•• Allen DB. The safety of inhaled corticosteroids in the treatment of asthma. *J Respir Dis* 2002, 23(suppl A):16–26.
This is an excellent review of the literature surrounding the side effects of ICS use.

40. Doull IJ, Freezer NJ, Holgate ST: Growth of prepubertal children with mild asthma treated with beclomethasone dipropionate. *Am J Respir Crit Care Med* 1995, 151:1715–1719.

41. Affrime MB, Kosoglou T, Thonoor CM, et al.: Mometasone furoate has minimal effects on the hypothalamic-pituitary-adrenal axis when delivered at high doses. *Chest* 2000, 118:1538–1546.

42. Ayers JG, Bateman ED, Lundback B, et al.: High dose fluticasone propionate, 1 mg daily versus fluticasone 2 mg daily or budesonide 1.6 mg daily in patients with chronic severe asthma. International Study Group. *Eur Respir J* 1995, 8:579–586.

43. Li JT, Goldstein MF, Gross GN, et al.: Effects of fluticasone propionate, triamcinolone acetonide, prednisone and placebo on the hypothalamic-pituitary-adrenal axis. *J Allergy Clin Immunol* 1999, 103:622–629.

44. Li JT, Ford LB, Chervinsky P, et al.: Fluticasone propionate powder and lack of clinically significant effects on hypothalamic-pituitary-adrenal axis and bone mineral density over 2 years in adults with mild asthma. *J Allergy Clin Immunol* 1999, 103:1062–1068.

45. Hodsman AB, Toogood JH, Jennings B, et al.: Differential effects of inhaled budesonide and oral prednisone on serum osteocalcin. *J Clin Endocrinol Metab* 1991, 72:530–540.

46. Villareal Ms, Klaustermeyer WB, Hahn TJ, et al.: Osteoporosis in steroid-dependent asthma. *Ann Allergy Asthma Immunol* 1996, 76:369–372.

47. Wong CA, Walsh LJ, Smith CJ, et al.: Inhaled corticosteroid use and bone mineral density on patients with asthma. *Lancet* 2000, 355:1399–1403.

48. Meeran K, Hattersley A, Burrin J, et al.: Oral and inhaled corticosteroids reduce bone formation as shown by plasma osteocalcin levels. *Am J Respir Crit Care Med* 1995, 151:333–336.

49. Tinkelman DG, Reed CE, Nelson HS, Offord KP: Aerosol beclomethasone dipropionate compared with theophylline as primary treatment of chronic, mild to moderately severe asthma in children [see comments]. Pediatrics 1993, 92:144–146.

50. Allen DB, Bronsky EA, LaForce CF, et al.: Growth in asthmatic children treated with fluticasone propionate: Fluticasone Propionate Asthma Study Group. *J Pediatrics* 1998, 132:472–477.

51.•• Price JF, Russell G, Hindmarsh PD, et al.: Growth during one year of treatment with fluticasone propionate or sodium cromoglycate in children with asthma. *Pediatr Pulmonol* 1997, 24:178–186.
This is a reassuring study of growth in ICS-treated children that is of long duration and is nicely controlled.

52. Agertoft L, Pedersen S: Effect of long term treatment with inhaled budesonide on adult height in children with asthma. *N Engl J Med* 2000, 343:1064–1069.

53. Toogood JH, Markov AE, Baskerville J, et al.: Association of ocular cataracts with inhaled and oral steroid therapy during long term treatment of asthma. *J Allergy Clin Immunol* 1993, 91:571–579.

54. Simons FE, Persaud MP, Gillespie CA, et al.: Absence of posterior subcapsular cataracts in patients treated with inhaled glucocorticoids. *Lancet* 1993, 342:776–778.

55. Dubus JC, Marguet C, Deschildre A, et al.: Local side effects of inhaled corticosteroids in asthmatic children: influence of drug, dose, age and device. *Allergy* 2001, 56:944–948.

56. Toogood JH, White FA, Baskerville JC, et al.: Comparison of the antiasthmatic, oropharyngeal and systemic glucocorticoid effects of budesonide administered through a pressurized aerosol plus spacer or the Turbuhaler dry powder inhaler. *J Allergy Clin Immunol* 1997, 99:186–193.

57. Toogood JH, Jennings B, Greenway RW, et al.: Candidiasis and dysphonia complicating beclomethasone treatment of asthma. *J Allergy Clin Immunol* 1980, 65:145–153.

58. Jenkins C, Woolcock AJ, Saarelainen P, et al.: Salmeterol/ fluticasone propionate combination therapy 50/250 twice daily is more effective than budesonide 800 mcg twice daily in treating moderate to severe asthma. *Respir Med* 2000, 94:715–723.

59. Nelson HS: Advair: combination treatment with fluticasone propionate/salmeterol in the treatment of asthma. *J Allergy Clin Immunol* 2001, 107:397–416.

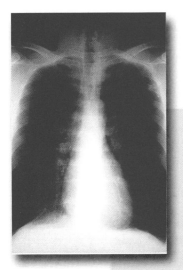

Short- and Long-acting Bronchodilators in Asthma

Robert Townley

PUTTING BRONCHODILATORS INTO PERSPECTIVE IN ASTHMA MANAGEMENT

The use of bronchodilators is a very important part of the pharmacologic therapy for patients with asthma. However, it is clear there are four essential components for the long-term control of asthma, and that pharmacologic therapy is only one of these. The other components include the assessment and monitoring of the symptoms of asthma, the spirometric or pulmonary function, and peak expiratory flow rate (PEFR) parameters. Other components include control of factors contributing to asthma severity and patient education for a partnership. The National Heart, Lung, and Blood Institute (NHLBI) guidelines [1] recommend establishing the patient–clinician partnership to address the patient's concerns, agree on the goals of asthma therapy, and create a written action plan for self-management. It is also important to treat asthma episodes promptly with the use of an inhaled short-acting inhaled β_2-agonist (SABA) and, if the episode is moderate to severe, a 3- to 10-day course of oral prednisone. If the symptoms are not controlled, an inhaled corticosteroids (ICS) can be added. The key is prompt communication and follow-up with the clinician to determine the effectiveness of the pharmacologic therapy. The effectiveness, of course, will be modified in the presence of inflammation caused by airway irritants, respiratory infections, and exposure to environmental allergens.

Another major recommendation is that all patients should monitor their symptoms. Patients with moderate to severe persistent asthma should also monitor their PEFR. Patients should be seen every 1 to 6 months, depending on the severity of their asthma and the degree of control. The need for repeated education is essential in terms of avoiding triggers and allergens, to determine the action plan with patients, and to determine if they are using their medications, especially their inhalers, properly.

Some of the goals of asthma therapy include prevention of chronic asthma symptoms and asthma exacerbations during the day and night, prevention of sleep disruption by asthma, reduction of missed school or work days attributed to asthma, and eliminating or reducing the need for emergency room visits or hospitalizations. This is in conjunction with the ability to maintain normal activity levels, including exercise and other physical activities, and to have normal or near-normal lung function. This is also while receiving optimal medications with no or minimal side effects. It is important that these goals be shared with the patient and the patient's family, and that a contract on these goals serve as the foundation for the treatment plan.

Although this chapter focuses on bronchodilators, it is still important to emphasize the role of long-term control medications that reduce airway inflammation, particularly ICSs, which are the most potent anti-inflammatory medications currently available. It also should be emphasized that β_2-adrenergic bronchodilators provide more effective relief when used in combination with ICSs than either agent alone. In fact, the combination of these two agents allows the patient to use a considerably lower dose of ICS.

The adrenal glands are situated so that the cortex and medulla that provide the corticosteroids and catecholamines for our own natural defense against asthma are intimately related anatomically and are associated with the production and release of both of these agents during periods of stress. The fact that the adrenal cortex and medulla are frequently activated simultaneously may provide insight into why the combination of β-agonists and ICSs is greater than the individual components and greater than the sum of the two components. There appears to be a synergistic as well as an additive effect of these two agents. Certain strains of mice and rats were much more sensitive to anaphylaxis, histamine, and serotonin after adrenalectomy or β-adrenergic blockade, or after pertussis toxin and catecholamines, including epinephrine [2–4]. β-agonists provided only minimal protection. Similarly, the injection of corticosteroids into these animals provided only minimal protection, even at fairly high doses. However, low doses of corticosteroid with low doses of β-agonists provided complete protection [2–5].

WHEN AND HOW TO USE BRONCHODILATORS

Quick-relief medications are used to provide prompt treatment of acute airway obstruction and its symptoms. These medications include SABAs and, in more severe cases, oral steroids. Anticholinergics may be used in special circumstances.

Asthma cannot be cured, but it can be controlled through pharmacotherapy and avoidance of specific triggers, irritants, and allergens. Nevertheless, all patients should have an inhaled SABA to use as needed for symptoms. Patients with mild, moderate, or severe persistent asthma require daily, long-term medications to control their asthma.

Devices that hold the aerosol medication so the patient can inhale it easily are called spacers or holding chambers. Use of spacers avoids the problem or the difficulty of coordinating the actuation of the metered-dose inhaler (MDI) with the inhalation, which occurs at all ages, but especially in young children and the elderly. All children 5 years of age or younger with acute or chronic asthma symptoms need a SABA administered by nebulizer (0.05 mg/kg in 2 to 3 mL of saline) or inhaler with facemask and spacer (2 to 4 puffs; for exacerbations, repeat every 20 minutes for

≤ 1 hour), or oral β_2-agonist. With viral respiratory infections, SABAs every 4 to 6 hours and up to 24 hours may be required. If this persists beyond 24 hours, treatment should move up to the next step for managing asthma in patients who are 5 years of age and younger.

The medication delivery devices should be selected according to the child's ability to use them. Nebulized therapy is preferred for administering SABAs to children 2 years of age or younger. An MDI with a spacer or holding chamber that has a facemask may be used to administer inhaled steroids. In children 3 to 5 years of age, MDIs plus spacers may be used; however, if therapeutic effects are not realized, then a nebulizer or an MDI plus a space-holding chamber with facemask may be required. Appropriately sized facemasks, spacers with facemasks, and holding chamber devices need to be provided after proper instruction of the parents or caregivers. Various step-up programs for children and adults are available to physicians at www.nhlbi.nih.gov [6].

In older adults, it may be necessary to make adjustments to avoid asthma medications that can aggravate other conditions. Theophylline and epinephrine may exacerbate underlying heart conditions, and clearance of theophylline is reduced in the older patients.

The methylxanthines, *eg*, theophylline, which were standard therapy for asthma for a number of decades, induce certain side effects such as inattentiveness and hyperactivity in susceptible children. These and other adverse effects caused theophylline to become less commonly prescribed since the 1990s. However, the most commonly prescribed class of asthma medication, the racemic β_2-agonist, also caused a number of reversible side effects that may be disturbing to patients. A recent study suggests that individuals with asthma are disturbed more by quality of life issues and medication side effects than clinicians realize [7]. In this survey, questionnaires regarding the severity of asthma, treatment, and medication side effects were answered by 1230 pediatric and 604 adult asthmatic patients. The unwanted side effects were from their bronchodilators, which were primarily associated with racemic albuterol in either generic or brand form. Side effects were even more common when these agents were administered by nebulizers in all ages of patients as well as in pediatric patients using oral β-agonists. The most common troublesome side effects were jitteriness (58%), restlessness (57%), tachycardia (56%), and cough (56%) in pediatric patients. In adults, the most common troublesome side effects were tachycardia (64%), jitteriness (60%), shaky hands (43%), and restlessness (42%). Because of these side effects, up to 30% of patients reduced their bronchodilator dose on their own, and approximately 25% of patients skipped doses to avoid unwanted side effects. When patients spoke to their physicians, the majority of whom were either allergists or pulmonologists, the most common response was to change the brand of medication, change the class of medication, or adjust the dose. Nevertheless, because most of these side effects are directly attributed to β-adrenergic stimulation and because the medications were necessary for the treatment, they were advised that the side effects were to be expected. The patients were advised to tolerate the side effects because the medications were necessary. It was observed that the side effects were significantly less with the use of MDIs than with nebulizers or oral β-adrenergic–agonist medications. These findings point out the importance of physicians maintaining a good understanding of patients' compliance and their ability to tolerate side effects, and further illustrate the need to develop better bronchodilators with fewer unwanted side effects.

β-Blockers, especially nonselective β-blockers, should be avoided. When considering the use of β-blockers, it is essential that the physician ask if the patient is using eyedrops for glaucoma, which can severely exacerbate asthma and frequently may be overlooked as a cause of either severe or chronic persistent asthma. Studies in patients with asthma demonstrate that even 1 mg of propranolol intravenously significantly increased airway reactivity to methacholine and decreased pulmonary function [8]. In some allergic rhinitis patients who have underlying airway hyperresponsiveness, the β-adrenergic–blockers may also increase airway responsiveness to methacholine [9]. In addition, β-adrenergic–blockers are contraindicated because of the risk of anaphylaxis, and blocking the effect of their endogenous as well as exogenous β-adrenergic–agonist can lead to deterioration of asthma.

For patients with exercise-induced asthma, the diagnosis may be confirmed by prevention of symptoms or decrease in PEFR by using a SABA 5 to 60 minutes before exercise. The effects of treatment should last 2 to 3 hours. An inhaled long-acting β-agonist (LABA) provides protection for up to 10 to 12 hours. Teachers and coaches must be made aware that a child may need inhaled medication before activity. For adult patients with moderate persistent asthma or severe persistent asthma, salmeterol (Serevent; GlaxoSmithKline, Research Triangle Park, NC) or formoterol (Foradil; Novartis Pharmaceuticals, New York) 2 puffs every 12 hours is recommended along with their inhaled steroids.

FUNCTION OF ADRENERGIC RECEPTORS

The therapeutic effects elicited by changes in the target organs of asthma and the allergic response occur by interaction of the β-agonist bronchodilator with cell membrane receptors that are coupled to intracellular guanine nucleotide-binding regulatory proteins, designated G proteins. These G proteins mediate the signal transduction resulting from the effect of adrenergic agents on the specific receptors (Fig. 16-1) [10]. The various adrenergic receptor subtypes are members of the G protein–coupled superfamily of receptors. The understanding of these G

protein–coupled receptor signal transduction events has markedly increased as a result of a great deal of basic research. These various adrenergic receptors are unique products of distinct genes.

The human β$_2$-adrenergic receptor was cloned in 1986. Since then, nine human adrenergic receptor genes have been identified. G proteins mediate the signal transduction generated from the effect of adrenergic agents on the specific receptors. The G proteins are composed of α, β, and γ subunits and have been extensively reviewed [11]. A given G protein may transduce signals to several different effectors. The expression of G proteins and effectors varies in different cell types. These effector systems include not only affects on adenylate cyclase and cAMP, but also several other systems, including effects of cGMP phosphodiesterase, ion channels, and phospholipases. This results in various metabolic and ion changes within the cell or on the cell surface, which have several physiologic consequences on airway smooth muscle cells (SMC), a wide variety of cells in the airway, and the inflammatory cells associated with the allergic response (Table 16-1).

All of the various adrenergic receptors have in common seven membrane-spanning amino acid sequences. The gene encoding the β$_1$-adrenergic receptor has been located on human chromosome 10q24-26, which is very close to the α$_{2A}$-adrenergic receptor gene. Whereas stimulation of the β$_2$-receptor results in the decrease in the adenylate cyclase and cAMP, stimulation of β-receptors stimulates adenylate cyclase and increases cAMP. The β$_2$-adrenergic receptor has been localized on human chromosome 5q31-32, which is in the same region as the gene for β$_{1B}$-receptor.

The β$_3$-adrenergic receptor appears to play a functional role in tissues such as muscle and adipose sites, with a particular distribution to brown and white adipose tissue. All three subtypes of β-receptor, *ie*, the β$_1$-, β$_2$-, and β$_3$-adrenergic receptor, are coupled to the G$_s$ adenylyl cyclase effective pathway and result in increases in intracellular cAMP after agonist binding. Stimulation of the β$_1$-adrenergic receptor results in increased inotropic and chronotropic responses in the heart. The β$_2$-adrenergic receptors are located primarily in the lung and on many different cell types and tissues involved in the allergic response.

REGULATION OF ADRENERGIC RECEPTORS

It has been known since the 1950s that patients with severe asthma who do not responding to epinephrine or β-agonists will regain the efficacy for these bronchodilating agents approximately 4 hours after administration of corticosteroids. However, it was not until 1979 that the effect of hydrocortisone was shown to increase the density and activity of β-adrenergic receptors [4]. Furthermore, after bilateral adrenalectomy, the density and function of these β-adrenergic receptors in the lung were markedly decreased, further illustrating the regulation of the density and the function of β-adrenergic receptors by corticosteroids [4,12]. Furthermore, the genes for the β-adrenergic receptors contain DNA-binding sites for the glucocorticoid receptors [13]. The effect of β-adrenergic agents on β-receptors and the desensitization of the receptors that occurs have important implications in asthma therapy. This is particularly true for the LABAs. There has been considerable controversy regarding the regular use of β-agonists versus intermittent or on-demand use, because prolonged exposure of β-receptors to β-agonists results in receptor phosphorylation and is associated with impaired receptor G protein coupling [14]. In addition to phosphorylation of β-receptors, the prolonged exposure may also increase their internalization from the cell surface, and, therefore, make them unavailable for activation by β-adrenergic agonists.

Desensitization of the β-adrenergic receptors can occur as a result of homologous desensitization through the prolonged exposure of β-agonist, and results in β-adrenergic receptor kinase (βARK) [15]. A second type of regulation of β-receptors is known as heterologous desensitization. This may be an important mechanism in the decreased cAMP response that occurs in lymphocytes of asthmatic patients after allergen challenge and is associated with the late allergic reaction and with airway hyperresponsiveness [16]. The recent advances in understanding the various diverse types of adrenergic receptors

and their genetic and molecular biologic functions provides important opportunities to improve our understanding of autonomic deregulation in asthma. Furthermore, the interaction of the inflammatory responses is a result of the allergic reaction, which is associated with heterologous downregulation and decreased response to either endogenous or exogenously administered β-agonist.

INTERACTION OF α- AND β-ADRENERGIC MECHANISMS

Studies of the skin, pupil, and blood pressure by several investigators [17,18] provide evidence of increased α- and decreased β-adrenergic function in patients with asthma. However, α-adrenergic–blocking agents have not shown clinical efficacy in the treatment of patients with asthma, with the exception of exercise-induced asthma [19]. In testing human trachea and bronchi in vitro, the airway SMCs were contracted by epinephrine in the presence of the nonspecific β-blocker propranolol [20]. Use of hydrocortisone or the α-adrenergic blockers phentolamine and phenoxybenzamine resulted in the reduction or elimination of the contracting effect of epinephrine [20]. In patients with chronic obstructive pulmonary disease (COPD), airway SMCs show a greater direct contraction responsiveness to α-agonists than airways from healthy patients [21]. In contrast, airway SMCs from normal individuals show α-adrenergic contraction

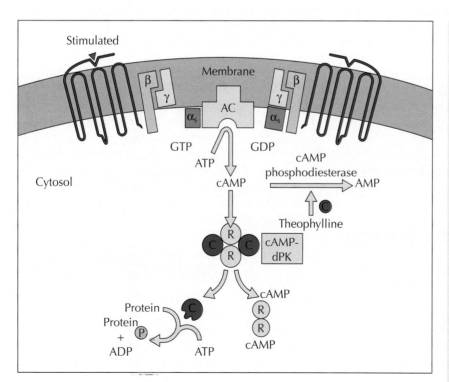

Figure 16-1.
Activation of adenylate cyclase (AC) and protein kinases. Shown are two β-adrenergic receptor molecules, each of which is composed of three transmembrane loops. Stimulation of the receptor (*left*) causes its activation, in which the α_s-protein binds guanosine triphosphate (GTP) and dissociates from the complex to the AC catalytic unit. Activated AC catalyzed the formation of cAMP, which binds to the regulatory units (R) of cAMP-dependent protein kinases (cAMP-dPK), thus freeing the catalytic units (C) to phosphorylate-specific proteins. The activated state exists only transiently; ATP hydrolysis to ADP leads to reassociation of the α_sBγ-complex of G_s, inactivation of AC, receptor regeneration, and the breakdown of AMP by phosphodiesterases. (*Adapted from* Holgate and Church [10].)

only when the SMCs were already partially depolarized by histamine or potassium chloride. This suggests that airway SMCs from subjects with asthma and some subjects with COPD are partially depolarized, and the effect of an α-agonist on contraction is enhanced. Human airways contain β_2-adrenergic receptors and may mediate an inhibition of cholinergic neurotransmission at the parasympathetic ganglia or at postganglionic parasympathetic nerve endings.

Antigen challenge in sensitized guinea pigs results in a diminution of the β_2-receptor and an increase in the α_1-receptor in lungs of animals exposed to a specific antigen [20,22].

SITE-DIRECTED MUTAGENESIS

Understanding of the structure and function of receptors has been markedly enhanced with the use of site-directed mutagenesis. Site-directed mutagenesis can affect agonist-binding affinity but not G_s activation. Studies in which stretches of the amino acid sequence are removed by deletion mutagenesis indicate that the third intracellular loop is critical for interaction between β_2-adrenergic receptors and G_s [23]. There are at least six different polymorphic forms of β_2-adrenergic–adrenergic receptors. These mutations are not the primary cause of asthma, but they may account for some of the clinical heterogeneity among patients with asthma as well as the response to β-agonists. Even single amino acid mutation of the β_2-adrenergic receptor can affect receptor function [24]. The lymphocytes of 56 healthy persons and 51 patients with moderately severe asthma were used to isolate the genomic DNA.

The distribution of β_2-adrenergic receptor mutations in the two populations is shown in Figure 16-2 [24]. Four mutations did cause changes in the encoded residues, and these occurred at amino positions 16, 27, 34, and 164. These investigators noticed a clustering of patients with ARG-16 to Gly polymorphism in 75% of patients who were corticosteroid-dependent (defined as the need for prednisone 20 mg/d for more 6 months). When these investigators compared this mutated receptor with the wild-type β_2-adrenergic receptor, they found several abnormalities [25].

A mutation of Gly-16 polymorphism of the β_2-adrenergic receptor results in enhanced downregulation of receptor number and is overrepresented in patients with nocturnal asthma [26]. In a separate study [27], investigators reported an association of Glu-27 β_2-adrenergic receptor polymorphism with a fourfold lower airway reactivity to methacholine compared with the wild-type Gln-27 genotype.

The Thr-164 to Ile-164 mutation results in affinities for β-agonist about four times lower than that of the wild type. This decreased binding affinity of catecholamines resulted in significant impairment of agonist-promoted signal transduction. With this mutation, the effect of epinephrine on adenylate cyclase was decreased about 50% in the Thr-164 to Ile-164 polymorphism. Thus, these mutations are not the primary cause of asthma but clearly could result in an altered severity of asthma or response to therapy according to the β_2-adrenergic genotype. A further understanding of receptor function and structure as well as knowing the receptor genotype of specific patients may be important in the development of new drugs that interact with the transcriptional and post-translational formation of receptors.

In a further study [28], these investigators found β_2-adrenergic receptor autoantibodies in 5% of healthy patients and in 40% of asthmatic patients. The presence of these antibodies resulted in a 40% inhibition of binding to β_2-receptors and a 50% attenuation of isoproterenol-

Table 16-1. CELLULAR EFFECTS OF β_2-ADRENERGIC RECEPTOR STIMULATION

Cell	Response
Airway SMC	Bronchodilation
Mast cells	Inhibition of mediator release
Eosinophils	Inhibition of mediator release and chemotaxis
Lymphocytes	Inhibition of activation
Skeletal muscle	Tremor
Metabolic	Hypokalemia, hyperglycemia
Mucous glands	Increased water content of mucus
Epithelial cells	Increased ciliary activity
Vascular endothelium	Decreased microvascular leakage
Alveolar type II cells	Increased surfactant secretion

SMC—smooth muscle cell.

stimulated cAMP production by these β_2-adrenergic receptor antibodies. The therapeutic response in such persons to β-agonists might be reduced considerably.

THE ROLE OF ION CHANNELS AND RELAXATION OF AIRWAY SMOOTH MUSCLE CELLS

Stimulation of β_2-adrenergic receptors causes hyperpolarization of airway SMCs and inhibits tension [20]. Conversely, stimulation of muscarinic receptors on airway SMCs causes depolarization and increases tension. β-adrenergic–agonist bronchodilators increase membrane conductance of potassium, and potassium channel blockers inhibit the hyperpolarization [29]. β-agonist stimulation of airway SMCs results in stimulation of calcium-activated potassium channels [30]. Stimulation of β-adrenergic receptors activates calcium-activated potassium channels by a second messenger, which results in phosphorylation of the channel protein and the opening of the potassium channel [31]. This is an important mechanism by which β-adrenergic receptors relax airway SMCs [32]. These β-adrenergic receptors are directly coupled to calcium-activated potassium channels through the guanine-nucleotide–binding protein. The inhibition of membrane voltage-dependent calcium channels may be an additional regulatory mechanism. Recent evidence suggests that the chloride channel may be an important regulatory mechanism of airway SMC function.

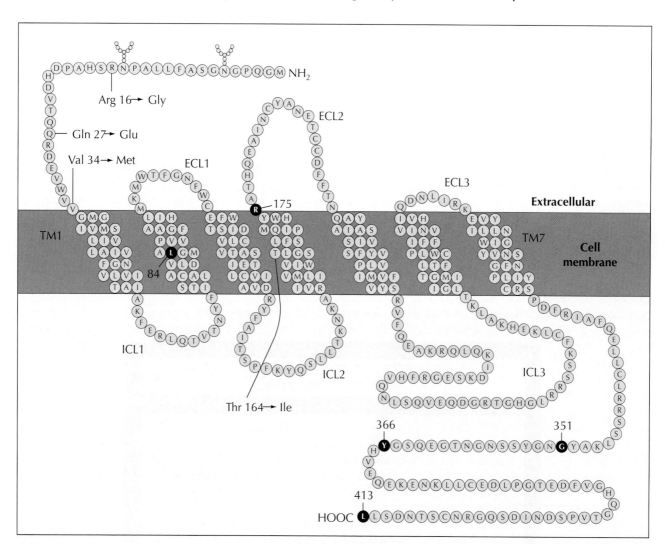

Figure 16-2.
Adrenergic receptor mutations found in patients with and without asthma. The *darkened circles* indicate where nucleic acid changes were detected. Regions of amino acid change ("missense mutations") are indicated by the amino acid substitutions (*eg*, Arg16→ Gly). Of the nine mutations found, five resulted in no amino acid changes, and four resulted in changes in the encoded residues indicated at amino acid positions 16, 27, 34, and 164. ECL1–ECL3—extracellular loops 1 to 3; ICL1–ICL3—intracellular loops; TM1 and TM7—transmembrane segments 1 and 7. (*Adapted from* Liggett [24].)

MECHANISMS INVOLVED IN RELAXATION OF AIRWAY SMOOTH MUSCLE CELLS

Bronchodilatation may involve at least three mechanisms. Elevation of tissue cAMP content, either by β-receptor activation or prostaglandin E stimulation of adenylate cyclase or by inhibiting the breakdown of cAMP with phosphodiesterase inhibitors, is one mechanism (*see* Fig. 16-1). The second mechanism is the elevation of tissue cGMP by agents such as nitric oxide or atrial natriuetic peptide. The third mechanism of relaxation is the direct action of drugs on ion channels, including voltage-operated calcium channel antagonists, which have a relatively weak effect, and potassium channel activators. There is significant crosstalk between second messenger pathways involving relaxation through the adenylate cyclase path and inositol phospholipids as a result of its formation in airway inflammatory cells and airway SMCs. An example is the effect of histamine, which induces inositol phosphate formation, which could be inhibited by β_2-adrenoceptor agonists in airway SMCs.

Patients with asthma are very sensitive to the inhalation of histamine. Because histamine is increased in the airways of asthmatic patients and contributes to airway tone, it seems potentially beneficial to inhibit its formation with LABAs. Airway SMC relaxation directly or indirectly involves and results from the reduction in intracellular calcium. Studies using isolated bronchial preparations or cultured cells show that inflammatory mediators and cytokines may alter calcium homeostasis in airway SMCs and render the cells nonspecifically hyperreactive to acetylcholine, histamine, and other bronchoconstrictor agents. The key events that modulate airway SMC shortening and contraction include increases in the cytosolic calcium concentration $(Ca^{2+})_i$ and phosphorylation of the light chains of myosin-2 by myosin light chain kinase [33]. An understanding of both the cellular and molecular mechanisms that promote airway SMC hyperresponsiveness is important in developing new strategies to treat patients with asthma. In this regard, an important area for investigation is agents that affect intracellular calcium in airway SMCs, *eg*, certain inflammatory mediators and cytokines. For example, inhalation of tumor necrosis factor-α (TNF-α) or interleukin-1β (IL-1β) can induce the nonspecific increase in bronchial responsiveness in humans [34,35]. Similarly, treatment of isolated tracheal rings with TNF-α or IL-1β increase SMC reactivity to a variety of stimuli, including histamine [36], carbachol [37], acetylcholine [38], and electric field stimulation [39].

Lysophosphatidic acid, a bioactive lipid released from activated platelets, increases contractile response to serotonin, substance P, and methacholine [40]. Bronchodilators, including β_2-agonists and other cAMP-elevating agents, are able to at least exert their bronchorelaxing effect through decreasing intracellular calcium. Current evidence points to calcium homeostasis in airway SMCs, which can be altered in vitro by a variety of extracellular stimuli that are relevant to the pathogenesis of asthma. However, the relationship between calcium dysfunction and airway SMC responsiveness in vitro is not clearly established. Nevertheless, the ability of extracellular stimuli such as proinflammatory cytokines TNF-α and IL-1β to enhance airway SMC responsiveness to agonists or to impair relaxation to β-agonists has important clinical implications. Modulation of calcium homeostasis in airway SMCs is a potential therapeutic target to inhibit airway hyperresponsiveness in asthma. β-adrenergic blocking agents cause bronchoconstriction in asthmatic patients but not in healthy individuals. In 1967, researchers suggested that there might be a defect in the β-adrenergic receptor function in individuals with asthma [2,41]. Human airways do not show functional adrenergic nerves to control airway SMCs; however, adrenergic nerves do influence cholinergic neurotransmission by prejunctional β-receptors [20,42]. It seems probable that circulating catecholamines would have a primary role in regulating bronchomotor tone through direct action on β-adrenergic receptors. It has been demonstrated that airways from asthmatic patients fail to relax normally to isoproterenol, suggesting a possible defect in β-receptor function in airway SMCs [20,43]. An abnormality in receptor coupling or in the biochemical pathways leading to relaxation has been implicated in the impaired response to β-adrenergic agonists [44].

CELLULAR EFFECTS OF β_2-ADRENERGIC RECEPTOR STIMULATION IN THE TARGET TISSUE OF ASTHMA

There is considerable evidence that the release of certain proinflammatory cytokines, as well as IL-13 and IL-4, results in modulation of G protein–coupled receptors and the associated calcium responses in airway SMCs [45–49]. The synthesis and release of certain cytokines and platelet activating factor (PAF) results in decreasing β-adrenergic response and increasing cholinergic response in the airways. Bronchial asthma might be partly caused by impaired β-adrenergic receptor function [41]. Several investigators [20,50] have observed downregulation of β-adrenergic receptors and upregulation of α-receptors in a guinea pig model of asthma. β-Adrenergic receptor function and circulating cat cholamines are the determining factors in the bronchodilating β-adrenergic receptor activity. The central and peripheral airway relaxation is mediated by β_2-adrenergic receptors, and the density of these receptors progressively increases from the trachea to the terminal bronchials [51]. It appears that β_2-receptors are regulated by circulating epinephrine and β_1-receptors are regulated by sympathetic nerves.

It is well demonstrated that β-agonists such as isoproterenol are more potent relaxants in the presence of intact airway epithelia and less potent when the epithelia has been damaged, as occurs after exposure to eosinophils in clinical asthma and in the late reaction [20]. Furthermore, the density of these β-receptors is higher in the epithelia than in the SMC itself [20]. Another contributing factor to the loss of the bronchodilating potency of β-agonists is the denudation of the airway epithelium with the loss of the epithelial-derived relaxant factor (EDRF) [20]. It is now clear that EDRF is nitric oxide, which is produced in airway epithelia constitutively and is induced as a result of the effect of certain proinflammatory cytokines (including TNF-α and IL-1α) on airway epithelium. Nitric oxide is increased in the exhaled air of asthmatic patients and is decreased to normal after administration of anti-IgE or corticosteroids [52]. $β_2$-Adrenergic receptors serve an important function in maintaining the integrity of the tight junctions between epithelial cells, thereby regulating the ion and fluid transport across epithelial cells. $β_2$-Adrenergic agents as well as phosphodiesterase type 4 inhibitors increase cAMP levels, and cAMP regulates the permeability of the airway mucosa as well as the vascular mucosa. $β_2$-Adrenergic receptor stimulation increases mucociliary clearance and increases the ciliary beat frequency [20] (Table 16-1).

$β_2$-Adrenergic receptors also exist on the cell membrane of human alveolar macrophages. These $β_2$-receptors may serve an important function because these macrophages contain several mediators, including leukotriene B4, leukotriene C4, PAF, IL-1, TNF, and superoxide anions. All of these mediators, as well as fibronectin-mediated phagocytosis and phagocytosis of microbes and immune complexes, can be modulated by cAMP. Furthermore, the release of lysosomal enzymes and mediators from alveolar macrophages is inhibited by increases in cAMP through activation of $β_2$-receptors [20,53] (*see* Table 16-1).

$β_2$-Agonists are the most potent agents for inhibiting mast cell degranulation and mast cell mediator release. Thus, in prevention and treatment of anaphylaxis, $β_2$-agonists are the most potent agents in inhibiting mast cell histamine release as well as certain mast cell-containing enzymes, cytokines such as TNF-α, and products of arachadonic acid, including the leukotrienes and prostaglandins [20] (*see* Table 16-1).

The release of oxygen radicals and lytic enzymes from neutrophils and eosinophils as well as alveolar macrophages may be partly under the control of β-adrenergics. It was observed that in the late-phase reaction, formoterol was very effective, not only in inhibiting the number of eosinophils and macrophages but also in inhibiting the production of superoxide from eosinophils [54]. In the late-phase reaction, the production of superoxide is markedly enhanced in eosinophils and macrophages 24 hours after antigen challenge. The therapeutic and anti-inflammatory effects of corticosteroids on leukocytes in the airways, where corticosteroids increase β-adrenergic responses, is consistent with these observations [20]. It is known that corticosteroids increase β-adrenergic responses and decrease α-adrenergic responses [20]. Conversely, the pretreatment with the β-adrenergic–blocking agent propranolol potentiates the bronchoconstriction caused by histamine, methacholine, acetylcholine, and cigarette smoke [55] in asthmatic patients [20]. However, these responses do not occur after use of propranolol in normal subjects [9,56]. In propranolol-induced bronchoconstriction, it is believed that the unopposed parasympathetic tone may be involved, because atropine prevents and partially reverses this effect in patients with mild asthma [57].

EFFECT OF THE ALLERGIC REACTION ON β-ADRENERGIC RESPONSES

A number of studies provide evidence suggesting a decrease in the adenylate cyclase response and cAMP production after antigen challenge. These findings have been reported both in sensitized animals and in asthmatic patients [20]. Although several groups of investigators have reported altered adrenergic responsiveness and decreased number of β-receptors in asthmatic patients, the evidence indicates a defect beyond the β-receptor itself [20]. The synthesis of certain cytokines and mediators after the allergic reaction, including PAF as well as TNF and IL-1, is associated with a decrease of β-adrenergic receptor function in the airway.

It was demonstrated that antigen challenge of sensitized guinea pigs in vivo resulted in diminished in vitro β-adrenergic agonist relaxation of airway SMCs [58]. Studies concluded that proinflammatory cytokines resulted in diminished β-adrenergic receptor function (Figs. 16-3 and 16-4) [58]. These authors also showed that IL-1 was able to induce G_i protein synthesis [58]. In endothelium cells, IL-1β produces increased mRNA levels of G_i proteins. Through inhibition of adenylate cyclase, decreased β-adrenergic response results from the induction G_i protein synthesis. Alternatively, IL-1β and TNF-α induce phospholipase A2 and increase production of lipid mediators, including leukotrienes and PAF. A reduced β-adrenergic response in experimental asthma can also occur as a result of phospholipase A2 [58]. PAF can cause bronchoconstriction, inflammation and edema, and chemotaxis of inflammatory cells, including neutrophils and eosinophils [48]. IL-1 causes the synthesis of PAF by vascular endothelial cells [20]. In vivo studies in guinea pigs demonstrated that PAF aerosol potentiated the increase in specific airway resistance produced by methacholine. Furthermore, the effect of isoproterenol or prostaglandin E_2 was diminished in these guinea pigs after PAF aerosol administration [59]. PAF-induced desensitization of β-adrenergic receptor responses could also be caused by an increase in phospholipase A_2 activity [20].

PAF and β-adrenergic receptor agonists can induce βARK translocation in blood lymphocytes; this suggests a functional role for the βARK mechanism of homologous receptor desensitization in immune cells [60]. The expression of βARK and several G protein–coupled receptor kinases in T lymphocytes results in β-adrenergic homologous desensitization [61]. These findings have important implications in the regulation of T lymphocyte subsets in the allergic inflammatory response. Some investigators have reported decreased lymphocyte β-receptor density as well as decreased β-adrenergic cAMP responsiveness of lymphocytes in asthmatic patients who have not used a β_2-agonist for at least 2 weeks [20]. Helper type 2 T cells play an important role in orchestrating the immune response in the airways. Th2 cytokines such as IL-3, IL-4, IL-5, IL-9, and IL-13, which are very important in mast cell, basophil, and eosinophil growth and differentiation, are important features of asthma.

The effect of these cytokines on airway SMCs is now being investigated vigorously by several laboratories. Use of isolated airway preparations provides investigators with a model to study both airway SMC contractile and relaxation responses. Human or rabbit airway SMCs passively sensitized with asthmatic serum exhibit the nonspecific increase in reactivity to agonists such as acetylcholine that stimulates specific G protein–coupled receptors and is associated with a decreased response to the β-agonist isoproterenol. These studies show that factors in the serum from patients with asthma, *eg*, cytokines and IgE, can interact to modulate airway SMC responsiveness. Furthermore, rhinovirus, an important

contributing factor to exacerbation of asthma, particularly rhinovirus 16, can increase the response to acetylcholine and decrease the response to isoproterenol in isolated airway SMCs [37,62] (Figs. 16-5 and 16-6). Studies of the effects of certain cytokines point to the in vivo model of asthma, which supports the in vitro findings of the effect of cytokines on airway SMCs [20,63].

In addition to uncoupling of the β-receptor from the G protein and decreased adenylate cyclase responsiveness, an additional mechanism is a decrease in cAMP response resulting from elevated phosphodiesterase activity [20,64]. The various subtypes of phosphodiesterase and their inhibitors, particularly inflammatory cells such as the eosinophil and alveolar macrophage in asthma, have been recently reviewed [65,66]. The development of specific phosphodiesterase IV inhibitors potentially has very significant therapeutic advantages over theophylline. Phosphodiesterase IV inhibitors are several orders of magnitude more potent than theophylline, particularly in the inflammatory cells in asthma, *eg*, monocytes, T lymphocytes, basophils, mast cells, and eosinophils.

TOLERANCE AND CONTINUOUS USE OF β-ADRENERGIC AGONISTS: CONTROVERSY AND CONFUSION

In the past, there was considerable confusion in the minds of the public as well as physicians about whether fatal or near-fatal asthma attacks are caused by under- or overtreatment with bronchodilators [20,67,68]. This has

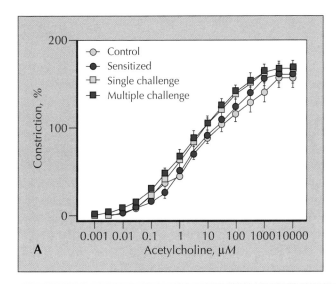

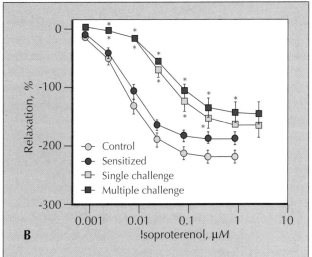

Figure 16-3.
Constriction-relaxation responses of tracheas isolated from guinea pigs sensitized with ovalbumin. The constrictor response (**A**) to acetylcholine and the relaxant response (**B**) to isoproterenol after preconstriction with 0.1 μM ET-1 were isometrically measured using tracheas

isolated from various animals: control, sensitized, single-challenged, and multichallenged guinea pigs, according to the method described in the text. Relaxation was expressed as percentage of the constriction produced by 50 mM KCl, a nonreceptor-mediated constriction. (*Adapted from* Wills-Karp *et al.* [58].)

resulted partly from reports of patients dying with bronchial asthma who were using twice the recommended number of inhalations per month of inhaled β-agonists before death. This question of undertreatment versus overtreatment is particularly important because of the recent availability of powerful new LABAs. Clearly, some of these deaths are associated with a lack of treatment or undertreatment of the inflammatory process; the overdependency and overuse of β-agonists may lead to temporary relief of symptoms without treating the underlying inflammation [20,68]. The nonspecific β-agonist isoproterenol is associated with cardiotoxicity, particularly in the presence of hypoxia in animals [69]. However, it has been difficult to assess this in patients with life-threatening asthma attacks. However, in a study of 10 asthmatic patients with respiratory arrest, it was concluded that undertreatment, rather than overtreatment, was the major factor involved in an increased number of deaths from asthma [67]. These authors concluded that

asphyxia, rather than cardiac complications of β-agonist therapy, was a cause of the majority of deaths in patients with bronchial asthma, at least in young and middle-aged patients. Concern about powerful new LABAs was raised by Sears *et al.* [70], who reported that on-demand inhaled bronchodilator therapy was more effective than regular use of inhaled bronchodilator therapy. In this placebo-controlled study, the placebo-treated group showed a higher percentage of patients who were able to reduce the need for oral prednisone and have lower bronchial reactivity, fewer nocturnal or daytime symptoms, and higher PEFRs than patients who continually used the inhaled β-agonist fenoterol. While 17 subjects had better control while taking formoterol four times a day, 40 patients showed better control of asthma during the placebo treatment and had received bronchodilator only on demand rather than on continuous use.

A mild increase in airway reactivity has been reported with regular use of inhaled β-agonists [71]. However, the

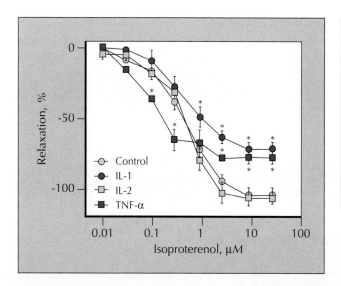

Figure 16-4.

Effects of proinflammatory cytokines on isoproterenol-induced relaxation of cultured tracheas. Relaxation was expressed as percentage of the maximal contraction to carbamylcholine. Isoproterenol responses were studied after no exposure to cytokines ($n = 12$) and incubation with IL-1β (4 ng/mL; $n = $=4), IL-2 (0.2 µg/mL; $n = 4$), and tumor necrosis factor-α (TNF-α) (0.1 µg/mL; $n = 4$). Data were the means ± SEM. The values marked were significantly different from the control value, as determined by analysis of variance (ANOVA) ($P \leq 0.05$). (*Adapted from* Wills-Karp *et al.* [58].)

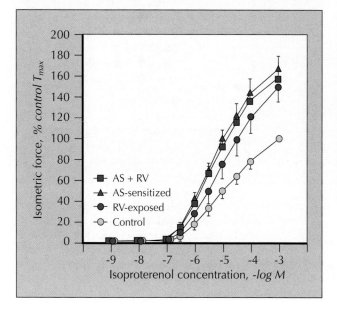

Figure 16-5.

Comparison of constrictor dose-response relationships to acetylcholine (Ach) in paired control serum-incubated, rhinovirus (RV)-inoculated, atopic asthmatic serum (AS)-sensitized, and AS-sensitized plus RV-inoculated (AS + RV) airway smooth muscle (ASM) tissue segments. T_{max}, maximal isometric contractile force. Data are means ± SE from eight paired experiments. Note that relative to control tissues, serum-incubated ASM, constrictor responses to Ach were significantly enhanced in the AS-sensitized, RV-inoculated, and AS + RV tissues. (*Adapted from* Grunstein *et al.* [62].)

LABA salmeterol actually decreased airway reactivity and completely protected against late bronchial reactions [72]. The marked downregulation of β-adrenergic responses in leukocytes with continued use of β₂-agonists suggests that LABAs only further downregulate these β-adrenergic responses. It is clear, however, that even though the β-receptors on leukocytes are the same as the β₂-receptors in the airway epithelium and airway SMCs, this appears to result in only a modest diminution of the response in the airways [73]. This is illustrated by the observation that prolonged administration of β₂-agonists in asthmatic patients usually results in no diminution of the bronchodilating effect. However, there is some decrease in the duration of the bronchodilation [20]. Additionally, the bronchoprotective effect of β-agonists does appear to be diminished with prolonged treatment or use of long-acting agents such as salmeterol and results in significant tolerance to its protective effect against the bronchoconstrictor stimulus of methacholine [74]. The clinical implication is that patients receiving regular monotherapy with β₂-agonists may become more susceptible to acute bronchoconstricting stimuli, which would occur with exposure to allergens. For this reason, the use of inhaled corticosteroids to prevent tolerance to the protective effect of a LABA is suggested.

Some confusion remains that the development of tolerance to the bronchoprotective effect may be related to the specific β-agonist used. In the report by Sears *et al.* [70], of the 26 patients who developed a significant increase in bronchial responsiveness to methacholine, 22 were more responsive with regular use of fenoterol. This raises the possibility that fenoterol has a greater potential to downregulate β-adrenergic responsiveness than other commonly used β-agonists [20]. In subjects treated with

albuterol, two puffs four times daily, there were more symptoms during the night, particularly 4 hours after the last inhalation of albuterol, than in patients treated with long-acting theophylline alone or a combination of long-acting theophylline and albuterol four times daily [75]. In one study [76], patients were maintained on theophylline; however, for the 2-week period that they received inhaled terbutaline, they did better in terms of all the variables of asthma control than when taking a matching placebo. It remains to be seen whether theophylline plays a role in preventing subsensitivity to β₂-agonists. Agents that increase cAMP, *eg*, β-adrenergic agents, result in increased phosphodiesterase IV and in increased metabolism of cAMP [77]. These findings need to be tested in vivo in patients to determine if a phosphodiesterase inhibitor in combination with β₂-agonist prevents the subsensitivity to β₂-agonists.

THE ROLE OF LONG-ACTING β₂-AGONISTS

Formoterol and salmeterol are both selective LABAs with effects that last at least 12 hours and up to 20 hours. In contrast to SABAs, both of these agents have a marked inhibitory effect on the late reaction.

Salmeterol

Salmeterol, 50 μg inhaled before allergen challenge, prevented both early- and late-phase bronchoconstriction [72]. Investigators also observed that salmeterol completely inhibited the allergen-induced increase in nonspecific bronchial responsiveness over a 24-hour period. The authors provided evidence that these effects were unrelated to prolonged bronchodilation or functional antagonism [72]. Radioligand-binding studies

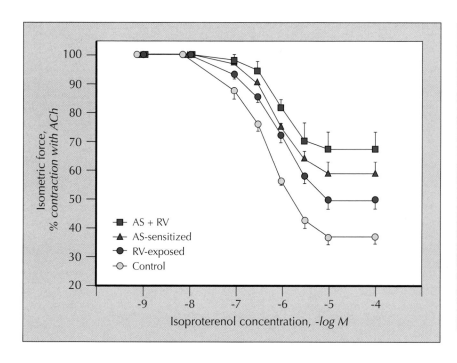

Figure 16-6.
Comparison of relaxation dose–response relationships to isoproterenol in paired control serum-incubated, rhinovirus (RV)-inoculated, asthmatic serum (AS)-sensitized, and AS + RV airway smooth muscle (ASM) tissue segments. Data are means ± SE from eight paired experiments. Note that relative to control tissues, serum-incubated ASM, relaxation responses to isoproterenol were significantly attenuated in the AS-sensitized and RV-inoculated tissues, and a near-additive attenuated effect on maximal relaxation was obtained in AS + RV ASM. (*Adapted from* Grunstein *et al.* [62].)

indicate that salmeterol has a high affinity (K_i = 33 nM) with little or no dissociation from its receptor. Whereas protection against methacholine challenge for 12 hours was demonstrated with salmeterol 50 µg, albuterol 200 µg by inhalation protected at 1 hour but not at 4 hours [20]. Nocturnal asthma was significantly decreased with salmeterol 50 µg twice a day, in a controlled study [78]. This was also associated with improved morning and daytime symptoms and PEFR in 667 subjects with mild to moderate asthma. In this study, salmeterol improved evening PEFR, decreased nocturnal asthma, and decreased the need for additional albuterol. In all of these parameters, salmeterol 50 µg twice a day was more effective than albuterol 200 µg four times a day [79]. Because of the late onset of action of salmeterol, it is essential that all patients carry with them a β_2-agonist inhaler with a quicker onset of action. Despite a warning in the salmeterol packet insert, 20 deaths and respiratory arrests were reported in 1994 related to the slow onset of action of salmeterol.

The comparative potency of β_2-receptors on airway SMCs demonstrated that isoproterenol has a potency of 1.00 versus albuterol's 0.55; salmeterol has a potency of 8.50 [20,80]. This resulted in a selective ratio of β_2 compared with β_1 of 85,000 for salmeterol versus one for isoproterenol.

However, in studies of the inhibition of mediator release from human lungs by β-adrenoceptor agonists, it was evident that isoproterenol was slightly more effective than salmeterol on the percent inhibition of release of histamine and leukotriene C4 and D4. Nevertheless, salmeterol was at least 1 log more potent in this regard than albuterol [81].

COMPARISON OF EFFICACY OF CORTICOSTEROIDS WITH SALMETEROL AND IN COMBINATION

In patients with moderate persistent asthma, salmeterol 50 µg twice a day plus beclomethasone 200 µg twice a day was compared with beclomethasone 500 µg twice a day plus albuterol in a 6-month treatment period [82] (Fig. 16-7). It was determined that adding salmeterol provided superior improvement of the morning PEFR versus increasing the dose of an ICS. The combination of salmeterol with the lower dose of ICS proved superior to increasing the dose of beclomethasone to 500 mg twice daily. The inclusion criteria for these asthmatic patients aged 18 to 75 years was that they were receiving 500 µg per day via MDI of beclomethasone and, despite that, had symptoms for 4 of 7 days during the baseline and a variation in their PEFR of greater than 15% during the baseline. The mean age for both groups was approximately 48 years. The morning PEFR measurements in the subjects receiving the lower dose of 200 µg twice a day of beclomethasone plus salmeterol showed a 30 L/min increase in the PEFR by 5 weeks. This was maintained throughout the 21-week, double-blind phase of the study. The morning PEFR was significantly higher from week one for the rest of the study compared with the subjects receiving 500 µg twice daily of beclomethasone [82] (*see* Fig. 16-7). The evening PEFR measurements were also significantly higher in the group receiving the combination of salmeterol plus beclomethasone for all weeks beginning at week one.

A separate study [83] was conducted to determine whether the addition of salmeterol to existing cortico-

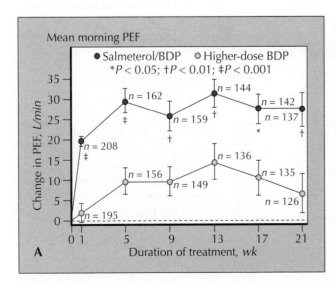

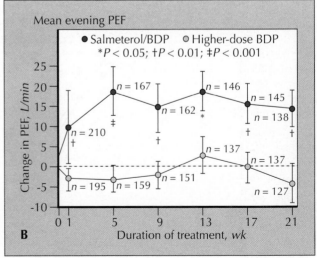

Figure 16-7.
Changes from baseline (± SE) in mean morning (**A**) and evening (**B**) peak expiratory flow (PEF) during 6 months' study treatment. (*Adapted from* Greening *et al.* [82].)

steroid therapy provides greater therapeutic benefit than doubling the dose of ICS in patients with symptomatic asthma. It was concluded that patients treated with salmeterol plus beclomethasone, 168 µg twice a day, had significantly greater improvement compared with beclomethasone 336 µg twice a day. This improvement was greater in terms of lung function, including the FEV_1 (forced expiratory volume in 1 second) and AM and PM PEFR, asthma symptom scores, percentage of symptom-free days, supplemental albuterol rescue use, and percentage of days and nights not requiring albuterol. This double-blind, parallel-group study of 514 patients included a 2-week run-in period followed by a 24-week treatment period. The subjects were 18 years or older with an FEV_1 range from 45% to 80% of predicted at the time of entry. They had an increase in FEV_1 of at least 12% after inhalation of 180 µg of albuterol. It was also required that they be symptomatic while taking inhaled beclomethasone 336 µg or triamcinolone 800 µg daily. The FEV_1 improved significantly from the baseline in both treatment groups. However, this effect was significantly greater in the salmeterol group receiving 50% of the dose of beclomethasone. In this group, the FEV_1 improved by 300 mL from baseline by week 4 and showed continued improvement throughout the 24-week period with the FEV_1 approximately 350 mL above baseline for the last 4 to 8 weeks. This is in comparison to approximately 200 mL above baseline in the group receiving twice the dose of inhaled corticosteroids [81]. Similar changes were noted in the improvement in PEFR, mean asthma symptoms score, and mean percent of symptom-free days. In these parameters, the salmeterol group was significantly greater than the subjects receiving placebo plus twice the dose of beclomethasone. This was also true for the mean daytime supplemental albuterol use and mean nighttime supplemental albuterol use (*ie*, the need for rescue with albuterol) in these subjects. There were no significant differences between treatment groups in the amount of sleep loss, asthma exacerbations, or adverse event frequency.

The efficacy and safety of adding salmeterol therapy to patients who remain symptomatic while receiving fluticasone compared with increasing the dose of fluticasone was studied [84]. In this double-blind, double-dummy, parallel-group study, 437 patients received fluticasone, 88 µg, during the screening phase for 2 to 4 weeks and were followed for an additional 24-week treatment period. These subjects were 12 years of age and older, demonstrated a 15% reversibility in FEV_1 with use of a bronchodilator, and had a baseline FEV_1 of 40% to 80% of predicted at the time of the screening. In this study, the change in morning PEFR was significantly greater in the group receiving salmeterol plus fluticasone 88 µg versus the group receiving fluticasone 220 µg. Similarly, there was a significantly greater improvement in the FEV_1 in the group receiving salmeterol plus 88 µg of fluticasone.

There was also statistically superior response with the addition of salmeterol compared with increasing the dose of fluticasone in terms of improved symptom control and reduction in albuterol use. Both treatments were well tolerated, and the total number of reported adverse events was similar between the groups.

Advair Diskus (GlaxoSmithKline, Research Triangle Park, NC) is the first product to treat effectively both the inflammation and the bronchoconstriction of asthma with fluticasone and salmeterol in a single device [85]. This combination provides a high level of symptom relief and control of asthma [86] (Fig. 16-8). The recommend dosage for Advair Diskus is one inhalation twice daily approximately 12 hours apart, which should not be exceeded. An additional advantage of this compound is that the patient does not need to carry several different MDIs. Its convenient dry powder dispenser is easy to use. This should presumably improve compliance, because asthmatic patients tend to use their bronchodilator because they feel relief with it; this is not true with the inhaled steroids, at least in the short term. Advair Diskus does not replace fast-acting inhalers to treat acute symptoms and should be used with caution in patients with cardiovascular disorders. This combination is further supported by evidence from nine clinical studies involving nearly 4000 patients demonstrating that greater clinical efficacy is achieved when salmeterol is added to the inhaled corticosteroid than when the inhaled corticosteroid dose is doubled [87].

Salmeterol: Comparison with Leukotriene-receptor Antagonists and Quality of Life

The use of an ICS plus salmeterol was compared with the use of monteleukast. An ICS was associated with a significant reduction in the need for SABAs, decreased hospital event rates, and significantly lower total asthma care costs than the montelukast group [88].

Salmeterol was compared with zafirlukast in the treatment of patients with persistent asthma [89]. This study concluded that salmeterol provided significantly greater improvement than oral zafirlukast in pulmonary lung function as measured by the morning PEFR. The safety profiles were similar, and both treatment groups were well tolerated. The AM PEFR increased approximately 30 L/min in the salmeterol group and approximately 15 L/min in the zafirlukast group [89].

The effect of salmeterol via MDI for the treatment of asthma on asthma-specific quality of life in patients experiencing significant nocturnal asthma was studied [90]. This study concluded, after 12 weeks of treatment, that salmeterol significantly improved pulmonary function, asthma symptom scores, percent of symptom-free days, and percentage of nights of no awakenings. Salmeterol also reduced the need for supplemental albuterol compared with placebo, and was well tolerated throughout the 12 weeks of treatment.

Chervinsky *et al.* [91] studied the long-term cardiovascular safety of salmeterol. The adverse events, including cardiovascular events, were monitored and collected for each visit, as was the pulse rate, blood pressure, and an ECG with a rhythm strip at screening day 1 and weeks 8, 20, and 48. Patients also had a Holter monitor evaluated by an independent cardiologist. There were no significant changes in the placebo group. Four patients taking salmeterol had

clinically significant changes on the ECG. Two of these were considered to be drug-related, with nonspecific ST-T wave changes; one patient had similar nonspecific ST-T wave changes and prolonged QTC interval. There were no significant differences in the treatment groups in terms of blood pressure or pulse rate. Overall, fewer than 2% of patients treated with salmeterol exhibited abnormal ECGs that were considered clinically significant. No patient

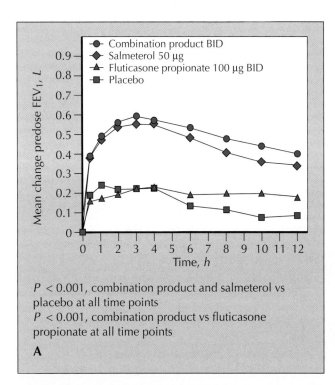

$P < 0.001$, combination product and salmeterol vs placebo at all time points
$P < 0.001$, combination product vs fluticasone propionate at all time points

A

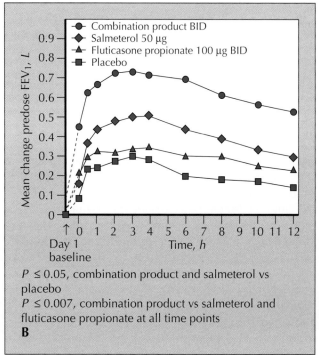

$P \leq 0.05$, combination product and salmeterol vs placebo
$P \leq 0.007$, combination product vs salmeterol and fluticasone propionate at all time points

B

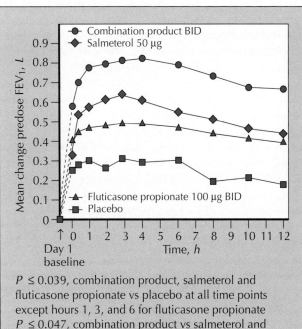

$P \leq 0.039$, combination product, salmeterol and fluticasone propionate vs placebo at all time points except hours 1, 3, and 6 for fluticasone propionate
$P \leq 0.047$, combination product vs salmeterol and fluticasone propionate at all time points

C

Figure 16-8.
Mean change from baseline (before randomization of study drug) in serial FEV_1 (forced expiratory volume in 1 second) over 12 hours at **A**, day 1, **B**, week 1, and **C**, week 12. BID—twice a day (*Adapted from* Kavuru *et al.* [86].)

discontinued treatment with the study medication, withdrew from the study, or required intervention for any ECG abnormality. The conclusion of this study is that long-term, twice-daily therapy with salmeterol powder was not associated with unfavorable clinically significant changes in cardiac function or with cardiovascular adverse events.

Salmeterol (Serevent; GlaxoSmithKline, Research Triangle Park, NC) by MDI is indicated for the maintenance treatment of asthma and the prevention of bronchospasm in patients age 12 years and older, including patients with nocturnal asthma who require regular treatment with inhaled SABAs. In patients whose asthma can be managed by occasional use of inhaled SABAs, salmeterol should not be used. For patients 4 years of age and older, Serevent Diskus inhalation powder is indicated for long-term, twice-daily administration in the maintenance treatment of asthma. Salmeterol should not be initiated in patients with significantly worsening or acutely deteriorating asthma, which might be a life-threatening condition. It is important to emphasize that salmeterol is not a substitute for inhaled or oral corticosteroids, and patients must be warned not to stop or reduce corticosteroid therapy without medical advice even if they feel better when they are being treated with salmeterol. Salmeterol should be used with caution in patients with cardiovascular disorders, especially coronary insufficiency and cardiac arrhythmias, and in patients with convulsive disorders or thyrotoxicosis and those who are unusually responsive to sympathomimetic amines.

Formoterol

Another new LABA is formoterol (Foradil; Novartis, East Hanover, NJ) [20,92]. Formoterol fumarate inhalation powder is a formylamino-substituted catecholamine. Although marketed in Japan as an oral formulation, it has also been developed for inhalation treatment. Formoterol's major advantage is that it shows rapid maximal bronchodilator effect within 5 minutes and duration of action of 12 hours. Because its time of onset is equivalent to that of albuterol, formoterol has an important advantage over salmeterol in rescue bronchodilation.

In comparative trials, formoterol solution aerosol 12 μg twice a day provided greater bronchodilator effects than albuterol 200 μg four times daily, terbutaline 250 μg, or fenoterol 200 μg three times daily. The side effects after inhalation of formoterol were similar in frequency to the other β_2-adrenergic drugs [92]. Formoterol is lipophilic, but not as lipophilic as salmeterol. Its ability to inhibit mast cell histamine release is quite potent, with an ED_{50} of 10^{-11} M (140). Tokuyama *et al.* [93] observed that formoterol is approximately 35 times more potent than albuterol in inhibiting both microvascular leakage and airflow obstruction induced by histamine aerosol. This finding is supported by another study [94] demonstrating that inhaled formoterol is approximately 40 times more potent than albuterol.

The mucosal thickening that occurs as a result of microvascular leak and edema in small airways could have a profound influence on the tendency of small airways to close. The relative ability of formoterol to protect against the microvascular leak led to a study of its effect on its bronchial responsiveness and the late reaction in a model of antigen-sensitized guinea pig [95]. Specific airway conductance was measured using a two-chambered body plethysmograph. Antigen challenge was done under cover of an H_1-receptor antagonist. Formoterol 10 μg/mL, isoproterenol 1 mg/mL, or saline was inhaled 15 minutes before challenge. The late allergic reaction resulted in a 52% decrease in pulmonary function from baseline 6 to 8 hours after antigen challenge. Bronchoalveolar lavage showed a significant increase in eosinophils as well as macrophages and increased bronchial response to histamine 24 hours after antigen challenge. In this study, formoterol completely inhibited the late allergic reaction and the cellular increase in bronchial alveolar cells, especially eosinophils. Although both β-agonists were equally protective against the early reaction, isoproterenol failed to prevent this late reaction and did not prevent the decrease in pulmonary function during the late reaction or the increase in eosinophils and histamine sensitivity. In contrast, formoterol did decrease the antigen-induced increase in bronchial reactivity to histamine. These findings in a guinea pig model suggest that formoterol inhibits the late reaction and the inflammatory process in terms of accumulation of eosinophils and macrophages.

In asthmatic children, formoterol was shown to decrease the methacholine responsiveness, even at 12 hours after inhalation [96]. Both formoterol and salmeterol given before antigen challenge can attenuate the late allergic reaction in asthmatic patients [20,72,97]. There is some controversy whether these effects of formoterol and salmeterol in the late reaction and the airway inflammation are caused by the long-persisting action of β_2-receptor stimulation or some additional anti-inflammatory mechanism. Nevertheless, it is important to emphasize that neither of the LABAs should be used in place of corticosteroids.

The Foradil Aerolizer contains formoterol fumarate powder for inhalation. Its indication and usage for the maintenance treatment of asthma include nocturnal asthma in adults and children age 5 years and older. It is also used for prevention of exercise-induced bronchospasm and for the maintenance treatment of chronic obstructive pulmonary disease (COPD).

Results of pivotal clinical studies in asthma show that the onset of bronchodilation with formoterol is similar to albuterol, 180 μg, with a maximum improvement generally occurring within 1 to 3 hours and lasting for at least 12 hours. This resulted in improvement in daytime and nocturnal symptom scores, nighttime awakenings, rescue medication usage during the night, and PEFRs [98].

The bronchoprotective effect of formoterol, as assessed by methacholine challenge, was studied in three large clinical trials after an initial dose of 24 μg and after 2 weeks of 24 μg twice a day in 19 adult subjects with mild asthma. Similar to salmeterol, tolerance to the bronchoprotective effect of formoterol was observed, as evidenced by a diminished bronchoprotective effect on FEV_1 after 2 weeks. No rebound bronchial hyperresponsiveness was observed after cessation of chronic formoterol therapy. The efficacy of formoterol versus placebo was maintained; however, a slightly reduced bronchodilator response was observed as measured by the 12-hour FEV_1 area under the curve. This was particularly noticeable with the 24 μg dose twice a day. A similar reduced FEV_1 area under the curve over time was noted with albuterol 180 μg four times a day by MDI [98].

CLINICAL TRIALS

In two pivotal, 12-week, multicenter, randomized, double-blind, parallel group studies, inahled formoterol fumarate powder was compared with albuterol, 180 μg four times a day by MDI and placebo in a total of 1095 adult and adolescent patients 12 years of age and older with mild to moderate asthma. Formoterol, 12 μg twice a day, resulted in significantly greater postdose bronchodilation throughout the 12-week treatment period in both studies [98] (Fig. 16-9).

In a pediatric asthma trial in a total of 518 children with asthma 5 to 12 years of age who required daily bronchodilators and anti-inflammatory treatment, efficacy was evaluated on the first day of treatment, at week 12, and at the end of the 12-month treatment. This was a randomized, double-blind, parallel-group study comparing formoterol with placebo. Formoterol twice a day

demonstrated a greater 12-hour FEV_1 area under the curve compared with placebo on the first day of treatment, after 12 weeks of treatment, and after 1 year of treatment [98].

Inhaled formoterol fumarate powder is indicated for acute prevention of exercise-induced bronchospasm in adults and children 12 years of age and older, when administered on an occasional, as-needed basis. It is also indicated for long-term administration for maintenance treatment of asthma and COPD in adults and children 5 years of age and older with reversible obstructive airway disease. It is not indicated for patients whose asthma can be managed by occasional use of inhaled short-acting β-agonists. Formoterol fumarate carries a warning label that it is not a substitute for inhaled or oral corticosteroids, and corticosteroids should not be stopped or reduced when formoterol fumarate use is begun. It also should not be initiated in patients with significantly worsening or acutely deteriorating asthma, which may be a life-threatening condition. Patients who have been using short-acting $β_2$-agonists on a regular basis should be instructed to discontinue the regular use of these drugs and use them only for symptomatic relief of acute symptoms of asthma. Patients should be advised to continue taking oral or inhaled corticosteroids for treatment of asthma if they are starting formoterol fumarate, even if they feel better because of formoterol fumarate treatment. Reduction in corticosteroid dosage should be made only after clinical evaluation. The cardiovascular effects of formoterol fumarate are similar to those of other $β_2$-agonists and may need to be discontinued if certain ECG changes occur, *eg*, flattening of T waves, prolongation of QTc interval, and ST segment depression.

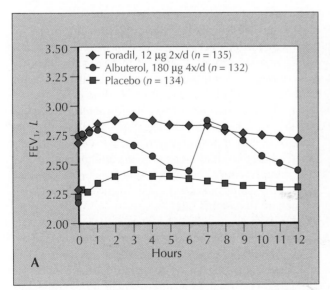
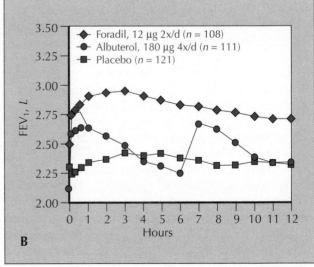
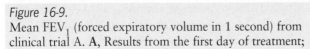

Figure 16-9.
Mean FEV_1 (forced expiratory volume in 1 second) from clinical trial A. **A,** Results from the first day of treatment; **B,** results from the last day of treatment. (*Adapted from* Novartis Pharmaceuticals Corporation [98].)

Formoterol fumarate should be used with caution in patients with cardiovascular disorders, especially those with coronary insufficiency, cardiac arrhythmias, and hypertension. This is consistent with warnings for other inhaled β_2-bronchodilators. Adverse effects are similar to those with other β_2-receptor-agonists. An incidence of adverse effects for inhaled formoterol fumarate 12 µg twice a day was at least 1% and greater than for placebo. For asthma, this included tremor, dizziness, and dysphonia. For COPD, it included pharyngitis, muscle cramps, increased sputum, dysphonia, myalgia, and tremor [98].

In several pivotal clinical studies, formoterol fumarate resulted in improvement in morning PEFRs, rescue medication usage, and quality of life in patients with COPD. This was accompanied by significant improvement in the FEV_1 and was maintained for 12 hours after either 12 or 24 µg twice a day. This improvement was greater than for ipratropium, 40 µg four times a day. This study involved approximately 194 subjects in each arm.

In a similar study [98] involving approximately 210 subjects in each arm, formoterol 12 µg and 24 µg twice daily, were compared with placebo and with slow-release theophylline 200 to 400 mg twice a day. In this study, formoterol 12 µg and 24 µg twice a day showed significantly greater pulmonary function improvement than theophylline. This improvement persisted for 12 weeks.

Levalbuterol Versus Racemic Albuterol

Racemic albuterol, similar to most other available β-agonist bronchodilators, is composed of two isomers whose activities are quite different. (R)-albuterol isomer, which is levalbuterol, is at least 100 times more potent in binding to the β_2-receptors than is the (S)-albuterol isomer. Whereas the (R)-isomer confers the bronchodilatory effect, the (S)-albuterol isomer has been reported to have several possible deleterious effects. (S)-albuterol has been reported by one investigator to have no bronchodilating activity and may enhance the calcium mobilization of SMCs [99]. The (S)-albuterol isomer has also been reported to facilitate acetylcholine release from dysfunctional prejunctional muscarinic receptors [100] and subsequently to enhance airway responsiveness to bronchoconstricting agents [101,102]. There is also evidence that (S)-albuterol in comparison with (R)-albuterol is metabolized slower and has plasma concentrations severalfold greater than the (R)-isomer.

The availability of the (R)-isomer, which is free of the (S)-isomer of albuterol and also free of preservatives, is available for the treatment of bronchospasm in children and adults. The (R)-isomer levalbuterol (Xopenex; Sepracor, Marlborough, MA) has been reported to show improved bronchodilation compared with racemic albuterol in patients with asthma [103]. Levalbuterol 0.31 mg and 0.63 mg produced FEV_1 reversibility comparable to racemic albuterol 2.5 mg and greater than the effect of 1.25 mg of the racemic mixture. Furthermore, in a study of children 3 to 11 years of age, it was associated with lower rates of β-adrenergic–mediated side effects, *ie*, a lower increase in heart rate and glucose and less decrease in serum potassium than a dose that was equally potent as a bronchodilator of the racemic mixture [104].

However, there is very little information about the lowest effective dose to provide adequate clinical response while minimizing side effects [1,105]. Because of the limited information, many pediatricians reduce the dose of racemic albuterol for patients younger than 12 years of age with the intent to decrease the β-adrenergic–mediated side effects.

Whereas the naturally occurring endogenous catecholamines are single isomers (the [R]-isomer), the (S)-isomer is not normally produced in humans. The US Food and Drug Administration has mandated the quantification of risk of the stereoisometric drugs [106].

Milgrom *et al.* [107] compared the effectiveness and safety of levalbuterol with racemic albuterol and placebo. These investigators studied 338 children 4 to 11 years of age whose FEV_1 was 40% to 85% of predicted. In this multicenter, randomized, double-blinded study, the children received 21 days of nebulized medication three times a day. They received levalbuterol 0.31 mg or 0.63 mg, racemic albuterol 1.25 mg or 2.50 mg, or placebo. In this five-way, parallel-group study, all active treatments significantly improved the primary endpoints in comparison with placebo. The immediate improvement in FEV_1 was significantly greater for the levalbuterol doses of 0.31 mg and 0.63 mg versus the racemic albuterol dose of 1.25 mg. The increase in FEV_1 was 19.0% and 18.1% for the 0.31 and 0.63 concentrations of levalbuterol and 12.4% and 15.6% increases for the racemic albuterol 1.25% and 2.50% mg, respectively. Levalbuterol 0.31 mg was the only treatment that did not differ from placebo for changes in ventricular heart rate, QTc interval, and blood glucose ($P > 0.05$). Serum potassium decreased with all active treatments from -0.30 to 0.60. The greatest decrease was with racemic albuterol, 2.50 mg, and was significantly greater than all other active agents in lowering serum potassium.

The effects of these therapeutic modalities on mean change, heart rate, mean decrease in serum potassium, and increase in blood sugar tended to decrease by day 21. However, there were no serious adverse events in these children. There were 146 adverse events in all, and the most common adverse events included fever, headache, asthma, pharyngitis, and rhinitis. There were no changes attributable to levalbuterol 0.31 mg compared with placebo in the QTc interval versus placebo. However, the QTc interval was significantly increased in all other active therapeutic agents versus placebo ($P < 0.001$). Racemic albuterol 2.50 mg causes significantly greater prolongation of the QTc than levalbuterol 0.31 mg. Levalbuterol 0.31 mg produced bronchodilation equivalent to that associated with racemic albuterol 2.50 mg, and was indistinguishable from placebo for most of the

β_2-adrenoceptor–mediated side effects. From these results, it was recommended that the starting dose of levalbuterol for children 4 to 11 years of age be 0.31 mg. Children who did not respond optimally to this dose might benefit from higher doses. Levalbuterol is an effective and safe alternative for bronchodilation in asthmatic children and has a more favorable therapeutic index than the standard or reduced dose of racemic albuterol. The pharmacokinetic analysis of this study showed the (S)-albuterol was fourfold higher compared with the (R)-albuterol in subjects receiving the racemic mixture. Furthermore, it has been demonstrated in other studies that the (S)-albuterol may persist up to 10 hours after a single dose and tends to accumulate with repeated dosing and be retained in the lungs [108]. Racemic albuterol 2.50 mg is the approved label dose and is recommended by the guidelines of the NHLBI and the American Academy of Allergy, Asthma and Immunology [1,105].

When racemic albuterol is administered with an MDI, the disposition of the (S)-enantiomer differs from that of the (R)-enantiomer. The plasma levels of the (S)-enantiomer were lower than those of the (R)-enantiomer for up to 4 hours. The systemic bioavailability of the (S)-enantiomer after inhalation of racemic albuterol in healthy subjects is caused by a preferential retention of the (S)-enantiomer in the lung [108]. This accumulation of (S)-albuterol may augment pulmonary tolerance. This tolerance is thought to represent downregulation of the β_2-receptor, with a loss of effect of β-agonist. It has been postulated that tolerance may actually represent the (S)-albuterol asthma-like effects noted as a result of progressive accumulation of (S)-albuterol. This (S)-albuterol accumulation could begin to oppose the bronchodilator effect of levalbuterol [109].

Nelson [110] reported in terms of clinical experience with levalbuterol and observed that single doses of levalbuterol provided more prolonged protection against methacholine challenge than the racemate; (S)-albuterol significantly increased sensitivity to methacholine. In a 4-week study in adults, equivalent amounts of pure levalbuterol provided greater bronchodilation than did similar amounts of levalbuterol given as racemic mixtures. After 4 weeks, the baseline morning FEV_1 was lower in those receiving the racemate than those receiving placebo or levalbuterol. These studies imply a deleterious response of (S)-albuterol on both the acute bronchodilator response and the baseline airway caliber. A mechanism of these effects of (S)-albuterol and its possible deleterious effects requires further investigation.

All β-adrenoceptor agonists, except for the pure isomers, exist as a pair of optical isomers (or mirror images), referred to as the (R)- and (S)-enantiomers, in a racemic mixture. Some β-agonists (eg, fenoterol, formoterol, and procaterol) have two asymmetric centers and there are four enantiomers: RR, SS, RS, and SR. It is clear that the activity lies predominantly in the (R)-enantiomer. For albuterol, the (R)-enantiomer is at least a hundredfold more potent as a β_2-agonist than the (S)-enantiomer [111]. For formoterol, the RR enantiomer has a thousandfold greater effect on β-receptors than the SS forms.

With salmeterol, there is still significant β_2-agonist activity in the (S)-enantiomer, which is only fortyfold less potent than the (R)-form and fifteenfold weaker than the racemic mixture. Both the (R)- and (S)-enantiomers of salmeterol are long-acting. There is no evidence that the (S)-isomer of salmeterol antagonizes the effects of the corresponding (R)-form [112].

The adverse effects of (S)-albuterol are most pronounced with chronic use because of the retention in the lung. The mechanism of the adverse event effects are not entirely known. The anti-inflammatory influences of (R)-isomers are negated in the presence of (S)-isomers. This has been demonstrated in human lymphocytes in which the anti-inflammatory effects of the (R)-isomer are masked by the additional presence of the (S)-isomer [113]. Another mechanism was recently reported showing that the protective effect of RR-formoterol in early and late allergic response and airway hyperresponsiveness in a mouse model of asthma is attenuated in the presence of SS-formoterol. There was a significant reduction in the early and late allergic bronchopulmonary responses by the RR- and RS-formoterol. The effect of RR-formoterol was much more pronounced than the RS-formoterol on the late-allergic response. SS-formoterol had no effect; instead, it increased the basal tone of the airways. RR-formoterol significantly attenuated the airway hyperresponsiveness to methacholine. There was a less pronounced effect of RS- or SS-formoterol on airway responsiveness to methacholine. These data suggest the possibility that the (S)-enantiomer present in racemic β-agonist may actually intensify the bronchoconstrictor response of asthmatic airways [114].

In a separate study [115], the production of granulocyte-macrophage colony-stimulating factor (GM-CSF) production by human airway SMCs treated with the (R)- and (S)-enantiomers of albuterol demonstrated that (R)-albuterol may provide some anti-inflammatory effect through downregulation of GM-CSF production by airway SMCs. The (S)-albuterol may amplify airway inflammation through upregulation of GM-CSF production. The production of GM-CSF may be important in airway inflammation. GM-CSF is a cytokine known to enhance eosinophil function. GM-CSF was increased 42% to 82% over control with 10 nM and 10 mM of (S)-albuterol.

A very intriguing aspect of the detrimental effect of SS-formoterol and S-albuterol has been reported to be associated with an increase in G_i-α_1 and G_i-α_3 proteins and activation of NF-κB in human airway SMCs. These detrimental effects were reported by Agrawal [116]. This report is consistent with the earlier studies by Agrawal in which although RR-formoterol and (R)-albuterol were protective in a mouse model of asthma, SS-formoterol and (S)-albuterol increased pulmonary responses to allergen challenge and increased bronchoalveolar lavage eosinophilia [114]. In this study on human airway SMCs, the cells were incubated with the enantiomers of both formoterol and albuterol. Expression of G_s and G_i proteins were analyzed by Western blot analysis, and NF-κB activity was assessed using antibodies specific to P65 unit of NF-κB. In addition to increasing the G_i-α1 and G_I-α3, both SS-formoterol and (S)-albuterol significantly increased intracellular calcium and potentiated the activity of NF-κB. In contrast, RR-formoterol and (R)-albuterol decreased intracellular calcium and had no effect on NF-κB activity. These findings suggest that the detrimental effects of SS-formoterol and (S)-albuterol on pulmonary function might be caused by an activation of proconstrictory and proinflammatory pathways in human airway SMCs. These latter studies are very recent, are in abstract form, and await confirmation.

REFERENCES AND RECOMMENDED READING

1. National Heart, Lung, and Blood Institute, National Asthma Education and Prevention Program: *Expert Panel Report 2: Guidelines for the Diagnosis and Management of Asthma.* Bethesda, MD: National Institutes of Health; Pub No. 97-4051; 1997.

2. Townley RG, Trapani IL, Szentivanyi A: Sensitization to anaphylaxis and to some of its pharmacological mediators by blockade of the beta adrenergic receptors. *J Allergy* 1967, 39:177–197.

3. Townley RG, Daley D, Selenke W: The effect of agents used in the treatment of bronchial asthma on carbohydrate metabolism and histamine sensitivity after beta adrenergic blockade. *J Allergy* 1970, 45:71–76.

4. Mano K, Akbarzadeh A, Townley RG: Effect of hydrocortisone on beta-adrenergic receptors in lung membranes. *Life Sci* 1979, 25:195.

5. Mano K, Akbarzadeh A, Ruprecht H, Townley R: Effect of *Bordetella pertussis* extracts on beta-adrenergic receptors in mouse lung. Presented at the Unified 1978 FASEB meetings, Atlantic City, NJ; April 10–14, 1978.

6. Asthma Management Model System. National Institutes of Health/ National Heart, Lung, and Blood Institute. http://www.nhlbi.nih.gov/health/prof/lung/asthma/am_fa99/am_fa99.pdf. Accessed September 19, 2002.

7. White MV, Sander N: Asthma from the perspective of the patient. *J Allergy Clin Immunol* 1999, 103(suppl):47–52.

8. Ryo UY, Townley RG: Comparison of respiratory and cardiovascular effects of isoproterenol, propranolol, and practolol in asthmatic and normal subjects. *J Allergy Clin Immunol* 1976, 57:12–24.

9. Townley RG, McGeady S, Bewtra A: The effect of beta-adrenergic blockade on bronchial sensitivity to acetyl-beta-methacholine in normal and allergic rhinitis subjects. *J Allergy Clin Immunol* 1976, 57:358–366.

10. Holgate ST, Church MK: *Allergy.* London: Gower Medical Publishing; 1993.

11. Fraser CM: Adrenergic agents. In *Allergy Principles and Practice.* Edited by Middleton E, Jr, Reed CE, Ellis EF, *et al.* St. Louis: CV Mosby; 1993:778–815.

12. Fraser CM, Venter JC: The synthesis of β-adrenergic receptors in cultured human lung cells: induction by glucocorticoids. *Biochem Biophys Res Commun* 1980, 94:390–397.

13. Malbon CC, Hadcock JR: Evidence that glucocorticoid response elements in the 5-noncoding region of the hamster β-adrenergic receptor gene are obligate for glucocorticoid regulation of receptor mRNA levels. *Biochem Biophys Res Commun* 1988, 154:676–681.

14. Sibley DR, Lefkowitz RJ: Molecular mechanisms of receptor desensitization using the β-adrenergic receptor-coupled adenylate cyclase systems as a model. *Nature* 1985, 317:124–129.

15. Benovic JL, Strasser RH, Caron MG, *et al.*: β-Adrenergic receptor kinase: identification of a novel protein kinase that phosphorylates the agonist-occupied form of the receptor. *Proc Natl Acad Sci U S A* 1986, 83:2797.

16. Meurs H, Kauffman HF, Timmermans A, *et al.*: Specific immunological modulation of lymphocyte adenylate cyclase in asthmatic patients after allergenic bronchial provocation. *Int Arch Allergy Appl Immunol* 1986, 81:224.

17. Henderson WR, Shelhamer JH, Reingold DG, *et al.*: α-Adrenergic hyperresponsiveness in asthma: analysis of vascular and papillary responses. *N Engl J Med* 1979, 300:642–647.

18. Davis PB: Pupillary responses and airway reactivity in asthma. *J Allergy Clin Immunol* 1986, 77:667–673.

19. Bleecker ER, Chahal KS, Mason P, *et al.*: The effect of α-adrenergic blockade in nonspecific airways reactivity and exercises induced asthma. *Eur J Respir Dis* 1983, 64(suppl):258.

20. Townley RG: Adrenergic receptors, mechanisms, and the late allergic reaction: therapeutic role of the new long-acting β-agonists. In *Immunopharmacology of Allergic Diseases.* Edited by Townley RG, Agrawal DK. New York: Marcel Dekker; 1996:491–521.

21. Kneussel MP, Richardson JB: α-Adrenergic receptors in human canine tracheal and bronchial smooth muscle. *J Appl Physiol* 1978, 45:307–311.

22. Barnes PJ, Dollery CT, Macdermot J: Increased pulmonary α-adrenergic and reduced β-adrenergic receptors in experimental asthma. *Nature* 1990, 285:569.

23. O'Dowd BF, Hantowich M, Regan JW, *et al.*: Site-directed mutagenesis of the cytoplasmic domains of the human β-adrenergic receptor. *J Biol Chem* 1988, 263:15985–15992.

24. Liggett SB: β-Adrenergic receptor structure and function. *J Respir Dis* 1994, 15:28–38.

25. Green SA, Cole G, Jacinto M, *et al.*: A polymorphism of the human β-adrenergic receptor within the fourth transmembrane domain alters ligand binding and functional properties of the receptor. *J Biol Chem* 1993, 268:23116–23121.

26. Turki J, Pak J, Green SA, *et al.*: Genetic polymorphisms of the β-adrenergic receptor in nocturnal and nonnocturnal asthma. *J Clin Invest* 1995, 95:1635–1641.

27. Hall IP, Wheatley A, Wilding P, Liggett SB: Association of Glu 27 β_2-adrenoceptor polymorphism with lower airway reactivity in asthmatic subjects. *Lancet* 1995, 345:1213–1214.

28. Turki J, Liggett SB: Receptor-specific functional properties of β-adrenergic receptor autoantibodies in asthma. *Am J Respir Cell Mol Biol* 1995, 12:531–539.

29. Allen SL, Beech DJ, Foster RW, *et al.*: Electrophysiological and other aspects of the relaxant action of isoprenaline in guinea-pig isolated trachealis. *Br J Pharmacol* 1985, 86:843–854.

30. Kume H, Takai A, Tokuno H, Tomita T: Regulation of CA2+-dependent K+-channel activity in tracheal myocytes by phosphorylation. *Nature* 1989, 341:152–154.

31. Ewald DA, Williams A, Levitan IB: Modulation of single CA2+-dependent K+-channel activity by protein phosphorylation. *Nature* 1985, 315:503–506.

32. Jones TR, Charette L, Garcia ML, Kaczorowski GJ: Selective inhibition of relaxation of guinea-pig trachea by charybdotoxin, a potent Ca2+ activated K+-channel inhibitor. *J Pharmacol Exp Ther* 1990, 255:697–706.

33. Amrani Y, Panettieri RA: Modulation of calcium homeostasis as a mechanism for altering smooth muscle responsiveness in asthma. *Curr Opin Allergy Clin Immunol* 2002, 2:39–45.

34. Tsukagoshi H, Robbins RA, Barnes PJ, Chung KF: Role of nitric oxide and superoxide anions in interleukin-1 beta-induced airway hyperresponsiveness to bradykinin. *Am J Respir Crit Care Med* 1994, 150:1019–1025.

35. Thomas PS, Yates DH, Barnes PJ: Tumor necrosis factor-alpha increases airway responsiveness and sputum neutrophilia in normal human subjects. *Am J Respir Crit Care Med* 1995, 152:76–80.

36. Pennings HJ, Kramer K, Bast A, et al.: Tumor necrosis factor-alpha induces hyperreactivity in tracheal smooth muscle of the guinea-pig in vitro. *Eur Respir J* 1998, 12:45–49.

37. Amrani Y, Chen H, Panettieri RJ: Activation of tumor necrosis factor receptor 1 in airway smooth muscle: a potential pathway that modulates bronchial hyper-responsiveness in asthma? *Respir Res* 2000, 1:49–53.

38. Sukkar MB, Hughes JM, Armour CL, Johnson PR: Tumor necrosis factor-alpha potentiates contraction of human bronchus in vitro. *Respirology* 2001, 6:199–203.

39. Anticevich SZ, Hughes JM, Black JL, Armour CL: Induction of human airway hyperresponsiveness by tumor necrosis factor-alpha. *Eur J Pharmacol* 1995, 284:221–225.

40. Toews ML, Ustinova EE, Schultz HD: Lysophosphatidic acid enhances contractility of isolated airway smooth muscle. *J Appl Physiol* 1997, 83:1216–1222.

41. Szentivanyi A: The beta adrenergic theory of the atopic abnormality in bronchial asthma. *J Allergy* 1968, 42:203–232.

42. Barnes PJ: Adrenergic regulation of airway function. In *The Airway Neural Control in Health and Disease*. Edited by Kaliner MA, Barnes PJ. New York: Marcel Dekker; 1988:57–85.

43. Cerrina J, Ladurie MIR, Labat C, et al.: Comparison of human bronchial muscle responses to histamine in vivo with histamine and isoproterenol agonists in vitro. *Am Rev Respir Dis* 1986, 134:57–61.

44. Bai TR: Abnormalities in airway smooth muscle in fatal asthma: a comparison between trachea and bronchus. *Am Rev Respir Dis* 1991, 143:441–443.

45. Townley RG, Hopp RG, Agrawal DK, Bewtra AK: Platelet-activating factor and airway reactivity. *J Allergy Clin Immunol* 1989, 83:997–1010.

46. Pype J, Xu H, Schuermans M, et al.: Mechanisms of interleukin 1β-induced human airway smooth muscle hyporesponsiveness to histamine: involvement of p38 MAPK NF-κB. *Am J Respir Crit Care Med* 2001, 163:1010–1017.

47. Yang C, Chien C, Wang C, et al.: Interleukin-1beta enhances bradykinin-induced phosphoinositide hydrolysis and CA2+ mobilization in canine tracheal smooth-muscle cells: involvement of the Ras/Raf/mitogen-activated protein kinase (MAPK) kinase (MEK)/MAPK pathway. *Biochem J* 2001, 354:439–446.

48. Hsu Y, Chiu C, Wang C, et al.: Tumor necrosis factor-alpha enhances bradykinin-induced signal transduction via activation of Ras/Raf/MEK/MAPK in canine tracheal smooth muscle cells. *Cell Signal* 2001, 13:633–643.

49. Madison J, Ethier M: Interleukin-4 rapidly inhibits calcium transients in response to carbachol in bovine airway smooth muscle cells. *Am J Respir Cell Mol Biol* 2001, 25:239–244.

50. Meurs H, Zaagsma J: Pharmacological and biochemical changes in airway smooth muscle in relation to bronchial hyperresponsiveness. In *Pharmacology and Toxicology: Inflammatory Cells and Mediators in Bronchial Asthma*. Edited by Agrawal DK, Townley RG. Boca Raton, FL: CRC Press; 1991:1–38.

51. Barnes PJ, Basbaum BJ, Nadel JA: Autoradiography localization of autonomic receptors in airway smooth muscle: marked differences between large and small airways. *Am Rev Respir Dis* 1983, 127:758.

52. Silkoff P, Romero FA, Townley RG, et al.: Exhaled nitric oxide in children with asthma receiving omalizumab, a monoclonal anti-IgE antibody. *Am J Respir Crit Care Med*; 2002, in press.

53. Rankin JA: Macrophages and their potential role in hyperreactive airways disease. In *Pharmacology and Toxicology: Inflammatory Cells and Mediators in Bronchial Asthma*. Edited by Agrawal DK, Townley RG. Boca Raton, FL: CRC Press; 1990:89–106.

54. Okada C, Sugiyama AH, Eda R, et al.: The effect of formoterol on superoxide anion generation from bronchoalveolar lavage cells after antigen challenge in guinea pigs. *Am J Respir Cell Mol Biol* 1993, 8:509–517.

55. Zuskin E, Mitchell CA, Bouhuys A: Interaction between effects of beta blockade and cigarette smoke on airways. *J Appl Physiol* 1974, 36:449–452.

56. Zaid G, Beall GN: Bronchial response to beta-adrenergic blockade. *N Engl J Med* 1966, 275:580–584.

57. Grieco MH, Pierson RN Jr: Mechanism of bronchoconstriction due to beta-adrenergic blockade. *J Allergy* 1971, 48:143–152.

58. Wills-Karp, Uchida Y, Lee JY, et al.: Organ culture with proinflammatory cytokines reproduces impairment of the β–adrenoceptor mediated relaxation in tracheas of a guinea pig antigen model. *Am J Respir Cell Mol Biol* 1993, 8:153–159.

59. Agrawal DK, Bergren DR, Byorth PJ, Townley RG: Platelet-activating factor induces non-specific desensitization to bronchodilators in guinea pigs. *J Pharmacol Exp Ther* 1991, 259:1–7.

60. Chuang TT, Sallese M, Ambrosini G, et al.: High expression of β-adrenergic receptor kinase in human peripheral blood leukocytes. Isoproterenol and platelet activating factor can induce kinase translocation. *J Biol Chem* 1992, 267:6886–6892.

61. DeBlasi A, Parruti G, Sallese M: Regulation of G protein coupled receptor kinase subtypes in activated T-lymphocytes. Selective increase of β-adrenergic receptor kinase 1 and 2. *J Clin Invest* 1995, 95:203–210.

62. Grunstein MM, Hakonarson H, Hodinka RL, et al.: Mechanism of cooperative effects of rhinovirus and atopic sensitization on airway responsiveness. *Am J Physiol Lung Cell Mol Physiol* 2001, 280(suppl L):229–238.

63. Horiba M, Townley RG: Different role of IL-1β and IL-13 on airway responsiveness and response to 2-agonist. *J Allergy Clin Immunol* 2001, 109.

64. Grewe SR, Chan SC, Hanifin JM: Elevated leukocyte cyclic AMP-phosphodiesterase in atopic disease: a possible mechanism for cyclic AMP-agonist hyporesponsiveness. *J Allergy Clin Immunol* 1982, 70:452–457.

65. Townley RG: Elevated cAMP-phosphodiesterase in atopic disease: cause or effect? [editorial]. *J Lab Clin Med* 1993, 121:15–17.

66. Giembycz MA, Souness JE: Phosphodiesterase IV inhibitors as potential therapeutic agents in allergic disease. In *Immunopharmacology of Allergic Disease*. Edited by Townley RG, Agrawal DK. New York: Marcel Dekker; 1996:523–559.

67. Molfino NA, Nannini LJ, Martelli AN, Slutky AS: Respiratory arrest in near fatal asthma. *N Engl J Med* 1991, 324:285–288.

68. Jackson R: Undertreatment and asthma deaths. *Lancet* 1985, 2:500.

69. Collins JM, McDevitt DG, Shanks RG, Swanton JG: The cardiotoxicity of isoprenaline during hypoxia. *Br J Pharmacol* 1969, 36:35–45.

70. Sears MR, Taylor DR, Print CG, *et al.*: Regular inhaled beta-agonist treatment in bronchial asthma. *Lancet* 1990, 336:1391.

71. Britton J, Hanley SP, Garrett HV, *et al.*: Dose-related effects of salbutamol and ipratropium bromide on airway caliber and reactivity in subjects with asthma. *Thorax* 1988, 43:300–305.

72. Twentyman OP, Finnerty JP, Harris A, *et al.*: Protection against allergen-induced asthma by salmeterol. *Lancet* 1990, 336:1338.

73. Weber RW, Smith JA, Nelson HS: Aerosolized terbutaline in asthmatics: development of subsensitivity with long-term administration. *J Allergy Clin Immunol* 1982, 70:417–422.

74. Cheng D, Timmers CM, Swinderman AH, *et al.*: Long term effects of a long-acting β$_2$-adrenoreceptor agonist, salmeterol, on airway hyperresponsiveness in patients with mild asthma. *N Engl J Med* 1992, 327:1198–1203.

75. Joad JP, Ahrens RC, Lindgren SD, Weinberger MM: Relative efficacy of maintenance therapy with theophylline, inhaled albuterol and the combination for chronic asthma. *J Allergy Clin Immunol* 1987, 79:78–85.

76. VandeWalker ML, Kray KT, Weber RW, Nelson HS: Addition of terbutaline to optimal theophylline therapy: double-blind crossover study in asthmatic patients. *Chest* 1986, 90:198–203.

77. Torphy TJ, Zhou HL, Cieslinski LB: Stimulation of beta adrenoceptors in a human monocyte cell line (u937) upregulates cyclic AMP-specific phosphodiesterase. *J Pharmacol Exp Ther* 1992, 263:1195–1205.

78. Britton MG: Salmeterol and salbutamol: large multicenter studies. *Eur Respir Rev* 1991, 1:288–292.

79. Pearlman DS, Chervinsky P, LaForce C, *et al.*: A comparison of salmeterol with albuterol in the treatment of mild-to-moderate asthma. *N Engl J Med* 1992, 327:1420–1425.

80. Johnson M, Butchers PR, Coleman RA, *et al.*: The pharmacology of salmeterol. *Life Sciences* 1993, 52:2131–2143.

81. Butchers PR, Vardey CJ, Johnson M: Salmeterol: a potent and long-acting inhibitor of inflammatory mediator release from human lung. *Br J Pharmacol* 1991, 104:672–676.

82. Greening AP, Ind PW, Northfield M, Shaw G: Added salmeterol versus higher-dose corticosteroid in asthma patients with symptoms on existing inhaled corticosteroid: Allen & Hanburys Limited UK Study Group. *Lancet* 1994, 334:219–224.

83. Murray JJ, Church NL, Anderson WH, *et al.*: Concurrent use of salmeterol with inhaled corticosteroids is more effective than inhaled corticosteroid dose increases. *Allergy Asthma Proc* 1999, 20:173–180.

84. Condemi JJ, Goldstein S, Kalberg C, *et al.* and the Salmeterol Study Group: The addition of salmeterol to fluticasone propionate versus increasing the dose of fluticasone propionate in patients with persistent asthma. *Ann Allergy Asthma Immunol* 1999, 82:383–389.

85. Boulet, LP *et al.*: Comparison of Diskus Inhaler, a new multi-dose powder inhaler, with Diskhaler inhaler for the delivery of Salmeterol to asthmatic patients. *J Asthma* 1995, 32:429–436.

86. Kavuru M, Melamed J, Gross G, LaForce C, *et al.*: Salmeterol and fluticasone propionate combined in a new powder inhalation device for the treatment of asthma: a randomized, double-blind, placebo-controlled trial. *J Allergy Clin Immunol* 2000, 105:1108–16.

87. Shrewsbury S, Pyke S, Britton M: Meta-analysis of increased dose of inhaled steroid or addition of salmeterol in symptomatic asthma. *Br Med J* 2000, 320:1368–1373.

88. Stempel DA, Mayer JW, O'Donnell JC: Inhaled corticosteroids plus salmeterol or montelukast: effect on resource utilization and costs. *J Allergy Clin Immunol* 2002, 109:433–439.

89. Busse W, Nelson H, Wolfe J, *et al.*: Comparison of inhaled salmeterol and oral zafirlukast in patients with asthma. *J Allergy Clin Immunol* 1999, 103:1075–1080.

90. Lockey RF, DuBuske LM, Friedman B, *et al.*: Nocturnal asthma: effect of salmeterol on quality of life and clinical outcomes. *Chest* 1999, 115:666–673.

91. Chervinsky P, Goldberg P, Galant S, *et al.*: Long-term cardiovascular safety of salmeterol powder pharmacotherapy in adolescent and adult patients with chronic persistent asthma: a randomized clinical trial. *Chest* 1999, 115:642–648.

92. Anderson GP: Formoterol: pharmacology, molecular basis of agonism and mechanism of long duration of a highly potent and selective β$_2$-adrenoceptor agonist bronchodilator. *Life Sci* 1993, 52:2145–2160.

93. Tokuyama K, Lotvall JO, Lofdahl CG, *et al.*: Inhaled formoterol inhibits histamine-induced airflow obstruction and airway microvascular leakage. *Eur J Pharmacol* 1991, 193:35–39.

94. Arvidsson P, Larsson S, Lofdahl CG, *et al.*: Formoterol, a new long-acting bronchodilator for inhalation. *Eur Respir J* 1989, 2:325–330.

95. Sugiyama H, Okada C, Bewtra AK, *et al.*: The effect of formoterol on the late asthmatic response in guinea pigs. *J Allergy Clin Immunol* 1992, 89:858–866.

96. Becker AB, Simons FER: Formoterol, a new long acting selective β$_2$-adrenergic receptor agonist: double blind comparison with salbutamol and placebo in children with asthma. *J Allergy Clin Immunol* 1989, 84:891–895.

97. Palmqvist M, Balder B, Lowhagen O, *et al.*: Late asthmatic reaction prevented by inhaled salbutamol and formoterol. *J Allergy Clin Immunol* 1989, 83:244.

98. Novartis Pharmaceuticals Corporation: Full prescribing information, Foradil Aerolizer: USA; 2001:1–35.

99. Mitra S, Ugur M, Ugur O, *et al.*: (S)-albuterol increases intracellular free calcium by muscarinic receptor activation and a phospholipase C-dependent mechanism in airway smooth muscle. *Mol Pharmacol* 1998, 53:347–354.

100. Zhang X, Zhu F, Olszewski MA, Robinson NE: Effects of enantiomers of 2 agonists on ACh release and smooth muscle contraction in the trachea. *Am J Physiol* 1998, 274:L32–L38.

101. Morley J: Anomalous effects of albuterol and other sympathomimetics in the guinea pig. *Clin Rev Allergy Immunol* 1996, 14:65–89.

102. Templeton A, Chapman I, Chilvers E, *et al.*: Effects of S-salbutamol on isolated human bronchus. *Pulmon Pharmacol Ther* 1998, 11:1–6.

103. Nelson H, Bensch G, Pleskow W, *et al.*: Improved bronchodilation with levalbuterol compared to racemic albuterol in patients with asthma. *J Allergy Clin Immunol* 1998, 102:943–952.

104. Gawchik S, Saccar C, Noonan M, *et al.*: The safety and efficacy of nebulized levalbuterol compared with racemic albuterol and placebo in the treatment of asthma in pediatric patients. *J Allergy Clin Immunol* 1999, 103:615–21.

105. Pediatric asthma: promoting best practice. In *Guide for Managing Asthma in Children*. Milwaukee, WI: American Academy of Asthma, Allergy, and Immunology; 1999.

106. US Department of Health and Human Services: FDA 1992 policy statement for the development of new stereoisomeric drugs. *Chirality* 1992, 4:338–440.

107. Milgrom H, Skoner DP, Bensch G, *et al.*: Low-dose levalbuterol in children with asthma: Safety and efficacy in comparison with placebo and racemic albuterol. *J Allergy Clin Immunol* 2001, 108:938–945.

108. Dhand R, Goode M, Reid R, *et al.*: Preferential pulmonary retention of (S)-albuterol after inhalation of racemic albuterol. *Am J Respir Crit Care Med* 1999, 160:1136–1141.

109. Handley D: The asthma-like pharmacology and toxicology of (S)-isomers of β-agonists. *J Allergy Clin Immunol* 1999, 104(suppl):69–76.

110. Nelson H: Clinical experience with levalbuterol. *J Allergy Clin Immunol* 1999, 104(suppl):77–84.

111. Perrin-Fayolle M: Salbutamol in the treatment of asthma. *Lancet* 1995 346:1101.

112. Johnson M: The β-adrenoceptor. *Am J Respir Crit Care Med* 1998, 158(suppl):146–153.

113. Baramki D, Koester J, Anderson AJ, Borish L: Modulation of T-cell function by R- and S-isomers of albuterol: anti-inflammatory influences of R-isomers are negated in the presence of the S-isomer. *J Allergy Clin Immunol* 2002, 109:449–454.

114. Agrawal DK: Protective effect of RR-formoterol in early- and late-allergic response and airway hyperresponsiveness in a mouse model of asthma. *Am J Respir Crit Care Med* 2001, 163(suppl A):590.

115. Ameredes KL, Hershman D, Brown B, *et al.*: GM-CSF production by human airway smooth muscle cells treated with the S-albuterol. *Am J Respir Crit Care Med* 2001, 163(suppl A):513.

116. Agrawal DK: Detrimental effect of (S, S)-formoterol and (S)-albuterol is due to an increase in Giα1 and Giα3 proteins and activation of NF-kB in human airway smooth muscle cells. *Am J Respir Crit Care Med* 2002, 165(suppl A):317.

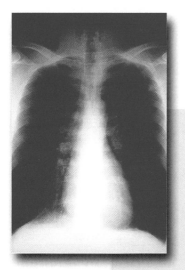

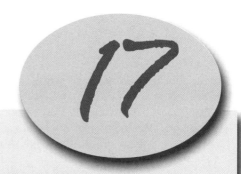

Theophylline

Peter J. Barnes

Because it is inexpensive, theophylline remains one of the most widely prescribed drugs for the treatment of airway diseases world-wide. In many industrialized countries, however, theophylline has become a third-line treatment used only in poorly controlled patients. This has been reinforced by various guidelines to therapy. Some have even questioned whether theophylline is indicated in any patients with asthma [1], although others have emphasized the special beneficial effects of theophylline which still give it an important place in management of asthma and chronic obstructive pulmonary disease (COPD) [2•]. However, the frequency of side effects and the relative low efficacy of theophylline have led to reduced usage, because inhaled β_2-agonists are far more effective as bronchodilators, and inhaled corticosteroids have a greater anti-inflammatory effect. Considerable uncertainty about the mode of action of theophylline in asthma and its logical place in therapy remain, despite its long-term use in asthma therapy. Because of problems with side effects, there have been attempts to improve on theophylline; recently, there has been increasing interest in selective phosphodiesterase (PDE) inhibitors. Selective PDE4 inhibitors, a cAMP-specific family that negatively regulates the function of almost all pro-inflammatory and immune cells and exerts widespread anti-inflammatory activity in animal models of asthma, have the possibility of improving the beneficial effects and reducing the adverse effects of theophylline, although existing inhibitors are limited by the same side effects as theophylline [3].

CHEMISTRY

Theophylline is a methylxanthine similar in structure to the common dietary xanthines caffeine and theobromine. Several substituted derivatives have been synthesized but none has any advantage over theophylline [4], apart from the 3-propyl derivative, enprofylline, which is more potent as a bronchodilator and may have fewer toxic effects [5]. Many salts of theophylline have also been marketed, the most common being aminophylline, the ethylene diamine salt used to increase solubility at neutral pH, so that intravenous administration is possible. Other salts, such as choline theophyllinate, do not have any advantage and others, *eg*, acepifylline, are virtually inactive [4].

MOLECULAR MECHANISMS OF ACTION

Although theophylline has been in clinical use since the 1940s, both its mechanism of action at a molecular level and its site of action remain uncertain. Several molecular mechanisms of action have been proposed, although many of these appear to occur only with higher concentrations of theophylline than are effective clinically (Table 17-1).

Phosphodiesterase Inhibition

Theophylline is a weak and nonselective inhibitor of PDEs, which break down cyclic nucleotides in the cell, thereby leading to an increase in intracellular cAMP and cGMP concentrations (Fig. 17-1). However, the degree of inhibition is small at therapeutically relevant concentrations of theophylline. Thus, total PDE activity in human lung extracts is inhibited by only 5% to 10% by therapeutic concentrations of theophylline [6]. There is convincing in vitro evidence that theophylline relaxes airway smooth muscle by inhibition of PDE activity, but relatively high concentrations are needed for maximal relaxation [7]. Similarly, the inhibitory effect of theophylline on mediator release from alveolar macrophages appears to be mediated by inhibition of PDE activity in these cells [8]. There is no evidence that airway smooth muscles of inflammatory cells concentrate theophylline to achieve higher intracellular than circulating concentrations. Inhibition of PDE should lead to synergistic interaction with β-agonists, but this has not been demonstrated convincingly in vivo. However, this might be because relaxation of airway smooth muscles by β-agonists may involve direct coupling of β-receptors via a stimulatory G protein to the opening of potassium channels, without the involvement of cAMP [9].

At least 12 isoenzyme families of PDE have now been recognized, and some (PDE3, PDE4, PDE5) are more important in smooth muscle relaxation [10,11]. However, there is no convincing evidence that theophylline has any greater inhibitory effect on the PDE isoenzymes involved in smooth

muscle relaxation. It is possible that PDE isoenzymes may have an increased expression in asthmatic airways, either as a result of the chronic inflammatory process or as a result of therapy. Elevation of cAMP by β-agonists may result in increased PDE activity, thus limiting the effect of β-agonists. Indeed, alveolar macrophages from asthmatic patients appear to have increased PDE activity [12]. This would mean that theophylline might have a greater inhibitory effect on PDE in asthmatic airways than in normal airways. Support for this is provided by the lack of bronchodilator effect of theophylline in healthy patients, compared to a bronchodilator effect in asthmatic patients [13].

Adenosine Receptor Antagonism

Theophylline is a potent inhibitor of adenosine receptors at therapeutic concentrations (both A_1- and A_2-receptors, although it is less effective against A_3 receptors), suggesting that this could be the basis for its bronchodilator effects [14]. Although adenosine has little effect on normal human airway smooth muscle in vitro, it constricts airways of asthmatic patients via the release of histamine and leukotrienes, suggesting that adenosine releases mediators from mast cells [15]. The receptor involved appears to be an A_3 receptor in rat mast cells [16], but in humans there is evidence for the involvement of an A_{2B} receptor [17]. Adenosine causes bronchoconstriction in asthmatic patients when given by inhalation [18]. The mechanism of bronchoconstriction is indirect and involves release of histamine from airway mast cells [15,19,20]. The bronchoconstrictor effect of adenosine is prevented by therapeutic concentrations of theophylline [18]. However, this only confirms that theophylline is capable of antagonizing the effects of adenosine at therapeutic concentrations; this does not indicate necessarily that this is important for its anti-asthma effect. However, adenosine antagonism is likely to account for some of the side effects of theophylline, *eg*, central nervous system stimulation, cardiac arrhythmias, gastric hypersecretion, gastroesophageal reflux, and diuresis.

Endogenous Catecholamine Release

Theophylline increases the secretion of adrenaline from the adrenal medulla [21], although the increase in plasma concentration is small and not sufficient to account for any significant bronchodilator effect [22].

Mediator Inhibition

Theophylline antagonizes the effect of some prostaglandins on vascular smooth muscle in vitro [23], but there is no evidence that these effects are seen at therapeutic concentrations or are relevant to its airway effects. Theophylline inhibits the secretion of tumor necrosis factor (TNF)-α by peripheral blood monocytes [24], and increases the secretion of the anti-inflammatory cytokine interleukin (IL)-10 [25]. However, these effects are not seen in alveolar macrophages obtained by bronchoalveolar lavage from patients treated with theophylline [26].

Table 17-1. MECHANISMS OF ACTION OF THEOPHYLLINE

Phosphodiesterase inhibition (nonselective)

Adenosine receptor antagonism (A_1, A_{2A}, A_{2B}-receptors)

Stimulation of catecholamine release

Mediator inhibition (prostaglandins, TNF-α)

Inhibition of intracellular calcium release

Inhibition of NF-κB (↓ nuclear translocation)

↑ Histone deacetylase activity
   (↑ efficacy of corticosteroids)

TNF—tumor necrosis factor.

Theophylline may also interfere with the action of TNF-α, which may be involved in inflammation in severe asthma. A related compound, pentoxifylline, prevents TNF-α–induced lung injury and enhanced hypoxic pulmonary vasoconstriction [27], but its mechanism of action is not yet understood.

Calcium Ion Flux

There is some evidence that theophylline may interfere with calcium mobilization in airway smooth muscle. Theophylline has no effect on entry of calcium ions (Ca^{2+}) via voltage-dependent channels, but it has been suggested that it may influence calcium entry via receptor-operated channels, release from intracellular stores, or have some effect on phosphatidylinositol turnover (which is linked to release of Ca^{2+} from intracellular stores). There is no direct evidence in favor of this, other than an effect on intracellular cAMP concentration due to its PDE inhibitory action. An early study suggesting that theophylline may increase Ca^{2+} uptake into intracellular stores has not been followed up [28].

Effect on Transcription

Theophylline prevents the translocation of the proinflammatory transcription factor NF-κB into the nucleus, thus potentially reducing the expression of inflammatory genes in asthma and COPD [29]. Recent studies suggest that low concentrations of theophylline increase the activity of histone deacetylases, which are recruited by corticosteroids to the transcription complex to switch off inflammatory genes [30]. This action of theophylline occurs at therapeutically relevant concentrations and is not mediated via PDE inhibition of adenosine antagonism. It predicts a synergistic action between theophylline and corticosteroids, and there is a marked synergy between theophylline and corticosteroids in suppressing the expression of inflammatory genes in vitro.

Effects on Apoptosis

Prolonged survival of granulocytes due to a reduction in apoptosis may be important in perpetuating chronic inflammation in asthma (eosinophils) and COPD (neutrophils). Theophylline inhibits apoptosis in eosinophils and neutrophils in vitro [31]. This is associated with a reduction in the anti-apoptotic protein bcl-2 [32]. This effect is not mediated via PDE inhibition, but in neutrophils it may be mediated by antagonism of adenosine A_{2A} receptors [33].

CELLULAR EFFECTS

Theophylline has several effects that may contribute to its clinical efficacy in the treatment of asthma and COPD (Fig. 17-2).

Airway Smooth Muscle Effects

The primary effect of theophylline is assumed to be relaxation of airway smooth muscle, and in vitro studies have shown that it is equally effective in large and small airways [34]. In airways obtained at lung surgery, approximately 25% of preparations fail to relax with a β-agonist, but all relax with theophylline [35]. The molecular mechanism of bronchodilatation is almost certainly related to PDE inhibition, resulting in an increase in cAMP [7]. The bronchodilator effect of theophylline is reduced in human airways by the toxin charybdotoxin, which inhibits large conductance Ca^{2+}-activated K^+ channels (maxi-K channels), suggesting that theophylline opens maxi-K channels via an increase in cAMP [36]. Theophylline acts as a functional antagonist and inhibits the contractile response of multiple spasmogens. In airways obtained postmortem from patients who have died from asthma, the relaxant response to β-agonists is reduced, whereas the bronchodilator response to theophylline is no different from that seen in normal

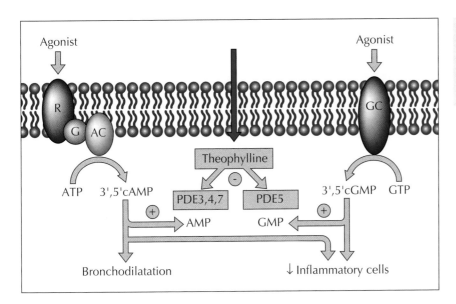

Figure 17-1.
Effect of phosphodiesterase (PDE) inhibitors in the breakdown of cyclic nucleotides in airway smooth muscle and inflammatory cells.

airways [37]. There is evidence that β-adrenoceptors in airway smooth muscle of patients with fatal asthma become uncoupled [38], and theophylline may therefore have a theoretical advantage over β-agonists in severe asthma exacerbations. However, theophylline is a weak bronchodilator at therapeutically relevant concentrations, suggesting that some other target cell may be more relevant for its anti-asthma effect. In human airways the median effective dose (EC_{50}) for theophylline is approximately $1.5 \times 10_{-4}$ M, which is equivalent to 67 mg/L assuming 60% protein binding [35]. However, as discussed above, it is important to consider the possibility that PDE activity may be increased in asthmatic airways, so theophylline may have a greater than expected effect.

In vivo intravenous aminophylline has an acute bronchodilator effect in asthmatic patients, which is most likely to be due to a relaxant effect on airway smooth muscle [39]. The bronchodilator effect of theophylline in chronic asthma is small in comparison with β-agonists, however. Several studies have demonstrated a small protective effect of theophylline on histamine, methacholine, or exercise challenge [40–43]. This protective effect does not correlate well with any bronchodilator effect, and it is interesting that in some studies the protective effect of theophylline is observed at plasma concentrations of less than 10 mg/L. These clinical studies suggest that theophylline may have anti-asthma effects unrelated to any bronchodilator action.

Anti-inflammatory Effects

Whether theophylline has significant anti-inflammatory effects in asthma or COPD is still unresolved [44]. Theophylline inhibits histamine release from human basophils in vitro [45] and mediator release from chopped human lung [46], although high concentrations are necessary and it is likely that this effect involves an increase in cAMP concentration due to PDE inhibition. Theophylline also has an inhibitory effect on superoxide anion release from human neutrophils [47] and inhibits the feedback stimulatory effect of adenosine on neutrophils in vivo [48]. At therapeutic concentrations, in vitro theophylline may *increase* superoxide release via an inhibitory effect on adenosine receptors, since endogenous adenosine may normally exert an inhibitory action on these cells [49]. Similar results are also seen in guinea pig and human eosinophils [50]. At therapeutic concentrations there is an increased release of superoxide anions from eosinophils, which appears to be mediated via inhibition of adenosine A_2-receptors and is mimicked by the adenosine antagonist 8-phenyltheophylline. Inhibition of eosinophil superoxide generation occurs only at high concentrations of theophylline ($> 10_{-4}$ M), which are likely to inhibit PDE. Similar results have also been obtained in human alveolar macrophages [8]. Macrophages lavaged from patients taking theophylline have been found to have a reduced oxidative burst response [51], but there is no reduction in the release of the proinflammatory cytokines tumor necrosis factor (TNF)-α or granulocyte-macrophage colony-stimulating factor (GM-CSF) [26]. Theophylline inhibits neutrophil chemotaxis via inhibition of adenosine A_{2A} receptors [33].

In vivo theophylline inhibits mediator-induced airway microvascular leakage in rodents when given in high doses [52], although this is not seen at therapeutically relevant concentrations [53]. Theophylline has an inhibitory effect on plasma exudation in nasal secretions induced by

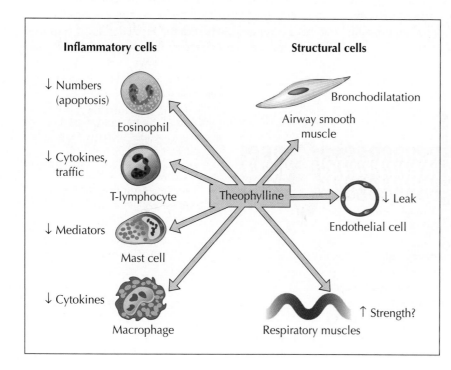

Figure 17-2.
Multiple effects of theophylline.

allergen in patients with allergic rhinitis, although this could be secondary to inhibition of mediator release [54].

In allergen challenge studies in asthmatic patients, intravenous theophylline inhibits the late response to allergen, while having relatively little effect on the early response [55]. A similar finding with allergen challenge has been reported after chronic oral treatment with theophylline [56]. This has been interpreted as an effect on the chronic inflammatory response. This finding is supported by a reduced infiltration of eosinophils into the airways after allergen challenge following low doses of theophylline [57]. In patients with nocturnal asthma, low-dose theophylline inhibits the influx of neutrophils and, to a lesser extent, eosinophils seen in the early morning [48]. Oral theophylline also inhibits the late response to toluene diisocyanate (TDI) in TDI-sensitive asthmatic patients [58], but has no effect on the subsequent increase in methacholine responsiveness. Similarly, theophylline has no effect on the increased airway responsiveness that follows allergen challenge [59], and does not reduce airway responsiveness in asthmatic patients after chronic administration [60]. These studies indicate that theophylline on its own may have effects on acute inflammation in the airways, but may be less effective on the chronic inflammatory process. However, a recent study in patients with mild asthma showed that low doses of theophylline reduced the numbers of eosinophils in bronchial biopsies, bronchoalveolar lavage, and induced sputum [61••]. There was no effect on exhaled nitric oxide, a non-invasive marker of airway inflammation.

In patients with COPD, theophylline reduces the proportion of neutrophils in induced sputum and reduces the concentration of IL-8, suggesting that it may have an anti-inflammatory effect unlike corticosteroids [62•]. This may be relevant in the treatment of more severe asthma, where there is a preponderance of neutrophils and an increase in IL-8 [63].

Immunomodulatory Effects

T lymphocytes are now believed to play a central role in coordinating the chronic inflammatory response in asthma. For many years theophylline has been shown to have several actions on T-lymphocyte function, suggesting that it might have an immunomodulatory effect in asthma. Theophylline has a stimulatory effect on suppressor (CD8+) T-lymphocytes, which may be relevant to the control of chronic airway inflammation [64,65], and has an inhibitory effect on graft rejection [66]. In vitro theophylline inhibits IL-2 synthesis in human T lymphocytes, an effect that is secondary to a rise in intracellular cAMP concentration [67]. At high concentrations, theophylline inhibits proliferation in CD4+ and CD8+ cells, an effect mediated via inhibition of PDE4 [68]. Theophylline also inhibits the chemotactic response of T lymphocytes, an effect that is also mediated through PDE inhibition [69]. In allergen-induced airway inflammation in guinea pigs,

theophylline has a significant inhibitory effect on eosinophil infiltration [70], suggesting that it may inhibit the T cell–derived cytokines responsible for this eosinophilic response. Theophylline has been reported to decrease circulating concentrations of IL-4 and IL-5 in asthmatic patients [71]. In asthmatic patients, low-dose theophylline treatment results in an increase in activated circulating CD4+ and CD8+ T cells but a decrease in these cells in the airways, suggesting that the treatment may reduce the trafficking of activated T cells into the airways [72]. This is supported by studies in allergen challenge, where low-dose theophylline decreases the number of activated CD4+ and CD8+ T cells in bronchoalveolar lavage fluid after allergen challenge, and is mirrored by an increase in these cells in peripheral blood [73]. These effects are seen even in patients treated with high doses of inhaled corticosteroids, indicating that the molecular effects of theophylline are likely to be different from those of corticosteroids. Theophylline induces apoptosis of T lymphocytes, thus reducing their survival [74]. This effect may be mediated via PDE4 inhibition, so it may not be relevant to clinical doses of theophylline. The therapeutic range of theophylline was based on measurement of immediate bronchodilatation in response to the acute administration of theophylline [39]. However, it is possible that the nonbronchodilator effects of theophylline, which may reflect some anti-inflammatory or immunomodulatory effect, may be exerted at lower plasma concentrations and that different molecular mechanisms may be involved [75•]. Indeed, the novel mechanism of action ascribed to theophylline involving activation of histone deacetylases is found at therapeutic concentrations of theophylline, but lost at the higher concentrations needed for PDE inhibition and bronchodilatation [30].

Extrapulmonary Effects

Theophylline may exert its effects in asthma and COPD via some action outside the airways. It may be relevant that theophylline is ineffective when given by inhalation until therapeutic plasma concentrations are achieved [76]. This may indicate that theophylline has effects on cells other than those in the airway. One possible target cell is the platelet; theophylline has been demonstrated to inhibit platelet activation.

An effect of theophylline that remains controversial is its action on respiratory muscles. Aminophylline increases diaphragmatic contractility and reverses diaphragm fatigue [77]. This effect has not been observed by all investigators, and there now are doubts about the relevance of these observations to the clinical benefit provided by theophylline in COPD [78].

PHARMACOKINETICS

There is a close relationship between the acute improvement in airway function and serum theophylline concentration. Below 10 mg/L, therapeutic effects (at least in terms of rapid improvement in airway function) are small, and above 25 mg/L, additional benefits are outweighed by side effects, so the therapeutic range was considered to be 10 to 20 mg/L (55–110 μM) [2•]. It is now apparent that nonbronchodilator effects of theophylline may be seen at plasma concentrations of less than 10 mg/L, and that clinical benefit may be derived from these lower concentrations of theophylline. This suggests that it is necessary to redefine the therapeutic range of theophylline based on anti-asthma effect, rather than the acute bronchodilator response that requires a higher plasma concentration. The dose of theophylline required to give therapeutic concentrations varies among subjects, largely because of differences in clearance. In addition, there may be differences in bronchodilator response to theophylline and, with acute bronchoconstriction, higher concentrations may be required to produce bronchodilatation [79].

Theophylline is rapidly and completely absorbed, but there are large interindividual variations in clearance due to differences in hepatic metabolism (Table 17-2). Theophylline is metabolized in the liver by the cytochrome P450/P448 microsomal enzyme system, and a large number of factors may influence hepatic metabolism. Theophylline is predominantly metabolized by the CYP1A2 enzyme, while at higher plasma concentrations CYP2E1 is also involved [80].

Increased Clearance

Increased clearance is seen in children ages 1 to 16 years, and in tobacco and marijuana smokers. Concurrent

---

Table 17-2. FACTORS AFFECTING CLEARANCE OF THEOPHYLLINE

Increased Clearance

Enzyme induction (rifampicin, phenobarbitone, ethanol)

Smoking (tobacco, marijuana)

High-protein, low-carbohydrate diet

Barbecued meat

Childhood

Decreased Clearance

Enzyme inhibition (cimetidine, erythromycin, ciprofloxacin, allopurinol, zileuton)

Congestive heart failure

Liver disease

Pneumonia

Viral infection and vaccination

High-carbohydrate diet

Old age

---

administration of phenytoin and phenobarbitone increases activity of P450, resulting in increased metabolic breakdown, so that higher doses may be required.

Reduced Clearance

Reduced clearance is found in liver disease, pneumonia, and heart failure, and doses need to be reduced to half and plasma levels monitored carefully [81]. Increased clearance is also seen with certain drugs, including erythromycin, certain quinolone antibiotics (ciprofloxacin, but not ofloxacin), allopurinol, cimetidine (but not ranitidine), serotonin uptake inhibitors (fluvoxamine), and the 5-lipoxygenase inhibitor zileuton, all of which interfere with CYP 1A2 function. Thus, if a patient on maintenance theophylline requires a course of erythromycin, the dose of theophylline should be halved. Viral infections and vaccination may also reduce clearance, and this may be particularly important in children. Because of these variations in clearance, individualization of theophylline dosage is required and plasma concentrations should be measured 4 hours after the last dose with slow-release preparations when steady state has been achieved. There is no significant circadian variation in theophylline metabolism [82], although there may be delayed absorption at night, which may relate to the supine posture [83].

ROUTES OF ADMINISTRATION

Intravenous

Intravenous aminophylline has been used for many years in the treatment of acute severe asthma. The recommended dose is now 6 mg/kg given intravenously over 20 to 30 min, followed by a maintenance dose of 0.5 mg/kg/h. If the patient is already taking theophylline, or there are any factors that decrease clearance, these doses should be halved and the plasma level checked more frequently.

Oral

Plain theophylline tablets and elixir, which are rapidly absorbed, give wide fluctuations in plasma levels and are not recommended. Several effective sustained-release preparations are available which are absorbed at a constant rate and provide steady plasma concentrations over a 12–24 hour period [84]. Although there are differences between preparations, these are relatively minor and of no clinical significance. Both slow-release aminophylline and theophylline are available and are equally effective, although the ethylene diamine component of aminophylline occasionally has been implicated in allergic reactions. For continuous treatment, twice-daily therapy (approximately 8 mg/kg twice daily) is needed, although some preparations are designed for once daily administration. For nocturnal asthma, a single dose of slow-release theophylline at night is often effective [85,86], and often more effective than an oral slow-release β-agonist preparation. Once optimal doses have been determined, plasma concentrations usually remain stable, providing no factors that alter clearance change.

Other Routes

Aminophylline may be given as a suppository, but rectal absorption is unreliable and proctitis may occur, so it is best avoided. Inhalation of theophylline is irritant and ineffective. Intramuscular injections of theophylline are very painful and should never be given. The inhaled route is ineffective.

CLINICAL USE

Acute Severe Asthma

Intravenous aminophylline has been used in the management of acute severe asthma since the 1950s, but this use has been questioned in view of the risk of adverse effects compared with nebulized β₂-agonists. In patients with acute asthma, intravenous aminophylline is less effective than nebulized β₂-agonists [87], and should therefore be reserved for those patients who fail to respond to β-agonists. There is some evidence that the use of aminophylline in the emergency room for patients with acute asthma reduces subsequent hospital admissions [88]. In a meta-analysis of 13 acceptably designed clinical trials to compare nebulized β-agonists with or without intravenous aminophylline, there was no overall additional benefit from adding aminophylline [89]. This indicates that aminophylline should not be added routinely to nebulized β-agonists. Indeed, addition of aminophylline may only increase side effects [90]. Several deaths have been reported after intravenous aminophylline. In one study of 43 asthma deaths in southern England, there was a significantly greater frequency of toxic theophylline concentrations (21%) compared with matched controls (7%) [91]. These concerns have led to the view that intravenous aminophylline should be reserved for the few patients with acute severe asthma who fail to show a satisfactory response to nebulized β₂-agonists. When intravenous aminophylline is used, it should be given as a slow intravenous infusion with careful monitoring, and a plasma theophylline concentration should be measured prior to infusion.

Chronic Asthma

In most guidelines for asthma management, theophylline is used as an additional bronchodilator if asthma remains difficult to control after high doses of inhaled corticosteroids and long-acting inhaled β₂-agonists. The introduction of long-acting inhaled β₂-agonists has further threatened the position of theophylline because the side effects of these agents may be less frequent that those associated with theophylline and long-acting inhaled β₂-agonists are more effective controllers than theophylline [92].

Whether theophylline has some additional benefit over its bronchodilator action is now an important consideration. In studies of patients with chronic asthma, oral theophylline appears to be as effective as cromolyn sodium in controlling young patients with allergic asthma [93] and it provides additional control of asthma symptoms even in patients talking inhaled steroids regularly [94]. Theophylline was almost as effective as a low dose of inhaled corticosteroids in both children and adults [95,96].

In one study of a group of adolescent patients with difficult to control asthma who were controlled with oral and inhaled steroids, nebulized β₂-agonists, inhaled anticholinergics, and cromones, in addition to regular oral theophylline, withdrawal of oral theophylline resulted in a marked deterioration of asthma control which could not be controlled by further increase in steroids and only responded to reintroduction of theophylline [97]. This suggests that there may be a group of patients with severe asthma who particularly benefit from theophylline. In a controlled trial of theophylline withdrawal in patients with severe asthma controlled only on high doses of inhaled corticosteroids, there was a significant deterioration in symptoms and lung function when placebo was substituted for the relatively low maintenance dose of theophylline [72]. There is also evidence that addition of theophylline improves asthma control to a greater extent than do β₂-agonists in patients with severe asthma treated with high-dose inhaled steroids [98]. This suggests that theophylline may have a useful place in the optimal management of patients with moderate to severe asthma and appears to provide additional control above that provided by high-dose inhaled steroids [99].

Theophylline may be a useful treatment for nocturnal asthma; a single dose of a slow-release theophylline preparation given at night may provide effective control of nocturnal asthma symptoms [85,100]. There is evidence that slow-release theophylline preparations are more effective than slow-release oral β₂-agonists and inhaled β₂-agonists in controlling nocturnal asthma [86,101,102]. Theophylline is approximately equal in efficacy to salmeterol in controlling nocturnal asthma, but the quality of sleep is better with salmeterol as compared with theophylline [103]. The mechanism of action of theophylline in nocturnal asthma may involve more than long-lasting bronchodilatation, and could involve inhibition of some components of the inflammatory response, which may increase at night [48].

Several studies have demonstrated that adding low-dose theophylline to inhaled corticosteroids in patients who are not controlled gives better asthma control than doubling the dose of inhaled corticosteroids. This has been demonstrated in patients with moderate to severe and mild asthma [104•,105–107]. Interestingly, there is a greater degree of improvement in forced vital capacity than FEV₁ (forced expiratory volume in 1 second), possibly indicating an effect on peripheral airways. Because the improvement in lung function was relatively slow, this suggests that the effect of the added theophylline may be anti-inflammatory rather than bronchodilatory, particularly because the plasma concentration of theophylline in these studies was less than 10 mg/mL. These studies suggest that low-dose theophylline may be preferable to increasing the dose of inhaled steroids when asthma is not controlled on moderate doses of inhaled steroids; such a therapeutic approach would be much less expensive than adding long-acting inhaled β_2-agonists. Several studies have documented steroid-sparing effects of theophylline [108].

Interaction with β-Agonists

If theophylline exerts its effects by PDE inhibition, then a synergistic interaction with β-agonists would be expected. Many studies have investigated this possibility, but while there is good evidence that theophylline and β-agonists have additive effects, true synergy is not seen [109,110]. This can now be understood in terms of the molecular mechanisms of action of β-agonists and theophylline. β-Agonists may cause relaxation of airway smooth muscle via several mechanisms. Classically they increase intracellular cAMP concentrations, which were believed to be an essential event in the relaxation response. It has recently become clear that β-agonists may cause bronchodilatation, at least in part, by opening maxi-K channels in airway smooth muscle cells [9,36]. Maxi-K channels are opened by low concentrations of β_2-agonists that are likely to be therapeutically relevant. There is now evidence that β-receptors may be coupled directly to maxi-K channels via the α-subunit of G_s [111], and therefore may induce relaxation without any increase in cAMP, thus accounting for a lack of synergy. Another reason for the lack if synergy may be that cells other than airway smooth muscle may be the main target for the anti-asthma effect of theophylline.

Repeated administration of β_2-agonists may result in tolerance. While this may be explained by down-regulation of β_2-receptors, an additional mechanism may involve up-regulation of PDE enzymes (especially PDE4D) which then break down cAMP more readily [112]. Theophylline may therefore theoretically prevent the development of tolerance, although this has not yet been studied clinically. Theophylline may provide useful additional bronchodilatation in patients with COPD, even when maximally effective doses of a β-agonist have been given. However, theophylline at therapeutic concentrations does not prevent the loss of the bronchoprotective effect of inhaled long-acting β_2-agonists [113].

SIDE EFFECTS

There is no doubt that theophylline provides clinical benefit in obstructive airway disease, but the main limitation to its use is the frequency of adverse effects [114]. Unwanted effects of theophylline are usually related to plasma concentration and tend to occur when plasma levels exceed 20 mg/L. However, some patients develop side effects even at low plasma concentrations. To some extent side effects may be reduced by gradually increasing the dose until therapeutic concentrations are achieved.

The most common side effects are headache, nausea and vomiting, abdominal discomfort, and restlessness. There may also be increased acid secretion, gastroesophageal reflux, and diuresis. There has recently been concern that theophylline, even at therapeutic concentrations, may lead to behavioral disturbance and learning difficulties in school children [115], although it is difficult to design adequate controls for such studies. At high concentrations convulsions and cardiac arrhythmias may occur, and there is concern that intravenous aminophylline administered in the emergency room may be a contributory factor to the deaths of some patients with severe asthma [91].

Some of the side effects of theophylline (central nervous system stimulation, gastric secretion, diuresis, and arrhythmias) may be due to adenosine receptors, and therefore these may be avoided by PDE inhibitors. The most common side effects of theophylline are nausea and headaches, which may be due to inhibition of certain PDEs (*eg*, PDE4 in the vomiting center) [116].

FUTURE OF THEOPHYLLINE

Although theophylline use has declined recently, it may come back into fashion for the treatment of chronic asthma given the recognition that it may have an anti-inflammatory and immunomodulatory effect when given in low doses (plasma concentration 5–10 mg/L) [75•]. At these low doses the drug is easier to use, side effects are uncommon, and the problems of drug interaction are less of a problem, thus making the clinical use of theophylline less complicated. Theophylline appears to have an effect that is different from that of corticosteroids, and it may therefore be a useful drug to combine with low-dose inhaled steroids. The molecular mechanism of anti-inflammatory effects of theophylline is now becoming clearer and it seems likely that there is a synergistic interaction with the anti-inflammatory mechanism of corticosteroids. This interaction may underlie the beneficial effects of theophylline when added to inhaled corticosteroids. Because slow-release theophylline preparations are cheaper than long-acting inhaled β_2-agonists and anti-leukotrienes, this may justify the choice of low-dose theophylline as the add-on therapy for asthma control. In addition, compliance with oral therapy is likely to be greater than with inhaled therapies [117]. This suggests that low-dose theophylline may find an important place in modern asthma management in patients with moderate asthma as well as in patients with severe asthma.

REFERENCES AND RECOMMENDED READING

Papers of particular interest, published recently, have been highlighted as:
- • Of importance
- •• Of major importance

1. Lam A, Newhouse MT: Management of asthma and chronic airflow limitation. Are methylxanthines obsolete? *Chest* 1990, 98:4–52.

2.• Weinberger M, Hendeles L: Theophylline in asthma. *N Engl J Med* 1996, 334:1380–1388.
Good review of theophylline in asthma.

3. Giembycz MA: Phosphodiesterase 4 inhibitors and the treatment of asthma: where are we now and where do we go from here? *Drugs* 2000, 59:193–212.

4. Weinberger M: The pharmacology and therapeutic use of theophylline. *J Allergy Clin Immunol* 1984, 73:525–540.

5. Persson CGA: Development of safer xanthine drugs for the treatment of obstructive airways disease. *J Allergy Clin Immunol* 1986, 78:817–824.

6. Poolson JB, Kazanowski JJ, Goldman AL, Szentivanyi A: Inhibition of human pulmonary phosphodiesterase activity by therapeutic levels of theophylline. *Clin Exp Pharmacol Physiol* 1978, 5:535–539.

7. Rabe KF, Magnussen H, Dent G: Theophylline and selective PDE inhibitors as bronchodilators and smooth muscle relaxants. *Eur Respir J* 1995, 8:637–642.

8. Dent G, Giembycz MA, Rabe KF, *et al.*: Theophylline suppresses human alveolar macrophage respiratory burst through phosphodiesterase inhibition. *Am J Respir Cell Mol Biol* 1994, 10:565–572.

9. Kume H, Hall IP, Washabau RJ, *et al.*: Adrenergic agonists regulate K_{Ca} channels in airway smooth muscle by cAMP-dependent and -independent mechanisms. *J Clin Invest* 1994, 93:371–379.

10. Beavo JA: Cyclic nucleotide phosphodiesterases: functional implications of multiple isoforms. *Physiol Rev* 1995, 75:725–748.

11. Rabe KF, Tenor M, Dent G, *et al.*: Phosphodiesterase isozymes modulating intrinsic tone in human airways: identification and characterization. *Am J Physiol* 1993, 264:L458–L464.

12. Bachelet M, Vincent D, Havet N, *et al.*: Reduced responsiveness of adenylate cyclase in alveolar macrophages from patients with asthma. *J Allergy Clin Immunol* 1991, 88:322–328.

13. Estenne M, Yernault J, De Troyer A: Effects of parenteral aminophylline on lung mechanics in normal humans. *Am Rev Respir Dis* 1980, 121:967–971.

14. Pauwels RA, Joos GF: Characterization of the adenosine receptors in the airways. *Arch Int Pharmacodyn Ther* 1995, 329:151–156.

15. Bjorck T, Gustafsson LE, Dahlen SE: Isolated bronchi from asthmatics are hyperresponsive to adenosine, which apparently acts indirectly by liberation of leukotrienes and histamine. *Am Rev Respir Dis* 1992, 145:1087–1091.

16. Fozard JR, Pfannkuche HJ, Schuurman HJ: Mast cell degranulation following adenosine A3 receptor activation in rats. *Eur J Pharmacol* 1996, 298:293–297.

17. Feoktistov I, Polosa R, Holgate ST, Biaggioni I: Adenosine A2B receptors: a novel therapeutic target in asthma? *Trends Pharmacol Sci* 1998, 19:148–153.

18. Cushley MJ, Tattersfield AE, Holgate ST: Adenosine-induced bronchoconstriction in asthma: antagonism by inhaled theophylline. *Am Rev Respir Dis* 1984, 129:380–384.

19. Cushley MJ, Holgate ST: Adenosine induced bronchoconstriction in asthma: role of mast cell mediator release. *J Allergy Clin Immunol* 1985, 75:272–278.

20. Björk T, Gustafsson LE, Dahlén SE: Isolated bronchi from asthmatics are hyperresponsive to adenosine, which apparently acts indirectly by liberation of leukotrienes and histamine. *Am Rev Respir Dis* 1992, 145:1087–1091.

21. Ishizaki T, Minegishi A, Morishita A, *et al.*: Plasma catecholamine concentrations during a 72-hour aminophylline infusion in children with acute asthma. *J Allergy Clin Immunol* 1988, 92:146–154.

22. Barnes PJ: Endogenous catecholamines and asthma. *J Allergy Clin Immunol* 1986, 77:791–795.

23. Horrobin DF, Manku MS, Franks DJ, Hamet P: Methylxanthine phosphodiesterase inhibitors behave as prostaglandin antagonists in a perfused rat mesenteric artery preparation. *Prostaglandins* 1977, 13:33–40.

24. Spatafora M, Chiappara G, Merendino AM, *et al.*: Theophylline suppresses the release of tumour necrosis factor-alpha by blood monocytes and alveolar macrophages. *Eur Respir J* 1994, 7:223–228.

25. Mascali JJ, Cvietusa P, Negri J, Borish L: Anti-inflammatory effects of theophylline: modulation of cytokine production. *Ann Allergy Asthma Immunol* 1996, 77:34–38.

26. Oliver B, Tomita K, Meah S, *et al.*: The effect of low dose theophylline on cytokine production from alveolar macrophages in patients with mild asthma. *Am J Respir Crit Care Med* 2000, 161:A614.

27. Liu S-F, Dewar A, Crawley DE, *et al.*: Effect of tumor necrosis factor on hypoxic pulmonary vasoconstriction. *J Appl Physiol* 1992, 72:1044–1049.

28. Kolbeck RC, Speir WA, Carrier GO, Bransome ED: Apparent irrelevance of cyclic nucleotides to the relaxation of tracheal smooth muscle induced by theophylline. *Lung* 1979, 156:173–183.

29. Tomita K, Chikumi H, Tokuyasu H, *et al.*: Functional assay of NF-κB translocation into nuclei by laser scanning cytometry: inhibitory effect by dexamethasone or theophylline. *Naunyn Schmiedebergs Arch Pharmacol* 1999, 359:249–255.

30. Ito K, Lim S, Caramori G, *et al.*: A molecular mechanism of action of theophylline: Induction of histone deacetylase activity to decrease inflammatory gene expression. *Proc Natl Acad Sci U S A* 2002, 99(13):8921–8926.

31. Yasui K, Hu B, Nakazawa T, *et al.*: Theophylline accelerates human granulocyte apoptosis not via phosphodiesterase inhibition. *J Clin Invest* 1997, 100:1677–1684.

32. Chung IY, Nam-Kung EK, Lee NM, *et al.*: The downregulation of bcl-2 expression is necessary for theophylline-induced apoptosis of eosinophil. *Cell Immunol* 2000, 203:95–102.

33. Yasui K, Agematsu K, Shinozaki K, *et al.*: Theophylline induces neutrophil apoptosis through adenosine A_{2A} receptor antagonism. *J Leuko Biol* 2000, 67:529–535.

34. Finney MJB, Karlson JA, Persson CGA: Effects of bronchoconstriction and bronchodilation on a novel human small airway preparation. *Br J Pharmacol* 1985, 85:29–36.

35. Guillot C, Fornaris M, Badger M, Orehek J: Spontaneous and provoked resistance to isoproterenol in isolated human bronchi. *J Allergy Clin Immunol* 1984, 74:713–718.

36. Miura M, Belvisi MG, Stretton CD, *et al.*: Role of potassium channels in bronchodilator responses in human airways. *Am Rev Respir Dis* 1992, 146:132–136.

37. Goldie RG, Spina D, Henry PJ, *et al.*: In vitro responsiveness of human asthmatic bronchus to carbachol, histamine, beta-adrenoceptor agonists and theophylline. *Br J Clin Pharmacol* 1986, 22:669–676.

38. Bai TR: Beta$_2$-adrenergic receptors in asthma: a current perspective. *Lung* 1992, 170:125–141.

39. Mitenko PA, Ogilvie RI: Rational intravenous doses of theophylline. *N Engl J Med* 1973, 289:600–603.

40. McWilliams BC, Menendez R, Kelly WH, Howick J: Effects of theophylline on inhaled methacholine and histamine in asthmatic children. *Am Rev Respir Dis* 1984, 130:193–197.

41. Cartier A, Lemire I, L'Archeveque J: Theophylline partially inhibits bronchoconstriction caused by inhaled histamine in subjects with asthma. *J Allergy Clin Immunol* 1986, 77:570–575.

42. Magnusson H, Reuss G, Jorres R: Theophylline has a dose-related effect on the airway response to inhaled histamine and methacholine in asthmatics. *Am Rev Respir Dis* 1987, 136:1163–1167.

43. Magnussen H, Reuss G, Jörres R: Methylxanthines inhibit exercise-induced bronchoconstriction at low serum theophylline concentrations and in a dose-dependent fashion. *J Allergy Clin Immunol* 1988, 81:531–537.

44. Persson CGA: Xanthines as airway anti inflammatory drugs. *J Allergy Clin Immunol* 1988, 81:615–617.

45. Lichtenstein LM, Margolis S: Histamine release in vitro: inhibition by catecholamines and methylxanthines. *Science* 1968, 161:902–903.

46. Orange RP, Kaliner MA, Laraia PJ, Austen KF: Immunological release of histamine and slow reacting substance of anaphylaxis from human lung. II. Influence of cellular levels of cyclic AMP. *Fed Proc* 1971, 30:1725–1729.

47. Nielson CP, Crawley JJ, Morgan ME, Vestal RE: Poly-morphonuclear leukocyte inhibition by therapeutic concentrations of theophylline is mediated by cyclic 3′,5′ adenosine aminophosphate. *Am Rev Respir Dis* 1988, 137:25–30.

48. Kraft M, Torvik JA, Trudeau JB, *et al.*: Theophylline: potential antiinflammatory effects in nocturnal asthma. *J Allergy Clin Immunol* 1996, 97:1242–1246.

49. Schrier DJ, Imre RM: The effects of adenosine antagonists on human neutrophil function. *J Immunol* 1986, 137:3284–3289.

50. Yukawa T, Kroegel C, Chanez P, *et al.*: Effect of theophylline and adenosine on eosinophil function. *Am Rev Respir Dis* 1989, 140:327–333.

51. O'Neill SJ, Sitar DS, Kilass DJ: The pulmonary disposition of theophylline and its influences on human alveolar macrophage bactericidal function. *Am Rev Respir Dis* 1988, 134:1225–1228.

52. Erjefalt I, Persson CGA: Pharmacologic control of plasma exudation into tracheobronchial airways. *Am Rev Respir Dis* 1991, 143:1008–1014.

53. Boschetto P, Roberts NM, Rogers DF, Barnes PJ: The effect of antiasthma drugs on microvascular leak in guinea pig airways. *Am Rev Respir Dis* 1989, 139:416–421.

54. Naclerio RM, Bartenfelder D, Proud D, *et al.*: Theophylline reduces histamine release during pollen-induced rhinitis. *J Allergy Clin Immunol* 1986, 78:874–876.

55. Pauwels R, van Revterghem D, van der Straeten M, *et al.*: The effect of theophylline and enprophylline on allergen-induced bronchoconstriction. *J Allergy Clin Immunol* 1985, 76:583–590.

56. Ward AJM, McKenniff M, Evans JM, *et al.*: Theophylline—an immunomodulatory role in asthma? *Am Rev Respir Dis* 1993, 147:518–523.

57. Sullivan P, Bekir S, Jaffar Z, *et al.*: Anti-inflammatory effects of low-dose oral theophylline in atopic asthma. *Lancet* 1994, 343:1006–1008.

58. Mapp C, Boschetto P, Dal Vecchio L, *et al.*: Protective effect of antiasthma drugs on late asthmatic reactions and increased airway responsiveness induced by toluene diisocyanate in sensitized subjects. *Am Rev Respir Dis* 1987, 136:1403–1407.

59. Cockroft DW, Murdock KY, Gore BP, *et al.*: Theophylline does not inhibit allergen-induced increase in airway responsiveness to methacholine. *J Allergy Clin Immunol* 1991, 83:913–920.

60. Dutoit JI, Salome CM, Woolcock AJ: Inhaled corticosteroids reduce the severity of bronchial hyperresponsiveness in asthma, but oral theophylline does not. *Am Rev Respir Dis* 1987, 136:1174–1178.

61.•• Lim S, Tomita K, Carramori G, *et al.*: Low-dose theophylline reduces eosinophilic inflammation but not exhaled nitric oxide in mild asthma. *Am J Respir Crit Care Med* 2001, 164:273–276.
A paper illustrating the anti-inflammatory effect of low-dose theophylline.

62.• Culpitt SV, de Matos C, Russell RE, *et al.*: Effect of theophylline on induced sputum inflammatory indices and neutrophil chemotaxis in COPD. *Am J Respir Crit Care Med* 2002, 165:1371–1376.
First investigation of an anti-inflammatory effect of theophylline in COPD.

63. Jatakanon A, Lalloo UG, Lim S, *et al.*: Increased neutrophils and cytokines, TNF-alpha and IL-8, in induced sputum of non-asthmatic patients with chronic dry cough. *Thorax* 1999, 54:234–237.

64. Shohat B, Volovitz B, Varsano I: Induction of suppressor T cells in asthmatic children by theophylline treatment. *Clin Allergy* 1983, 13:487–493.

65. Fink G, Mittelman M, Shohat B, Spitzer SA: Theophylline-induced alterations in cellular immunity in asthmatic patients. *Clin Allergy* 1987, 17:313–316.

66. Guillou PJ, Ramsden C, Kerr M, *et al.*: A prospective controlled clinical trial of aminophylline as an adjunct immunosuppressive agent. *Transplant Proc* 1984, 16:1218–1220.

67. Didier M, Aussel C, Ferrua B, Fehlman M: Regulation of interleukin 2 synthesis by cAMP in human T cells. *J Immunol* 1987, 139:1179–1184.

68. Giembycz MA, Corrigan CJ, Seybold J, *et al.*: Cyclic AMP phosphodiesterases 3,4 and 7 in human CD4+ and CD8+ T-lymphocytes: role in regulating proliferation and the generation of interleukin-2. *Am J Respir Crit Care Med* 1996, 153:A144.

69. Hidi R, Timmermans S, Liu E, *et al.*: Phosphodiesterase and cyclic adenosine monophosphate-dependent inhibition of T-lymphocyte chemotaxis. *Eur Respir J* 2000, 15:342–209.

70. Sanjar S, Aoki S, Kristersson A, *et al.*: Antigen challenge induces pulmonary eosinophil accumulation and airway hyperreactivity in sensitized guinea pigs: the effect of anti-asthma drugs. *Br J Pharmacol* 1990, 99:679–686.

71. Kosmas EN, Michaelides SA, Polychronaki A, *et al.*: Theophylline induces a reduction in circulating interleukin-4 and interleukin-5 in atopic asthmatics. *Eur Respir J* 1999, 13:53–58.

72. Kidney J, Dominguez M, Taylor PM, *et al.*: Immunomodulation by theophylline in asthma: demonstration by withdrawal of therapy. *Am J Respir Crit Care Med* 1995, 151:1907–1914.

73. Jaffar ZH, Sullivan P, Page C, Costello J: Low-dose theophylline modulates T-lymphocyte activation in allergen-challenged asthmatics. *Eur Respir J* 1996, 9:456–462.

74. Ohta K, Yamashita N: Apoptosis of eosinophils and lymphocytes in allergic inflammation. *J Allergy Clin Immunol* 1999, 104:14–21.

75.• Barnes PJ, Pauwels RA: Theophylline in asthma: time for reappraisal? *Eur Respir J* 1994, 7:579–591.
A review of the non-bronchodilatory effects of theophylline.

76. Cushley MJ, Holgate ST: Bronchodilator actions of xanthine derivatives administered by inhalation in asthma. *Thorax* 1985, 40:176–179.

77. Aubier M, De Troyer A, Sampson M, *et al*.: Aminophylline improves diaphragmatic contractility. *N Engl J Med* 1981, 305:249–252.

78. Moxham J: Aminophylline and the respiratory muscles: an alternative view. *Clin Chest Med* 1988, 2:325–340.

79. Vozeh S, Kewitz G, Perruchoud A, *et al*.: Theophylline serum concentration and therapeutic effect in severe acute bronchial obstruction: the optimal use of intravenously administered aminophylline. *Am Rev Respir Dis* 1982, 125:181–184.

80. Zhang ZY, Kaminsky LS: Characterization of human cytochromes P450 involved in theophylline 8-hydroxylation. *Biochem Pharmacol* 1995, 50:205–211.

81. Jusko WJ, Gardner MJ, Mangiore A, *et al*.: Factors affecting aminophylline clearance: age, tobacco, marijuana, cirrhosis, congestive heart failure, obesity, oral contraceptives, benzodiazepines, barbiturates and ethanol. *J Pharm Sci* 1979, 68:1358–1366.

82. Taylor DR, Ruffin D, Kinney CD, McDevitt DG: Investigation of diurnal changes in the disposition of theophylline. *Br J Clin Pharmacol* 1983, 16:413–416.

83. Warren JB, Cuss F, Barnes PJ: Posture and theophylline kinetics. *Br J Clin Pharmacol* 1985, 19:707–709.

84. Weinberger M, Hendeles L: Slow-release theophylline: rationale and basis for product selection. *N Engl J Med* 1983, 308:760–763.

85. Barnes PJ, Greening AP, Neville L, *et al*.: Single dose slow-release aminophylline at night prevents nocturnal asthma. *Lancet* 1982, 1:299–301.

86. Heins M, Kurtin L, Oellerich M, *et al*.: Nocturnal asthma: slow-release terbutaline versus slow-release theophylline therapy. *Eur Respir J* 1988, 1:306–310.

87. Bowler SD, Mitchell CA, Armstrong JG: Nebulised fenoterol and i.v. aminophylline in acute severe asthma. *Eur Respir J* 1987, 70:280–283.

88. Wrenn K, Slovis CM, Murphy F, Greenberg RS: Aminophylline therapy for acute bronchospastic disease in the emergency room. *Ann Intern Med* 1991, 115:241–247.

89. Littenberg B: Aminophylline treatment in severe acute asthma: a meta-analysis. *JAMA* 1988, 259:1678–1689.

90. Fanta CH, Rossing TH, McFadden ER: Treatment of acute asthma—is combination therapy with sympathomimetics and methylxanthines indicated? *Am J Med* 1986, 80:5–10.

91. Eason J, Makowe HLJ: Aminophylline toxicity—how many hospital asthma deaths does it cause? *Respir Med* 1989, 83:219–226.

92. Wilson AJ, Gibson PG, Coughlan J: Long acting beta-agonists versus theophylline for maintenance treatment of asthma. *Cochrane Database Syst Rev* 2000:CD001281.

93. Furukawa CT, Shapiro SG, Bierman CW, *et al*.: A double-blind study comparing the effectiveness of cromolyn sodium and sustained release theophylline in childhood asthma. *Pediatrics* 1984, 74:453–459.

94. Nassif EG, Weinburger M, Thompson R, Huntley W: The value of maintenance theophylline in steroid-dependent asthma. *N Engl J Med* 1981, 304:71–75.

95. Tinkelman DG, Reed CE, Nelson HS, Offord KP: Aerosol beclomethasone diprionate compared with theophylline as primary treatment of chronic, mild to moderately severe asthma in children. *Pediatrics* 1993, 92:64–77.

96. Reed CE, Offord KP, Nelson HS, *et al*.: Aerosol beclomethasone dipropionate spray compared with theophylline as primary treatment for chronic mild-to-moderate asthma. The American Academy of Allergy, Asthma and Immunology Beclomethasone Dipropionate-Theophylline Study Group. *J Allergy Clin Immunol* 1998, 101:14–23.

97. Brenner MR, Berkowitz R, Marshall N, Strunk RC: Need for theophylline in severe steroid-requiring asthmatics. *Clin Allergy* 1988, 18:143–150.

98. Rivington RN, Boulet LP, Cote J, *et al*.: Efficacy of slow-release theophylline, inhaled salbutamol and their combination in asthmatic patients on high-dose inhaled steroids. *Am J Respir Crit Care Med* 1995, 151:325–332.

99. Barnes PJ: The role of theophylline in severe asthma. *Eur Respir Rev* 1996, 6(rev 34):154S–159S.

100. Martin RJ, Pak J: Overnight theophylline concentrations and effects on sleep and lung function in chronic obstructive pulmonary disease. *Am Rev Respir Dis* 1992, 145:540–544.

101. Zwilli CW, Neagey SR, Cicutto L, *et al*.: Nocturnal asthma therapy: inhaled bitolterol versus sustained-release theophylline. *Am Rev Respir Dis* 1989, 139:470–474.

102. Fairfax AJ, Clarke R, Chatterjee SS, *et al*.: Controlled release theophylline in the treatment of nocturnal asthma. *J Int Med Res* 1990, 18:273–281.

103. Selby C, Engleman HM, Fitzpatrick MF, *et al*.: Inhaled salmeterol or oral theophylline in nocturnal asthma? *Am J Respir Crit Care Med* 1997, 155:104–108.

104.• Evans DJ, Taylor DA, Zetterstrom O, *et al*.: A comparison of low-dose inhaled budesonide plus theophylline and high-dose inhaled budesonide for moderate asthma. *N Engl J Med* 1997, 337:1412–1418.
A paper demonstrating the add-on effect of low-dose theophylline.

105. Ukena D, Harnest U, Sakalauskas R, *et al*.: Comparison of addition of theophylline to inhaled steroid with doubling of the dose of inhaled steroid in asthma. *Eur Respir J* 1997, 10:2754–2760.

106. Lim S, Jatakanon A, Gordon D, *et al*.: Comparison of high dose inhaled steroids, low dose inhaled steroids plus low dose theophylline, and low dose inhaled steroids alone in chronic asthma in general practice. *Thorax* 2000, 55:837–841.

107. Lim S, Groneberg D, Fischer A, *et al*.: Expression of heme oxygenase isoenzymes 1 and 2 in normal and asthmatic airways. effect of inhaled corticosteroids. *Am J Respir Crit Care Med* 2000, 162:1912–1918.

108. Markham A, Faulds D: Theophylline. A review of its potential steroid sparing effects in asthma. *Drugs* 1998, 56:1081–1091.

109. Handslip PDJ, Dart AM, Davies BTI: Intravenous salbutamol and aminophylline in asthma: a search for synergy. *Thorax* 1981, 36:741–744.

110. Jenne JW: Theophylline as a bronchodilator in COPD and its combination with inhaled beta-adrenergic drugs. *Chest* 1987, 92:7S–14S.

111. Kume H, Kotlikoff MI: K_{ca} in tracheal smooth muscle cells are activated by the beta subunit of stimulatory G protein 1 Gs. *Am Rev Respir Dis* 1992, 145:A204.

112. Giembycz MA: Phosphodiesterase 4 and tolerance to β_2-adrenocep-tor agonists in asthma. *Trends Pharmacol Sci* 1996, 17:331–336.

113. Cheung D, Wever AM, de Goej JA, *et al.*: Effects of theophylline on tolerance to the bronchoprotective actions of salmeterol in asthmatics in vivo. *Am J Respir Crit Care Med* 1998, 158:792–796.

114. Barnes PJ: Current therapies for asthma: promise and limitations. *Chest* 1997, 111:17S–22S.

115. Rachelefsky GS, Wo J, Adelson J, *et al.*: Behaviour abnormalities and poor school performance due to oral theophylline use. *Pediatrics* 1986, 78:1113–1138.

116. Nicholson CD, Challiss RAJ, Shahid M: Differential modulation of tissue function and therapeutic potential of selective inhibitors of cyclic nucleotide phosphodiesterase isoenzymes. *Trends Pharmacol Sci* 1991, 12:19–27.

117. Kelloway JS, Wyatt RA, Adlis SA: Comparison of patients' compliance with prescribed oral and inhaled asthma medications. *Arch Intern Med* 1994, 154:1349–1352.

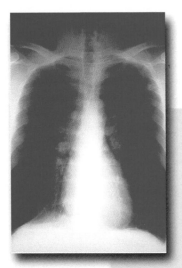

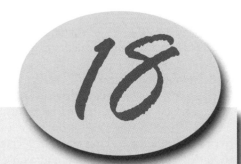

Anticholinergic Bronchodilators

Nicholas J. Gross

Anticholinergic agents are among the oldest known bronchodilators. They have been used for many centuries in the Indian subcontinent in the form of the leaves of *Datura stramonium* [1]. The active ingredients were identified by German chemists in the mid-19th century as the alkaloids, atropine and scopolamine, among others. These naturally occurring anticholinergic agents were widely used throughout Europe until they were replaced by adrenergic agents and methylxanthines in the early 20th century. In part, their disappearance was due to their rapid absorption from mucosal surfaces and the skin, which caused undesirable side effects.

Anticholinergic bronchodilators returned to clinical use when the role of the parasympathetic system in controlling airway tone was better understood, and with the development of synthetic congeners of atropine that were much less prone to produce side effects [2].

RATIONALE AND MECHANISM OF ACTION

The predominant nerve supply to the airways is derived from the vagus nerves, which are cholinergic branches of the parasympathetic system [3]. Their actions are to stimulate contraction of peribronchial smooth muscle; to promote the release of mucus from mucous glands; and to accelerate ciliary beat frequency by the release of their mediator, acetylcholine. This action, at rest, results in a low level of bronchomotor tone. But a variety of stimuli can also result in phasic augmentation of cholinergic activity (*ie*, bronchoconstriction) through neural reflex mechanisms. The bronchoconstriction caused by mechanical irritation of the airways, particle deposition, some irritant gases and aerosols, cold and dry air, and a variety of specific mediators is in part caused by such vagally mediated action [4,5]. There is also evidence that cholinergic bronchomotor tone is increased in both asthma [6] and chronic obstructive pulmonary disease (COPD) [7]. All such cholinergically mediated actions are, in theory, amenable to inhibition by anticholinergic agents. However, they do not inhibit other mediators of bronchoconstriction (*eg*, leukotrienes) or other mechanisms of airway obstruction (*eg*, airway inflammation), and airflow is not usually normalized by anticholinergic agents.

At least three of the many closely related muscarinic receptor genes (*ie*, M_1, M_2, and M_3) are expressed in the human lung and have different functions. Of these, M_1 receptors are believed to facilitate the amplification and transmission of cholinergic traffic to postganglionic nerves, and M_3 receptors, which are located on smooth muscle cells (SMCs) and submucosal glands, mediate SMC contraction and mucus secretion [8] (Fig. 18-1). Their inhibition thus is desirable in alleviating airway obstruction. By contrast, M_2 receptors located on postganglionic nerves act to inhibit further acetylcholine release from nerve terminals, tending to limit vagal bronchoconstriction by negative feedback. Their inhibition would be undesirable in treating airway obstruction.

The relevance of this scheme for the clinical use of anticholinergic agents is twofold. First, all naturally occurring anticholinergic agents and synthetic anticholinergic agents such as ipratropium and oxitropium are not selective for muscarinic receptor subtypes, inhibiting M_2 receptors as well as M_1 and M_3 receptors. Second, M_2 receptors may be selectively damaged by certain respiratory viruses, possibly accounting for the bronchospasm associated with viral infections in children [9,10]. Some eosinophil products may have a similar, selective effect on M_2 receptors, which would limit the efficacy of current anticholinergic agents in asthma. A selective anticholinergic agent that is functionally selective for M_1 and M_3 receptors, tiotropium, has been developed and may be more efficacious [11–13].

Anticholinergic agents do not inhibit other mediators of bronchospasm (*eg*, leukotrienes), and they do not have any known action against other mechanisms of airway obstruction (*eg*, airway inflammation). Consequently, airflow is not usually normalized by anticholinergic agents.

PHARMACOLOGY

All currently approved anticholinergic bronchodilators are quaternary ammonium alkaloids. Unlike naturally occurring molecules such as atropine, which are tertiary, quaternary agents are very poorly absorbed.

Quaternary agents such as ipratropium retain their anticholinergic action at the site of deposition. For example, they dilate the pupil if delivered to the eye or dilate the airways when inhaled. However, their systemic absorption from these sites is insufficient to produce significant systemic effects, even when delivered in much higher than recommended dosage [14]. Agents such as ipratropium and tiotropium thus can be regarded for practical purposes as topical forms of atropine. This group includes ipratropium bromide, oxitropium bromide, atropine methonitrate, glycopyrrolate bromide, and tiotropium bromide. Of these, ipratropium and tiotropium are approved for use as bronchodilators in the United States.

Tiotropium is of particular interest. Besides being functionally selective for muscarinic receptor subtypes that are believed to mediate bronchoconstriction, it is also extremely long acting, which allows for once-daily dosing [11,12]. Its prolonged action may provide protection against nocturnal bronchoconstriction, which is largely mediated by cholinergic mechanisms. In a recent randomized, 3-month trial of 288 patients with stable COPD, tiotropium was more effective than ipratropium in improving trough, average, and peak FEV_1 (forced expiratory volume in 1 second) [15•]. Subsensitivity or tachyphylaxis has not been convincingly demonstrated for any anticholinergic agent, nor would subsensitivity be expected for receptor antagonists.

Regarding pharmacokinetics, serum levels after using inhaled ipratropium are very low, with a peak at about 1 to 2 hours and a half-life of about 4 hours. Most of the drug is excreted unchanged in the urine. Very little reaches the central nervous system. Its bronchodilator effect after inhalation is 4 to 6 hours. Most of an oral dose is recovered unchanged in the feces, and a small amount is recovered as inactive metabolites in the urine. A similar distribution is likely for tiotropium, although its duration of action is much longer.

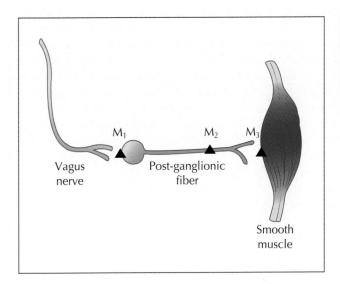

Figure 18-1.
Representation of the location of the three muscarinic receptor subtypes in the airways. *Triangles* represent receptor subtypes.

CLINICAL EFFICACY

Dose–Response

Dose–response data for a variety of anticholinergic agents given by various inhalational methods are provided in a previous review [16]. For ipratropium by nebulized solution, the optimal dose is 500 µg in adults and 125 to 250 µg in children. By metered-dose inhaler (MDI), its optimal dose is 40 to 80 µg in young adults with asthma and 160 µg in older patients with stable COPD who tend to have more severe airway obstruction [17]. The optimal dose by dry powder inhaler (DPI) may be lower by half than that by MDI [18]. The optimal dose of tiotropium by DPI in patients with stable COPD is 18 µg [12,19•]. Tiotropium is not available as an MDI.

Protection Against Specific Stimuli

Anticholinergic agents provide variable protection against bronchospastic stimuli. They protect well against cholinergic agonists such as methacholine, as expected, and against bronchospasm induced by β-blocking agents and by psychogenic factors [2]. Against most other stimuli (*eg*, histamine, prostaglandins, nonspecific dusts, irritant aerosols), exercise, and hyperventilation with cold and dry air, they provide only partial protection at best [20,21]. In most of the latter cases, adrenergic agents usually provide greater protection. Ipratropium has no prophylactic effect against leukotriene (LTD4)-induced bronchospasm [22].

Stable Asthma

A large number of studies have compared the bronchodilator effect of anticholinergic agents with those of adrenergic agents in patients with stable asthma. In general, the anticholinergic agent takes longer to reach peak effect: 30 to 90 minutes for ipratropium compared with 10 to 15 minutes for most adrenergic agents. The peak effect of ipratropium is typically less than that after an adrenergic agent, but it

tends to be slightly longer acting than an adrenergic agent such as albuterol (Fig. 18-2) [23]. However, the response varies considerably among individuals.

The bronchodilator effect of ipratropium is constant or may even increase with age, in contrast to that of adrenergic agents, which tends to decrease with age [24]. However, children between 10 and 18 years of age have been shown to respond to anticholinergic use [25]. Asthmatic patients with intrinsic asthma and those with longer duration of asthma may also respond better to an anticholinergic agent than do individuals with extrinsic asthma [26]. Other than these general observations, it has not been possible to predict which asthmatic patients will respond to an anticholinergic agent. In the United States, ipratropium has not been approved by the Food and Drug Administration for the treatment of patients with asthma.

Acute Severe Asthma (Status Asthmaticus)

The consensus is that β-adrenergic agonists are the bronchodilators of choice for patients with acute severe asthma, and that an anticholinergic agent should not be used as the sole initial bronchodilator for individuals with the condition. However, several studies suggest it may add to the bronchodilatation achieved by an adrenergic agent. Thus, the combination of 500 µg nebulized ipratropium with 1.25 mg nebulized fenoterol (a β-adrenergic agent) resulted in significantly more bronchodilatation over the first 90 minutes of treatment than either agent alone, and patients with more severe airway obstruction obtained the greatest benefit from the combination [27]. In a meta-analysis [28] of 10 clinical studies (total of 1377 patients), the addition of ipratropium to a β-agonist reduced hospital admissions by 27% and increased FEV_1 by about 100 mL more than in patients receiving adrenergic agents alone. The benefit of including ipratropium in the bronchodilator regimen was both statistically and clinically significant, particularly in the initial treatment of patients with more severe airflow obstruction [29].

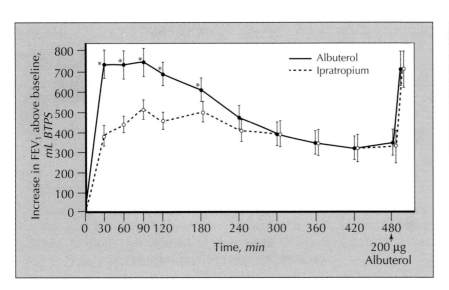

Figure 18-2.
Increase in FEV_1 (forced expiratory volume in 1 second) of 25 patients with asthma after inhalation of 200 µm albuterol or 36 µm ipratropium, both by metered-dose inhaler on separate days. (*Adapted from* Ruffin *et al.* [23].)

Pediatric Airways Disease

In children with acute severe asthma, the addition of ipratropium to a β-agonist accelerated the rate of improvement of airflow in some studies [30,31] but not in others [32–35]. A review of 10 studies concluded that the addition of ipratropium to adrenergic therapy was safe, improved lung function more effectively, and reduced hospitalization rates in children with acute severe asthma [36]. Therefore, as for adult status asthmaticus, the addition of ipratropium to an adrenergic agent is probably more effective than adrenergic monotherapy, particularly in severe exacerbations.

The role of ipratropium in stable pediatric asthma is less clear. Two consensus reports concluded that ipratropium was safe for the pediatric population, but that it was not as potent as an adrenergic agent [37,38].

Reports of the use of ipratropium in other pediatric conditions such as cystic fibrosis, viral bronchiolitis, exercise-induced bronchospasm, and bronchopulmonary dysplasia provide only inconsistent evidence for the benefit of ipratropium over alternative bronchodilators. Ipratropium has not been approved in the United States for pediatric use.

Stable Chronic Obstructive Pulmonary Disease

The main role of anticholinergic agents—and their only approved indication in the United States—is in the management of patients with stable COPD. A large number of studies [39,40] have compared anticholinergic agents with other bronchodilators. In most of these reports, patients with COPD responded as well to an anticholinergic agent as to an adrenergic agent. The current recommended dose of ipratropium (36 μg) is suboptimal for patients with COPD [17] and can safely be increased by a factor of 2 to 4. With larger, cumulative doses of a similar anticholinergic agent, atropine methylnitrate, all the possible bronchodilation in the COPD population was achieved [41]. Note that anticholinergic agents are clearly less effective than adrenergic agents in patients with asthma but are at least as effective as adrenergic agents in patients with COPD. The reasons for this are unknown but may be related to the fact that airway obstruction in asthma is caused by numerous factors, such as airway inflammation and mucosal edema, that are at least partially addressed by adrenergic agents but not by anticholinergic agents. In COPD, the major reversible component is bronchomotor tone, which is best reversed by an anticholinergic agent. Ipratropium is currently recommended as first-line treatment for maintenance therapy of stable COPD in almost all guidelines and statements [42,43••].

Anticholinergic agents have no effect on the airways apart from the temporary relief of airways obstruction. The Lung Health Study [44••] showed that regular use of ipratropium over a 5-year period had no discernible effect on the age-related decline in lung function of smokers. A smaller retrospective review suggested a small improvement in

baseline FEV_1 after 3 months of regular use [45]. The effects of regular ipratropium use that are presumably secondary to its bronchodilator action include modest improvements in exercise tolerance and health status (quality of life) and improvement in quality of sleep [46].

Acute Exacerbations of Chronic Obstructive Pulmonary Disease

Studies comparing the efficacy of bronchodilators in acute exacerbations of COPD do not show a difference in efficacy between adrenergic and anticholinergic agents or their combination [27,47–49]. Published guidelines from the American Thoracic Society [42], European Respiratory Society [43••], and British Thoracic Society [50] recommend combination therapy with both adrenergic and anticholinergic agents in the initial management of acute exacerbations of COPD.

Combinations with Other Bronchodilators

The combination of different classes of bronchodilators often provides more bronchodilation than do single agents. Because the recommended doses of bronchodilators are rarely the optimal doses, the greater efficacy of a combination may be attributable to an additive rather than potentiating effect. Different classes of bronchodilators work by different mechanisms, have different pharmacokinetic properties, and affect different-sized airways; therefore, their combination is rational. Moreover, because unfavorable interactions among the various classes of bronchodilators do not appear to occur, the greater bronchodilation resulting from their use in combination is achieved without an increase in the risk of side effects.

In practice, the simultaneous use of adrenergic plus anticholinergic agents to manage severe airway obstruction is endorsed by all current guidelines. Combinations of ipratropium and the β-agonist fenoterol have been widely used in many countries, but neither of these combinations has been available in the United States. More recently, a combination MDI containing ipratropium and albuterol has been developed (Combivent; Boehringer Ingelheim Pharmaceuticals, Inc., Ingelheim, Germany). For patients who need more than one bronchodilator, a single MDI containing both agents is not only more potent [51–53], but it has the potential advantages of lower expense [54], greater convenience and, thus, greater patient compliance. A nebulized form of this combination (DuoNeb; Dey, LP, Napa, CA) showed similar clinical benefits [55].

SIDE EFFECTS

The principal advantage of quaternary anticholinergic agents is that they are very poorly absorbed from mucosal surfaces, so the risk of systemic side effects is relatively small. Inhalational ipratropium has very few systemic atropine-like side effects [56]. It can, for example, be given to patients with narrow-angle glaucoma without affecting intraocular tension, provided care is taken to avoid spraying it directly into the eye [2,57]. Additionally, it does not have appreciable effects on urinary flow in older men. Numerous laboratory studies [2,58] show that it does not alter the viscosity or elasticity of respiratory mucus and does not impair mucociliary clearance, as does atropine. Its effects on ventilation, hemodynamics, and the pulmonary circulation are likewise trivial [59,60]. Anticholinergic agents do not significantly lower arterial oxygen tensions as do adrenergic agents [61–63], a potentially important consideration in exacerbations of asthma and COPD.

In clinical trials, the only side effects that occurred more commonly with ipratropium than with placebo were dry mouth and, sometimes, a brief coughing spell. Neither effect resulted in patient withdrawal from the studies. Other than these, extensive clinical investigation and the worldwide use of ipratropium for more than two decades demonstrate a very low incidence of undesirable side effects. There is no place for atropine as a bronchodilator in current clinical practice.

CLINICAL RECOMMENDATIONS

The main role of the currently available anticholinergic agent ipratropium in clinical practice is for the long-term management of stable COPD, in which it is probably the single most efficacious bronchodilator. It is best used on a regular, maintenance basis rather than as needed because of its relatively slow action. (A β-agonist such as albuterol is more appropriate for rapid relief of dyspnea.) The recommended dose of ipratropium, two 18-μg puffs, is suboptimal for most patients with COPD and can safely be doubled or quadrupled if necessary [64]. Combinations of ipratropium with albuterol, Combivent MDI, or DuoNeb nebulized solution are appropriate for patients who require more than one bronchodilator. Clinical studies suggest that tiotropium may find an important role as first-line therapy for stable COPD on a once-daily basis [65•].

Anticholinergic agents can and probably should be used in combination with adrenergic agents in the treatment of acute exacerbations of both COPD and status asthmaticus, particularly when they are severe.

REFERENCES AND RECOMMENDED READING

Papers of particular interest, published recently, have been highlighted as:
• Of importance
•• Of major importance

1. Gandevia B: Historical review of the use of parasympatholytic agents in the treatment of respiratory disorders. *Postgrad Med J* 1975, 51(suppl):13–20

2. Gross NJ, Skorodin SM: Anticholinergic, antimuscarinic bronchodilators. *Am Rev Respir Dis* 1984, 129:856–870.

3. Richardson JB: The innervation of the lung. *Eur J Respir Dis* 1982, 117(suppl):13–31.

4. Widdicombe JG: The parasympathetic nervous system in airways disease. *Scand J Respir Dis* 1979, 103(suppl):38–43.

5. Nadel JA: Autonomic regulation of airway smooth muscle. In *Physiology and Pharmacology of the Airways*. Edited by Nadel JA. New York: Marcel Dekker; 1980:217–257.

6. Shah PK, Lakhotia M, Mehta S, *et al.*: Clinical dysautonomia in patients with bronchial asthma: study with seven autonomic function tests. *Chest* 1990, 98:1408–1413.

7. Gross NJ, Co E, Skorodin MS: Cholinergic bronchomotor tone in COPD: estimates of its amount in comparison with that in normal subjects. *Chest* 1989, 96:984–987.

8. Gross NJ, Barnes PJ: A short tour around the muscarinic receptor. *Am Rev Respir Dis* 1988, 138:765–767.

9. Fryer AD, Jacoby DB: Parainfluenza virus infection damages inhibitory M2 muscarinic receptors on pulmonary parasympathetic nerves in the guinea-pig. *Br J Pharmacol* 1991, 102:267–271.

10. Fryer AD, Jacoby DB: Effect of inflammatory cell mediators on M2 muscarinic receptors in the lungs. *Life Sci* 1993, 52:529–536.

11. O'Connor BJ, Towse LJ, Barnes PJ: Prolonged effect of tiotropium bromide on methacholine-induced bronchoconstriction in asthma. *Am J Respir Crit Care Med* 1996, 154(4 pt 1):876–880.

12. Maesen FP, Smeets JJ, Sledsens TJ, *et al.*: Tiotropium bromide, a new long-acting antimuscarinic bronchodilator: a pharmacodynamic study in patients with chronic obstructive pulmonary disease (COPD): Dutch Study Group. *Eur Respir J* 1995, 8:1506–1513.

13. Barnes PJ, Belvisi MG, Mak JC, *et al.*: Tiotropium bromide (Ba 679 BR), a novel long-acting muscarinic antagonist for the treatment of obstructive airways disease. *Life Sci* 1995, 56:853–859.

14. Gross NJ, Skorodin MS: Massive overdose of atropine methonitrate with only slight untoward effects [letter]. *Lancet* 1985, 2:386.

15.• Van Noord JA, Bantje TA, Eland ME: A randomised controlled comparison of triotropium and ipratropium in the treatment of chronic obstructive pulmonary disease. *Thorax* 2000, 55:289–294.
This is an informative introduction into the properties and actions of this important new anticholinergic agent.

16. Gross NJ, Skorodin M: Anticholinergic agents. In *Drug Therapy*. Edited by Jenne JW, Murphy S. New York: Marcel Dekker; 1987:615–668.

17. Gross NJ, Petty TL, Friedman M, *et al.*: Dose response to ipratropium as a nebulized solution in patients with chronic obstructive pulmonary disease: a three-center study. *Am Rev Respir Dis* 1989, 139:1188–1191.

18. Bollert FG, Matusiewicz SP, Dewar MH, *et al.*: Comparative efficacy and potency of ipratropium via Turbuhaler and pressurized metered-dose inhaler in reversible airflow obstruction. *Eur Respir J* 1997, 10:1824–1828.

19.• Littner MR, Ilowite JS, Tashkin DP, *et al.*: Long-acting bronchodilation with once-daily dosing of tiotropium in stable chronic obstructive pulmonary disease. *Am J Respir Crit Care Med* 2000, 161:1136–1142.
This is an informative introduction into the properties and role of this new anticholinergic agent in clinical practice.

20. Ayala LE, Ahmed T: Is there loss of protective muscarinic receptor mechanism in asthma? *Chest* 1989, 96:1285–1291.

21. Azevedo M, da Costa JT, Fontes P, *et al.*: Effect of terfenadine and ipratropium bromide on ultrasonically nebulized distilled water-induced asthma. *J Int Med Res* 1990, 18:37–49.

22. Ayala LE, Choudry NB, Fuller RW: LTD4-induced bronchoconstriction in patients with asthma: lack of a vagal reflex. *Br J Clin Pharmacol* 1988, 26:110–112.

23. Ruffin RE, Fitzgerald JD, Rebuck AS: A comparison of the bronchodilator activity of Sch 1000 and salbutamol. *J Allergy Clin Immunol* 1977, 59:136–141.

24. Ullah MI, Newman GB, Saunders KB: Influence of age on response to ipratropium and salbutamol in asthma. *Thorax* 1981, 36:523–529.

25. Vichyanond P, Sladek WA, Sur S, *et al.*: Efficacy of atropine methylnitrate alone and in combination with albuterol in children with asthma. *Chest* 1990, 98:637–642.

26. Jolobe OM: Asthma vs. non-specific reversible airflow obstruction: clinical features and responsiveness to anticholinergic drugs. *Respiration* 1984, 45:237– 242.

27. Rebuck AS, Chapman KR, Abboud R, *et al.*: Nebulized anticholinergic and sympathomimetic treatment of asthma and chronic obstructive airways disease in the emergency room. *Am J Med* 1987, 82:59–64.

28. Stoodley RG, Aaron SD, Dales RE: The role of ipratropium bromide in the emergency management of acute asthma exacerbation: a meta-analysis of randomized clinical trials. *Ann Emerg Med* 1999, 34:8–18.

29. Brophy C, Ahmed B, Bayston S, *et al.*: How long should Atrovent be given in acute asthma? *Thorax* 1998, 53:363–367.

30. Beck R, Robertson C, Galdes-Sebaldt M, Levison H: Combined salbutamol and ipratropium bromide by inhalation in the treatment of severe acute asthma. *J Pediatr* 1985, 107:605–608.

31. Reisman J, Galdes-Sebalt M, Kazim F, *et al.*: Frequent administration by inhalation of salbutamol and ipratropium bromide in the initial management of severe acute asthma in children. *J Allergy Clin Immunol* 1988, 81:16–20.

32. Ducharme FM, Davis GM: Randomized controlled trial of ipratropium bromide and frequent low doses of salbutamol in the management of mild and moderate acute pediatric asthma. *J Pediatr* 1998, 133:479–485.

33. Schuh S, Johnson DW, Callahan S, *et al.*: Efficacy of frequent nebulized ipratropium bromide added to frequent high-dose albuterol therapy in severe childhood asthma. *J Pediatr* 1995, 126:639–645.

34. Zorc JJ, Pusic MV, Ogborn CJ, *et al.*: Ipratropium bromide added to asthma treatment in the pediatric emergency department. *Pediatrics* 1999, 103(4 pt 1):748–752.

35. Qureshi F, Pestian J, Davis P, Zaritsky A: Effect of nebulized ipratropium on the hospitalization rates of children with asthma. *N Engl J Med* 1998, 339:1030–1035.

36. Plotnick L, Ducharme F: Should inhaled anticholinergics be added to β2 agonists for treating acute childhood and adolescent asthma? A systematic review. *Br Med J* 1998, 317:971–977.

37. Warner JO, Gotz M, Landau LI, *et al.*: Management of asthma: a consensus statement. *Arch Dis Child* 1989, 64:1065–1079.

38. Hargreave FE, Dolovich J, Newhouse MT: The assessment and treatment of asthma: a conference report. *J Allergy Clin Immunol* 1990, 85:1098–1111.

39. Thiessen B, Pedersen OF: Maximal expiratory flows and forced vital capacity in normal, asthmatic and bronchitic subjects after salbutamol and ipratropium bromide. *Respiration* 1982, 43:304–316.

40. Passamonte PM, Martinez AJ: Effect of inhaled atropine or metaproterenol in patients with chronic airway obstruction and therapeutic serum theophylline levels. *Chest* 1984, 85:610–615.

41.•• Gross NJ, Skorodin MS: Role of the parasympathetic system in airway obstruction due to emphysema. *N Engl J Med* 1984, 311:421–425.
This study shows that optimal dosage of an anticholinergic agent provides all the available bronchodilation in COPD.

42. Siafakas NM, Vermeire P, Pride NB, *et al.*: Optimal assessment and management of chronic obstructive pulmonary disease (COPD): the European Respiratory Society Task Force. *Eur Respir J* 1995, 8:1398–1420.

43.•• American Thoracic Society: Standards for the diagnosis and care of patients with chronic obstructive pulmonary disease. *Am J Respir Crit Care Med* 1995, 152(5 pt 2):S77–121.
This is the current document on optimal management of COPD in the United States. It provides specific recommendations that are still appropriate.

44.•• Anthonisen NR, Connett JE, Kiley JP, *et al.*: Effects of smoking intervention and the use of an inhaled anticholinergic bronchodilator on the rate of decline of FEV1: the Lung Health Study. *JAMA* 1994, 272:1497–1505.
This is the definitive study on the importance of smoking cessation in COPD, its effect on subsequent airflow, and the lack of long-term benefit of iratropium.

45. Rennard SI, Serby CW, Ghafouri M, *et al.*: Extended therapy with ipratropium is associated with improved lung function in patients with COPD: a retrospective analysis of data from seven clinical trials. *Chest* 1996, 110:62–70.

46. Martin RJ, Bucher-Bartleson BL, Smith P, *et al.*: Effect of ipratropium bromide treatment on oxygen saturation and sleep quality in COPD. *Chest* 1999, 115:1338–1345.

47. Karpel JP, Pesin J, Greenberg D, Gentry E: A comparison of the effects of ipratropium bromide and metaproterenol sulfate in acute exacerbations of COPD. *Chest* 1990, 98:835–839.

48. Patrick DM, Dales RE, Stark RM, *et al.*: Severe exacerbations of COPD and asthma: incremental benefit of adding ipratropium to usual therapy. *Chest* 1990, 98:295–297.

49. Koutsogiannis Z, Kelly A: Does high dose ipratropium bromide added to salbutamol improve pulmonary function for patients with chronic obstructive airways disease in the emergency department? *Aust N Z J Med* 2000, 0:38–40.

50. British Thoracic Society: Guidelines for the management of chronic obstructive pulmonary disease. *Thorax* 1996, 52(suppl):1–28.

51. Petty TL: In chronic obstructive pulmonary disease, a combination of ipratropium and albuterol is more effective than either agent alone: an 85-day multicenter trial: Inhalation Aerosol Study Group. *Chest* 1994, 105:1411–1419.

52. Ikeda A, Nishimura K, Koyama H, Izumi T: Bronchodilating effects of combined therapy with clinical dosages of ipratropium bromide and salbutamol for stable COPD: comparison with ipratropium bromide alone. *Chest* 1995, 07:401– 405.

53. The COMBIVENT Inhalation Solution Study Group: Routine nebulized ipratropium and albuterol together are better than either alone in COPD. *Chest* 1997, 112:1514–1521.

54. Friedman M, Serby CW, Menjoge SS, *et al.*: Pharmacoeconomic evaluation of a combination of ipratropium plus albuterol compared with ipratropium alone and albuterol alone in COPD. *Chest* 1999, 115:635–641.

55. Gross N, Tashkin D, Miller R, Oren J, *et al.*: Inhalation by nebulization of albuterol-ipratropium combination (Dey combination) is superior to either agent alone in the treatment of chronic obstructive pulmonary disease. *Respiration* 1998, 65:354–362.

56. Gross NJ: Ipratropium bromide. *N Engl J Med* 1988, 319:486–494.

57. Watson WT, Shuckett EP, Becker AB, Simons FE: Effect of nebulized ipratropium bromide on intraocular pressures in children. *Chest* 1994, 105:1439–1441.

58. Pavia D, Bateman JR, Sheahan NF, Clarke SW: Effect of ipratropium bromide on mucociliary clearance and pulmonary function in reversible airways obstruction. *Thorax* 1979, 34:501–507.

59. Tobin MJ, Hughes JA, Hutchison DC: Effects of ipratropium bromide and fenoterol aerosols on exercise tolerance. *Eur J Respir Dis* 1984, 65:441–446.

60. Chapman KR, Smith DL, Rebuck AS, Leenen FH: Haemodynamic effects of inhaled ipratropium bromide, alone and combined with an inhaled beta 2-agonist. *Am Rev Respir Dis* 1985, 132:845–847.

61. Ashutosh K, Dev G, Steele D: Nonbronchodilator effects of pirbuterol and ipratropium in chronic obstructive pulmonary disease. *Chest* 1995, 107:173–178.

62. Gross NJ, Bankwala Z: Effects of an anticholinergic bronchodilator on arterial blood gases of hypoxaemic patients with chronic obstructive pulmonary disease: comparison with a beta-adrenergic agent. *Am Rev Respir Dis* 1987, 36:1091–1094.

63. Koukhaz G, Gross NJ: Effects of salmeterol on arterial blood gases in patients with stable chronic obstructive pulmonary disease: comparison with albuterol and ipratropium. *Am J Respir Crit Care Med* 1999, 160:1028–1030.

64. Leak A, O'Connor T: High dose ipratropium bromide: is it safe? *Practitioner* 1988, 232:9–10.

65. Samter M, Beers RF Jr: Intolerance to aspirin. Clinical studies and consideration of its pathogenesis. *Ann Intern Med* 1968, 68(5):975–983.

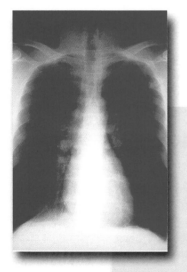

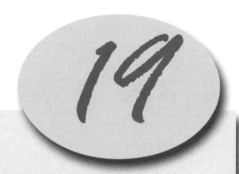

Leukotriene Modifiers in the Treatment of Asthma

Jonathan Sadeh and Elliot Israel

Asthma is a chronic inflammatory disease associated with variable airflow obstruction. The mechanisms that lead to airflow obstruction in asthma are bronchoconstriction, mucosal edema, increased secretion of mucus, and an inflammatory infiltrate that is rich in eosinophils. Leukotrienes (LTs) B4, C4, D4, and E4 have been shown experimentally to play a role in each of these inflammatory processes and mimic the pathologic changes seen in asthma [1,2]. LTC4, D4, and E4 have potent effects on airway smooth muscle, submucosal glands, epithelial cells, and blood vessels, where they cause contraction, mucus secretion, and changes in vascular permeability leading to edema. LTs are the most potent endogenous constrictors of airway smooth muscle that have been identified. Inhalation of LTD4 results in the same degree of airway obstruction as inhalation of solutions of histamine or methacholine that are 1,000 to 10,000 times as concentrated [3]. LTB4 can recruit neutrophils to the airways, thereby further promoting inflammation.

Further evidence of the role of LTs in the pathophysiology of asthma comes from studies showing elevated levels in the blood, urine, sputum, nasal secretions, and bronchoalveolar lavage fluid of patients with asthma and during asthma exacerbations [4,5]. These observations led to the development of agents with the capacity to inhibit the synthesis or action of LTs in an attempt to better control and treat asthma. Herein we review the biochemistry of LT formation, the effects of agents developed to modify their action, and their role in the management of the asthmatic patient.

LEUKOTRIENE SYNTHESIS

Leukotrienes are produced by various cells involved in the asthmatic response including eosinophils, mast cells, and neutrophils. Given the appropriate stimuli, LTs are formed through the arachidonic acid cascade (Fig. 19-1). This cascade begins with the initial cleavage of arachidonic acid from membrane phospholipids by the action of cytosolic phospholipase A2. The freed arachidonic acid is presented to the enzyme 5-lipoxygenase (5-LO) by a nuclear membrane protein known as the 5-lipoxygenase-activating protein (FLAP), with resultant formation of 5-hydroperoxyeicosatetraenoic acid (5-HPETE). 5-LO also catalyzes the conversion of 5-HPETE to an unstable intermediate, LTA4. LTA4 is rapidly converted to either LTC4 or LTB4, depending on the cell type where the reaction is occurring. In eosinophils, mast cells, and alveolar macrophages, LTA4 is converted to

LTC4 by LTC4 synthase, which adducts glutathione in the C-6 position of LTA4. LTC4 is exported from the cell cytosol to the extracellular space through a specific membrane transporter. In the extracellular space, glutamic acid is cleaved from LTC4 to form LTD4, which is further cleaved by extracellular dipeptidases to form LTE4. Since LTC4, LTD4, and LTE4 all contain the amino acid cysteine, they are referred to as cysteinyl LTs. LTs are also formed in neutrophils, where LTA4 is converted to LTB4 by the action of LTA4 epoxide hydrolase.

LEUKOTRIENE RECEPTORS

Leukotrienes exert their biologic effects by binding to LT receptors present on cell membranes. The cysteinyl LTs (LTC4, LTD4, LTE4) activate CysLT receptors 1 and 2 (CysLT1 and CysLT2), while LTB4 activates the B LT receptor (BLT). BLT has been cloned and belongs to the family of seven transmembrane G protein-coupled receptors [6]. The CysLT1 receptor has also been cloned and also belongs to the family of seven transmembrane G

protein-coupled receptors and is expressed in several organs, including the lung, where it is found mainly in smooth muscle cells and macrophages [7]. The CysLT2 receptor mediates constriction of pulmonary vascular smooth muscle in humans, although its actions are not as well defined as those of the CysLT1 receptor [8].

LEUKOTRIENE SYNTHESIS IN ASTHMA

Leukotriene production is increased in asthmatic patients. One study reported that blood eosinophils from asthmatic patients synthesize five- to tenfold greater amounts of cysteinyl LTs than healthy patients [9]. In patients presenting with an asthma exacerbation, the principal urinary metabolite of the cysteinyl luekotrienes, LTE4, is also significantly increased in the urine [4]. Multiple studies have shown increased levels of cysteinyl LTs in bronchoalveolar lavage (BAL) fluid and urine samples of patients with asthma after allergen challenge [10,11], as well as aspirin-intolerant patients after exposure to aspirin [12].

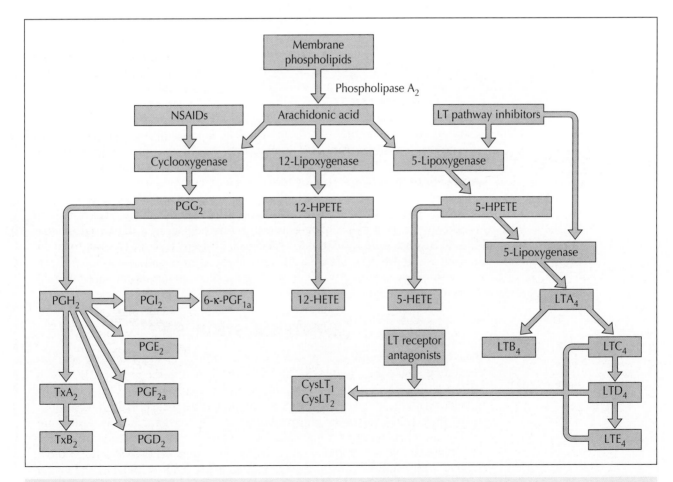

Figure 19-1.

The arachidonic acid cascade describes the site of activity for the leukotriene (LT) pathway inhibitors and the LT receptor antagonists. HETE—hydroxyeicosatetraenoic acid; HPETE—hydroperoxy eicosatetraenoic acid; PG—prostaglandin; TX—thromboxane.

Because of the potential importance of LTs in asthma, several agents which modify their formation or action have been developed by the pharmaceutical industry. Three such agents have been approved for clinical use in the United States (Table 19-1). Montelukast (Singulair; Merck, West Point, PA) and zafirlukast (Accolate; AstraZeneca, Wilmington, DE) inhibit cysteinyl LT action at the CysLT1 receptor through competitive antagonism at this receptor, while zileuton (Zyflo; Abbott, Abbott Park, IL) is an inhibitor of LT synthesis through inhibition of the LT biosynthetic enzyme 5-lipoxygenase. As a class, we refer to the CyLT1 antagonists and the LT synthesis inhibitors as LT modifiers.

EFFECTS OF LEUKOTRIENE MODIFIERS ON STIMULI TO BRONCHOCONSTRICTION

The best evidence that leukotrienes play a role in mediating airway narrowing that occurs after provocative stimuli comes from observations that LT modifiers markedly reduce bronchoconstrictor responses after such exposures. The data supporting the use of LT modifiers in asthma and reducing the responses to such stimuli in asthmatic patients is reviewed here.

Allergen-induced Bronchoconstriction

When patients with atopic asthma inhale a specific allergen, the result is degranulation of mast cells, release of preformed mediators such as histamine and proteases, and synthesis of mediators such as cytokines, prostaglandins, and cysteinyl LTs. In some patients, immediate bronchoconstriction progresses over the next 2 to 6 hours and patients develop a late-phase asthmatic response. This late-phase response is associated with increased airway responsiveness that can last for days. The early-phase airway response most likely is caused by release and synthesis, by cells residing in the lung, of bronchoconstrictor mediators such as LTs, prostaglandins, and histamines. The late-phase asthmatic response is charac-

terized by an inflammatory response consisting of airway perivascular edema, mucus plugging and infiltration composed of eosinophils, neutrophils, and monocytes in the airways.

LT antagonists significantly reduce bronchoconstriction during the early asthmatic response and attenuate it during the early period of the late asthmatic response [13,14]. In other studies, cysteinyl LT antagonists alone have not been shown to be effective in controlling allergen-induced bronchoconstriction 24 hours after an allergen challenge [15], suggesting they offer less protection in the late-phase asthmatic response. In addition, it appears that combining cysteinyl LT antagonists with other selected anti-mediators may produce even greater effects. In one report, pretreatment of asthmatic patients with a LT modifier and an antihistamine before allergen exposure eliminated both the early and late responses [16]. However, other data suggests only a blunting of the response [13].

Aspirin-induced Bronchoconstriction

Aspirin- and NSAID-induced asthma occurs in 3% to 8% of patients with asthma. In these patients, ingestion of an inhibitor of cyclooxygenase-1 can cause significant bronchoconstriction as well as naso-occular, dermal, and gastrointestinal responses. Inhibition of cyclooxygenase-1 results in increased production of LTs [17]. LTs are critical mediators of this aspirin-induced response. Even in the absence of aspirin challenge, elevated levels of cysteinyl LTs can be seen in most aspirin-sensitive patients, and pretreatment with a CysLT1 receptor antagonist or a 5-LO inhibitor prevents the physiologic response after aspirin administration [18]. In aspirin-sensitive patients, LT modifiers improve symptoms and pulmonary function in patients already taking moderate to high doses of glucocorticoids [19,20]. These results suggest LTs are important mediators of aspirin-sensitive asthma and that LT-modifying drugs play an essential role in the treatment of these patients.

Table 19-1. LEUKOTRIENE-MODIFYING DRUGS

Name	Recommended Oral Dose	Comments
Leukotriene-receptor antagonists		
Montelukast	Adults: 10 mg at night; children 6–12 y, 5 mg at night; children 2–5 y, 4 mg at night	Pediatric pills are chewable
Zafirlukast	20 mg BID	Take 1 h before or 2 h after eating
5-LO inhibitor		
Zileuton	600 mg QID	Check LFTs before treatment and periodically thereafter

BID—twice a day; LFTs—liver function tests; QID—four times a day.

Exercise-induced Bronchoconstriction

Exercise and hyperventilation stimulates bronchospasm in 70% to 80% of patients with asthma. Investigators have recovered cysteinyl LTs from the BAL fluid and urine of patients after exercise- and hyperventilation-induced bronchospasm [21]. LT modifiers have been shown to reduce the maximal bronchoconstrictor response after exercise and hyperventilation by 50% to 80% [22–24]. These data suggest that LTs play a role in mediating exercise-induced bronchoconstriction.

Clinically, LT modifiers appear to provide a degree of protection against exercise-induced bronchoconstriction over a prolonged period of time. Zafirlukast also has been shown to protect against exercise-induced bronchoconstriction for at least 8 hours after administration [25]. As compared with salmeterol, montelukast maintained its bronchoprotective effects for a longer period, especially as compared with chronic use of salmeterol (Fig. 19-2) [26]. These studies support the use of LT modifiers in the treatment of exercise-induced bronchoconstriction, although the degree of protection achieved varies among patients [27].

LEUKOTRIENE-MODIFYING DRUGS IN THE TREATMENT OF CHRONIC PERSISTENT ASTHMA

Many clinical trials have established the efficacy of LT-modifying drugs in the treatment of chronic persistent asthma. They have been shown to be superior to placebo in the treatment of mild to moderate asthma. They improve FEV_1 (forced expiratory volume in 1 second) by 10% to 15%, decrease symptoms, and decrease the use of β-agonists [28–30]. They have also been shown to decrease exacerbations that require steroid rescue by up to 80% [28].

The efficacy of LT-modifying drugs has also been compared to that of inhaled corticosteroids. In general, inhaled corticosteroids produce a greater improvement in lung function than LT modifiers, although in most cases their effect on indices of asthma control including exacerbations have been similar [31–33]. LT modifiers improve outcomes in patients already taking inhaled corticosteroids [20,34,35]. They have also been shown to permit a reduction in inhaled corticosteroid dose of up to 50% in patients who were stable on inhaled corticosteroids [33,36]. In patients poorly controlled on inhaled corticosteroids, substituting an LT modifier alone will generally not improve asthma control [34].

In patients poorly controlled on a stable dose of inhaled corticosteroids, adding a LT modifier produces improvements equivalent to doubling the inhaled corticosteroid dose [36]. In these patients, the improvement in lung function is not as great as that seen when adding the long-acting β-agonist salmeterol. Adding salmeterol in these patients also appears to improve symptoms more than an LT modifier does, but in most cases did not produce a significant difference in the effect of asthma exacerbations [37–39].

SAFETY AND DRUG INTERACTIONS

There is now substantial experience in the use of LT modifiers in the treatment of asthma. Overall they are very safe and generally well tolerated. The 5-lipoxygenase inhibitor zileuton can produce a 2% to 5% incidence of elevated transaminases, which reverses with drug withdrawal. Liver function tests should be checked at the onset of treatment and periodically thereafter with this drug. Zafirlukast, at its recommended dose of 20 mg twice a day, has a very low incidence of transaminitis. Three cases of liver failure in patients receiving

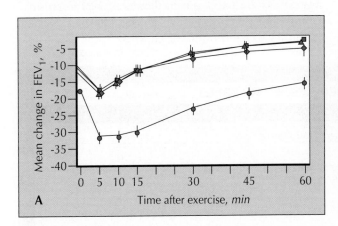

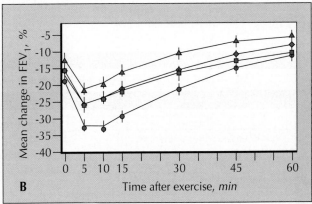

Figure 19-2.
Montelukast versus salmeterol protection against exercise-induced bronchospasm. The postexercise FEV_1 (forced expiratory volume in 1 second) in patients who received montelukast (**A**) and salmeterol

(**B**) is compared. The mean response curves are shown for percentage change in FEV_1 at baseline (*circles*) and days 1 to 3 (*triangles*), week 4 (*squares*), and week 8 (*diamonds*) after treatment.

zafirlukast were reported [40], but no further cases have been forthcoming. Routine measurement of liver function is not recommended. Montelukast has not been shown to cause liver function abnormalities.

After the introduction of the LT modifiers, case reports appeared describing a syndrome of systemic vasculitis with peripheral eosinophilia, pulmonary infiltrates, and myocarditis, in many cases meeting the criteria for the Churg-Strauss syndrome [41,42]. While initially thought to be associated with LT-modifier therapy, the prevalence of such episodes appears to be the same as expected in asthmatic patients [43].

No drug interactions have been reported for montelukast. Warfarin metabolism is reduced by zafirlukast and zileuton, and dosage reductions and monitoring of warfarin effects are recommended with concomitant administration. Additionally, zileuton increases theophylline levels and the effects of propranolol, and the doses of these drugs should be adjusted appropriately.

FUTURE DEVELOPMENTS

Analysis of the improvement in FEV_1 in response to LT modifiers as compared to inhaled corticosteroids showed that the large difference in mean response was driven by a small fraction of patients with substantial improvement in lung function in the inhaled corticosteroid group [31]. Further, it was clear that a significant proportion of patients did not respond to beclomethasone and an even larger group did not respond to montelukast. This variability in response among patients, recently confirmed in the case of inhaled corticosteroids [44], has spurred research into genetic factors that might influence the variability of response. In the case of LT modifiers, a polymorphism associated with downregulation of 5-LO expression (which occurs in 5% of people) has been associated with reduced responses to a 5-LO inhibitor [45]. It also appears that a polymorphism in the promoter of the LTC4 synthase enzyme may increase the response to LT modifiers [46]. These findings suggest that genetic

differences in the function and expression of drug targets may affect therapeutic response. Research is also currently underway examining the therapeutic effects of inhibiting CysLT2-mediated effects. Drug development is being targeted at the introduction of additional LT-synthesis inhibitors.

CONCLUSIONS

Leukotrienes play an important role in the pathogenesis of asthmatic inflammation. The LT modifiers have been shown to prevent asthma attacks and improve asthma control. Their exact role in asthma management has been a topic of debate. Potential uses of LTs are summarized in Table 19-2. LT modifiers are clearly indicated in the treatment of patients with aspirin-induced asthma. Their oral availability confers an advantage, especially in children where long-term use of steroids is of more concern. In patients with mild persistent asthma who use β-agonists only and require chronic therapy, LT modifiers may be an effective initial alternative to inhaled steroid therapy. If a satisfactory response is achieved, the agent should be continued. If not, inhaled steroids should be instituted as described in previously published guidelines by the National Heart, Lung, and Blood Institute [50].

LT modifiers can also be added to the regimen of patients with moderate persistent asthma who are poorly controlled on inhaled steroids alone. As compared with inhaled long-acting β-agonists as add-on therapy, LT modifiers may offer comparable improvement in symptoms but will not improve lung function to the same degree. In these patients, LT modifiers can allow a significant reduction in inhaled steroid dose. As monotherapy, they are not an effective substitute for inhaled steroids in patients who require moderate to high doses for asthma control.

In summary, LT modifiers are the newest class of generally available asthma controller medications. They provide additional options in the treatment of all classes of asthma patients.

Table 19-2. INDICATIONS FOR LEUKOTRIENE-MODIFYING DRUG USE

Treatment of mild-persistent asthma
    (try before using inhaled steroids [28,47,48])

Treatment of moderate to severe-persistent asthma
    (as an adjunct to inhaled and oral steroids,
    can allow decrease in steroids dose [31,33,34])

Treatment of aspirin-induced asthma
    (first-line agent [19,49])

Prophylaxis of exercise-induced asthma [25]

REFERENCES AND RECOMMENDED READING

1. Panettieri RA, Tan EM, Ciocca V, *et al.*: Effects of LTD4 on human airway smooth muscle cell proliferation, matrix expression, and contraction in vitro: differential sensitivity of cysteinyl leukotriene receptor antagonists. *Am J Respir Cell Mol Biol* 1998, 19:453–461.

2. Mulder A, Gauvreau GM, Watson RM, O'Byrne PM: Effect of inhaled leukotriene D4 on airway eosinophilia and airway hyperresponsiveness in asthmatic subjects. *Am J Respir Crit Care Med* 1999, 159(5 Pt 1):1562–1567.

3. Adelroth E, Morris MM, Hargreave FE, O'Byrne PM: Airway responsiveness to leukotrienes C4 and D4 and to methacholine in patients with asthma and normal controls. *N Engl J Med* 1986, 315:480–484.

4. Drazen JM, O'Brien JB, Sparrow D, *et al.*: Recovery of leukotriene E4 from the urine of patients with airway obstruction. *Am Rev Respir Dis* 1992, 146:104–108.

5. Taylor GW, Taylor I, Black P, *et al.*: Urinary leukotriene E4 after antigen challenge and in acute asthma and allergic rhinitis. *Lancet* 1989, 1:584–588.

6. Yokomizo T, Izumi T, Chang K, *et al.*: A G-protein–coupled receptor for leukotriene B4 that mediates chemotaxis. *Nature* 1997, 387(6633):620–624.

7. Sarau HM, Ames RS, Chambers J, *et al.*: Identification, molecular cloning, expression, and characterization of a cysteinyl leukotriene receptor. *Mol Pharmacol* 1999, 56(3):657–663.

8. Drazen JM, Israel E, O'Byrne PM: Treatment of asthma with drugs modifying the leukotriene pathway. *N Engl J Med* 1999, 340:197–206.

9. Bruijnzeel PL, Virchow JC, Jr., Rihs S, *et al.*: Lack of increased numbers of low-density eosinophils in the circulation of asthmatic individuals. *Clin Exp Allergy* 1993, 23(4):261–269.

10. Wenzel SE, Larsen GL, Johnston K, *et al.*: Elevated levels of leukotriene C4 in bronchoalveolar lavage fluid from atopic asthmatics after endobronchial allergen challenge. *Am Rev Respir Dis* 1990, 142:112–119.

11. Smith CM, Christie PE, Hawksworth RJ, *et al.*: Urinary leukotriene-E4 levels after allergen and exercise challenge in bronchial asthma. *Am Rev Respir Dis* 1991, 144:1411–1413.

12. Kumlin M, Dahlen B, Bjorck T, *et al.*: Urinary excretion of leukotriene E4 and 11-dehydro-thromboxane B2 in response to bronchial provocations with allergen, aspirin, leukotriene D4 and histamine in asthmatics. *Am Rev Respir Dis* 1992, 146:96–103.

13. Taylor IK, O'Shaughnessy KM, Fuller RW, Dollery CT: Effect of cysteinyl-leukotriene receptor antagonist ICI 204.219 on allergen-induced bronchoconstriction and airway hyperreactivity in atopic subjects. *Lancet* 1991, 337:690–694.

14. Diamant Z, Grootendorst DC, Veselic-Charvat M, *et al.*: The effect of montelukast (MK-0476), a cysteinyl leukotriene receptor antagonist, on allergen-induced airway responses and sputum cell counts in asthma. *Clin Exp Allergy* 1999, 29:42–51.

15. Hamilton AL, Watson RM, Wyile G, O'Byrne PM: Attenuation of early and late phase allergen-induced bronchoconstriction in asthmatic subjects by a 5-lipoxygenase activating protein antagonist, BAYx 1005. *Thorax* 1997, 52(4):348–354.

16. Roquet A, Dahlen B, Kumlin M, *et al.*: Combined antagonism of leukotrienes and histamine produces predominant inhibition of allergen-induced early and late phase airway obstruction in asthmatics. *Am J Respir Crit Care Med* 1997, 155:1856–1863.

17. Sestini P, Armetti L, Gambaro G, *et al.*: Inhaled PGE2 prevents aspirin-induced bronchoconstriction and urinary LTE4 excretion in aspirin-sensitive asthma. *Am J Respir Crit Care Med* 1996, 153:572–575.

18. Israel E, Fischer AR, Rosenberg MA, *et al.*: The pivotal role of 5-lipoxygenase products in the reaction of aspirin-sensitive asthmatics to aspirin. *Am Rev Respir Dis* 1993, 148:1447–1451.

19. Dahlen SE, Malmstrom K, Nizankowska E, *et al.*: Improvement of aspirin-intolerant asthma by montelukast, a leukotriene antagonist: a randomized, double-blind, placebo-controlled trial. *Am J Respir Crit Care Med* 2002, 165(1):9–14.

20. Dahlen B, Nizankowska E, Szczeklik A, *et al.*: Benefits from adding the 5-lipoxygenase inhibitor zileuton to conventional therapy in aspirin-intolerant asthmatics. *Am J Respir Crit Care Med* 1998, 157:1187–1194.

21. Pliss LB, Ingenito EP, Ingram RH, Jr., Pichurko B: Assessment of bronchoalveolar cell and mediator response to isocapnic hyperpnea in asthma. *Am Rev Respir Dis* 1990, 142:73–78.

22. Leff JA, Busse WW, Pearlman D, *et al.*: Montelukast, a leukotriene-receptor antagonist, for the treatment of mild asthma and exercise-induced bronchoconstriction. *N Engl J Med* 1998, 339:147–152.

23. Israel E, Dermarkarian R, Rosenberg M, *et al.*: The effects of a 5-lipoxygenase inhibitor on asthma induced by cold, dry air. *N Engl J Med* 1990, 323:1740–1744.

24. Meltzer SS, Hasday JD, Cohn J, Bleecker ER: Inhibition of exercise-induced bronchospasm by zileuton: a 5-lipoxygenase inhibitor. *Am J Respir Crit Care Med* 1996, 153:931–935.

25. Dessanges JF, Prefaut C, Taytard A, *et al.*: The effect of zafirlukast on repetitive exercise-induced bronchoconstriction: the possible role of leukotrienes in exercise-induced refractoriness. *J Allergy Clin Immunol* 1999, 104(6):1155–1161.

26. Edelman JM, Turpin JA, Bronsky EA, *et al.*: Oral montelukast compared with inhaled salmeterol to prevent exercise-induced bronchoconstriction. *Ann Intern Med* 2000, 132:97–104.

27. Finnerty JP, Wood-Baker R, Thomson H, Holgate ST: Role of leukotrienes in exercise-induced asthma. Inhibitory effect of ICI 204219, a potent leukotriene D4 receptor antagonist. *Am Rev Respir Dis* 1992, 145:746–749.

28. Israel E, Rubin P, Kemp J, *et al.*: The effect of inhibition of 5-lipoxygenase by zileuton in mild to moderate asthma. *Ann Intern Med* 1993, 119:1059–1066.

29. Reiss TF, Altman LC, Chervinsky P, *et al.*: Effects of montelukast (MK-0476), a new potent cysteinyl leukotriene (LTD4) receptor antagonist, in patients with chronic asthma. *J Allergy Clin Immunol* 1996, 98:528–534.

30. Spector SL, Smith LJ, Glass M: Accolate Asthma Trialists Group. Effects of 6 weeks of therapy with oral doses of ICI 204,219, a leukotriene D4 receptor antagonist, in subjects with bronchial asthma. *Am J Respir Crit Care Med* 1994, 150:618–623.

31. Malmstrom K, Rodriguez-Gomez G, Guerra J, *et al.*: Oral montelukast, inhaled beclomethasone, and placebo for chronic asthma. *Ann Intern Med* 1999, 130:487–495.

32. Reiss TF, Sorkness CA, Stricker W, *et al.*: Effects of montelukast (MK-0476), a potent cysteinyl leukotriene receptor antagonist, on bronchodilation in asthmatic subjects treated with and without inhaled corticosteroids. *Thorax* 1997, 52:45–48.

33. Lofdahl CG, Reiss TF, Leff JA, *et al.*: Randomised, placebo controlled trial of effect of a leukotriene receptor antagonist, montelukast, on tapering inhaled corticosteroids in asthmatic patients. *BMJ* 1999, 319:87–90.

34. Laviolette M, Malmstrom K, Lu S, *et al.*: Montelukast added to inhaled beclomethasone in treatment of asthma. *Am J Respir Crit Care Med* 1999, 160:1862–1868.

35. Virchow JC, Jr., Prasse A, Naya I, *et al.*: Zafirlukast improves asthma control in patients receiving high-dose inhaled corticosteroids. *Am J Respir Crit Care Med* 2000, 162:578–585.

36. Tamaoki J, Kondo M, Sakai N, *et al.*: Leukotriene antagonist prevents exacerbation of asthma during reduction of high-dose inhaled corticosteroid. *Am J Respir Crit Care Med* 1997, 155:1235–1240.

37. Busse W, Nelson H, Wolfe J, *et al.*: Comparison of inhaled salmeterol and oral zafirlukast in patients with asthma. *J Allergy Clin Immunol* 1999, 103:1075–1080.

38. Nelson HS, Busse WW, Kerwin E, *et al.*: Fluticasone propionate/salmeterol combination provides more effective asthma control than low-dose inhaled corticosteroid plus montelukast. *J Allergy Clin Immunol* 2000, 106(6):1088–1095.

39. Fish JE, Israel E, Murray JJ, *et al.*: Salmeterol powder provides significantly better benefit than montelukast in asthmatic patients receiving concomitant inhaled corticosteroid therapy. *Chest* 2001, 120(2):423–430.

40. Reinus JF, Persky S, Burkiewicz JS, *et al.*: Severe liver injury after treatment with the leukotriene receptor antagonist zafirlukast. *Ann Intern Med* 2000, 133(12):964–968.

41. Wechsler ME, Garpestad E, Flier SR, *et al.*: Pulmonary infiltrates, eosinophilia, and cardiomyopathy following cortico-steroid withdrawal in patients with asthma receiving zafirlukast. *JAMA* 1998, 279:455–457.

42. Tuggey JM, Hosker H: Churg-Strauss syndrome associated with montelukast therapy. *Thorax* 2000, 55:805–806.

43. Wechsler ME, Finn D, Gunawardena D, *et al.*: Churg-Strauss syndrome in patients receiving montelukast as treatment for asthma. *Chest* 2000, 117:708–713.

44. Szefler SJ, Martin RJ, King TS, *et al.*: Significant variability in response to inhaled corticosteroids for persistent asthma. *J Allergy Clin Immunol* 2002, 109(3):410–418.

45. Drazen JM, Yandava CN, Dube L, *et al.*: Pharmacogenetic association between ALOX5 promoter genotype and the response to anti-asthma treatment. *Nat Genet* 1999, 22:168–170.

46. Sampson AP, Siddiqui S, Buchanan D, *et al.*: Variant LTC(4) synthase allele modifies cysteinyl leukotriene synthesis in eosinophils and predicts clinical response to zafirlukast. *Thorax* 2000, 55(Suppl 2):S28–S31.

47. Reiss TF, Chervinsky P, Dockhorn RJ, *et al.*: Montelukast, a once-daily leukotriene receptor antagonist, in the treatment of chronic asthma. *Arch Intern Med* 1998, 158:1213–1220.

48. Drazen JM, Israel E: Should antileukotriene therapies be used instead of inhaled corticosteroids in asthma? Yes. *Am J Respir Crit Care Med* 1998, 158:1697–1698.

49. Dahlen B, Margolskee DJ, Zetterstrom O, Dahlen SE: Effect of the leukotriene receptor antagonist MK-0679 on baseline pulmonary function in aspirin sensitive asthmatic subjects. *Thorax* 1993, 48:1205–1210.

50. National Heart, Lung, and Blood Institute, National Asthma Education and Prevention Program: *Expert Panel Report 2: Guidelines for the Diagnosis and Management of Asthma.* Bethesda, MD: National Institutes of Health, Pub. No. 97-4051; 1997.

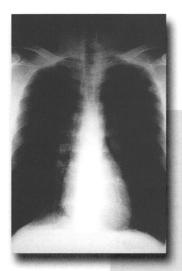

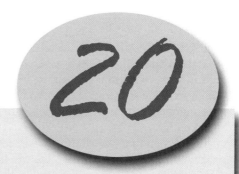

Allergen Avoidance

G. Daniel Brooks and Robert K. Bush

The association between allergen exposure and worsening asthma has been well established. Asthmatic subjects given an inhalant allergen challenge have increased airway inflammation and obstruction, and patients with sensitization to seasonal allergens often have a seasonal worsening of their disease. Because allergens have such adverse effects for sensitized patients with asthma, it is reasonable to reduce exposure to these provoking factors. Strategies have evolved to reduce indoor allergen exposure, including dust mite, animal, cockroach, and mold allergen exposures. This chapter reviews the evidence that specific strategies can attain meaningful reductions in allergen levels or clinical symptoms. These strategies should be reserved for patients with proven sensitization by skin test or radioallergosorbent test (RAST) IgE level [1•].

DUST MITE REDUCTION MEASURES

House dust mites are microscopic arachnids that live inside homes, primarily in bedding, carpeting, and upholstery. These animals feed on organic debris, most notably human skin scales, which accounts for the populations in bedding. Dust mites absorb water from moisture in the air and do not reproduce well in environments of low humidity or low temperature, such as found during the winter season in northern climates [2••]. Two species of dust mites, *Dermatophagoides farinae* and *Dermatophagoides pteronyssinus*, are common within temperate climates and are the primary source of allergens. The major dust mite allergens (Der f 1 and Der p 1) are digestive enzymes excreted into mite feces. Immunoassays allow measurement of these allergen levels in the home environment for the purpose of clinical trials.

Diagnosing dust mite hypersensitivity based on clinical history is nearly impossible. Patients may have perennial or seasonal symptoms, depending on variations in humidity and temperature. Symptoms provoked during cleaning or dust exposure are often caused by an irritant effect in non-allergic individuals, and confirmation of dust mite–specific IgE by either skin test or RAST is necessary for an accurate diagnosis. Still, these tests should be reserved for individuals with underlying asthma, atopic dermatitis, or allergic rhinoconjunctivitis because the significance of allergen-specific IgE in asymptomatic patients is unknown.

More allergic individuals are sensitized to dust mites than any other allergen, particularly in humid climates [2••], and convincing evidence suggests that dust mite allergen exposure is a significant risk factor for dust mite sensitivity and allergic asthma [1•,3]. Therefore, successful dust mite allergen reduction is an attractive goal for intervention, and many strategies have been used to reduce dust mite numbers, allergen levels, and patient exposure to allergen (Table 20-1).

Mattress and pillows are significant reservoirs of dust mites and serve as the primary site of allergen exposure within the home. Dust mite allergen–impermeable coverings can be made from plastic or from finely woven cloth, which is vapor permeable and more comfortable. Encasing mattresses and pillows in protective coverings has been shown to significantly reduce dust mite allergen levels on the bed surface [4•,5,6]. Synthetic pillows appear to offer no advantage over feather pillows and may even accumulate allergens more quickly [7].

The most successful trials of mattress encasements have also incorporated weekly laundering of bedding [4•,8]. Dust mites can be killed by washing in hot water (130°F) or drying at high temperatures (130°F), and dust mite allergen can be removed by washing in any temperature of water [2••,9]. Care must be taken in houses with children because 130°F water can be associated with serious burns.

Because house dust mites absorb most of their water from the air, decreasing humidity has the potential to reduce dust mite populations. Maintaining a relative humidity below 50% prevents population growth in laboratory dust mite cultures [10], so air conditioners and dehumidifiers have both been tried to replicate this effect in the home environment. One trial [11] demonstrated that houses with a relative humidity below 50% have a 50-fold decrease in live mites and a fourfold decrease in major allergen levels over 17 months without special cleaning measures. However, lowering the relative humidity below 50% was difficult: 14 of 19 homes with high-efficiency dehumidifiers reached the target, but only seven of 26 homes with only an air conditioner reached the target. Unfortunately, high-efficiency dehumidification units are expensive, and the role of single-room dehumidification has not been clearly established [12]. If humidity control is planned, it should be directed by measurements of relative humidity, not the blind use of humidity-removing devices [11].

Various acaricides have been successful at killing house dust mites in laboratory cultures; however, these chemicals have been less successful at killing mites in the home environment. It is difficult to deliver the acaricides to some of the key dust mite reservoirs such as inside a mattress or deep within carpet pile. In addition, the possible effects of these chemicals on human health must be considered, particularly if applying the materials to bedding. A recent meta-analysis [13•] of chemical mite control measures suggests they may have an adverse impact on asthma.

Removal of carpets and upholstery is often recommended because these are known reservoirs for the dust mites. This approach is logical, but it has not been well studied, and the degree of allergen reduction to expect is unknown. Of course, carpet removal is an expensive proposition, and this advice is generally reserved for people who are already planning to move, redecorate, or trade bedrooms.

Vacuuming carpets may help to reduce the reservoir of dust mite allergen, but it must be done in combination with other control methods. Dust mites are often found deep within the carpet pile, and vacuum cleaners do not remove live mites effectively. Vacuum high-efficiency particulate air (HEPA) filters and two-layer vacuum bags retain dust mite allergen well but do not reduce allergen levels without performing other dust mite eradication measures [14].

A new method of killing dust mites in mattresses has been investigated [15]. A hot metal probe is inserted into the mattress followed by steam treatments of the surface. Houses in the treatment group had reduced allergen levels for 6 months, and subjects in the treatment group had

Table 20-1. DUST MITE REDUCTION MEASURES

Intervention	Recommended?	Comments
Bedding encasements	Yes, strongly	Controlled trials suggest decreased allergen, improved airway responsiveness
Wash bedding weekly	Yes, strongly	Used in successful encasement trials
Keep humidity < 50%	Yes	Kills mites, but difficult to implement; high-efficiency dehumidifiers expensive
Weekly vacuuming (HEPA filter or double bag)	Yes	Reduces allergen reservoir; does not remove live mites
Remove carpets	Yes	Costly; recommend if already planning a move or renovation
Chemical acaricides	No	No benefit, may be harmful
Air filters or duct cleaning	No	Dust mite allergen does not circulate well

HEPA—high-efficiency particulate air.

reduced bronchial hyperresponsiveness (BHR) at 9 months. This approach to dust mite reduction is promising but still unavailable clinically.

Patients often ask about purchasing air filtration units or cleaning out the ducts in their house. Because dust mite allergen particles are large and settle relatively quickly, they do not circulate well in the air. Therefore, ducts contain little allergen, and air filtration units are of minimal benefit.

Clinical Effects of Dust Mite Reduction

Because dust mite allergen levels correlate with asthma severity, it is reasonable to hypothesize that reducing dust mite levels will lead to clinical benefit. However, studies of specific reduction measures have had variable results. A Cochrane meta-analysis [16] was published in 1998 and reported no asthma improvement in subjects assigned to dust mite reduction measures versus control subjects. An updated version of this meta-analysis [13•] includes more recent studies and now indicates that nonchemical methods (*eg*, mattress encasements and dehumidifiers) show a significant benefit. It is important to note that the majority of the studies included in this analysis did not include a measurement of allergen reduction, and many of the studies used reduction measures that have since been abandoned because of lack of efficacy.

The approach most strongly recommended includes covering the mattress, boxspring, and pillows in dust mite–impermeable encasements and washing bedding weekly. Studies of this approach have shown some of the best clinical results, including improvements in symptom scores and BHR [4•,8]. Reducing humidity below 50% decreases mite allergen levels, but the clinical response to this intervention is not well documented.

CONTROL OF ANIMAL ALLERGENS

New studies suggest that the presence of a cat in the home from birth may protect children from developing cat sensitization [17,18]. However, for patients with established cat sensitization, exposure to cat allergen is a significant risk factor for developing asthma [19], and for patients who have both cat sensitization and allergic asthma, cat allergen can act as a potent trigger of symptoms or exacerbations.

The major cat allergen, Fel d 1, is primarily produced in the sebaceous glands and squamous epithelium of all cats [20•]. Individual cats shed different quantities of allergen, but the notion that some breeds of cat secrete less allergen is probably not correct [21]. Androgens can affect allergen production: females and castrated males produce less Fel d 1 [22]. Cat allergen has electrostatic charges that make it adhere to clothing, walls, and carpets, and at least 15% of the allergen is found on small particles that can remain airborne for some time [20•].

The optimal avoidance strategy for cat allergy is to avoid bringing cats into the home and find a new home for any cats already in the home. Homes with a cat can have 100-fold higher levels of Fel d 1 than homes without a cat [23]. Even after a cat is removed from the environment, despite regular cleaning, the cat allergen may persist for more than 6 months [24]. Thus, a short trial of removing a pet from the home is not helpful. In fact, allergen can persist in the mattress for years after removal of a cat, and new mattresses or bed encasements may be required [25,26]. Although removing a cat from the home is clearly the best way to reduce cat allergen exposure, many families are unwilling to part with a beloved pet, so other strategies of allergen reduction have been investigated (Table 20-2).

Washing a cat weekly decreases the quantity of airborne cat allergen [27], but the effect does not last a whole week, and long-term reductions have not been demonstrated [28,29]. Cats generally dislike bathing, and it is difficult to justify this recommendation. Private companies have developed and marketed special formulations for removing allergens from pets, most notably Allerpet (Allerpet Inc., New York, NY). Allerpet is a solution that is applied to a washcloth and used to wipe the animal, with the intention of removing allergen. However, clinical investigations suggest that any allergen decrease is transient, erratic, no greater than wiping with water, and, in one study, compa-

---

Table 20-2. CAT ALLERGEN REDUCTION MEASURES

Intervention	Recommended?	Comments
Remove cat from home	Yes, strongly	May take > 6 mo for allergen to be removed
HEPA filter plus exclude cat from bedroom	Yes	Not as good as pet removal
Bathing cat	No	Poorly tolerated by cats; allergen decrease is transient
Allerpet*	No	No significant effect on airborne allergens
Acepromazine	No	No effect on allergen production

Allerpet, Inc., New York, NY.
HEPA—high-efficiency particulate air

rable to not washing at all [28,30]. Acepromazine, an animal tranquilizer, is sometimes prescribed by veterinarians in an attempt to reduce cat allergen production, but it also appears to have no effect on Fel d 1 levels [28].

Because a significant proportion of cat allergen is located on particles that remain airborne, it can be removed with a HEPA air cleaner. The two trials [31,32] that evaluated this intervention have arrived at different conclusions. Wood *et al.* [31] found that the combination of cat exclusion from the bedroom, mattress and pillow encasements, and placement of an air cleaner with HEPA filter in the bedroom for 3 months led to a decrease in Fel d 1 levels; however, there was no significant effect on nasal symptom scores, chest symptom scores, medication usage, peak flow rates, or methacholine reactivity. Cat exclusion and encasements with dummy air filters did not affect Fel d 1 levels. Van der Heide *et al.* [32] studied 20 children with cat or dog allergy using air cleaner units in the bedroom and living room with either HEPA or sham filters for 3 months. In this study, children with HEPA filters had reduced peak flow variability and reduced adenosine responsiveness. The better results in the Van der Heide study may indicate that children are more likely to respond than adults or that living room filters significantly affect clinical exposure.

Vacuum cleaners with HEPA filtration features reduce cat allergen leakage, although significant leakage still occurs [33]. This probably helps to reduce the allergen reservoir [14], particularly after a cat has been removed from the environment, but it does not protect the person who is vacuuming from allergen exposure during vacuuming [34].

Sensitization to dog is generally less common than to cat, although it has been associated with asthma [35]. The major dog allergen is Can f 1, which is also found on small particles that remain airborne. There have been significantly fewer trials investigating dog allergen reduction than for cat allergen, but existing trials suggest a similar approach. Washing a dog reduces recoverable allergen from the dog, but the effects only last 3 days [36], and the small decrease in airborne Can f 1 is of questionable clinical benefit [36]. A double-thickness vacuum bag may help decrease allergen load in carpets, and HEPA air cleaners reduce Can f 1 levels in homes [37,38]. The clinical benefits of these measures are unknown.

If a pet remains in the home, any allergen-control measures are of questionable benefit. Allergen levels are often only decreased modestly, particularly when compared with homes without a pet [23,31,32,36,39]. Thus, physicians and sensitized patients must understand that the continued presence of an indoor animal can lead to worsening asthma, increased medication requirements, or both [40••].

Cockroach Abatement

In the United States, cockroach allergy prevalence ranges from 17% to 41% in studies of both children and adults [41••]. Both cockroach sensitization and increased cockroach allergen levels have been associated with asthma

morbidity in children and increased airway obstruction in adults [42–44]. The two most common species in the United States are the German cockroach (*Blatella germanica*) and the American cockroach (*Periplaneta americana*). The German cockroach is about 16 mm long and brown, and the American cockroach is 38 mm long and has reddish-brown wings [45••].

Inside the home, cockroaches prefer to hide in dark, humid, and warm microenvironments. They often hide in tiny cracks near sources of water or food [45••], and come out at night to drink and feed. If they are visible during the daylight hours, it is an indication of a more severe infestation. Other evidence of infestation may include the presence of cockroach feces (black pellets the size of a grain of sand) in the kitchen [45••].

German cockroach allergen levels (Bla g 1 or Bla g 2) are typically measured in studies of cockroach-associated asthma morbidity [42–44]. The major cockroach allergens are present in both the feces and the body of the cockroach. Similar to dust mite allergen, cockroach allergen is primarily found on relatively large particles that require disturbance to be detected in the air [41••]. Cockroach allergen levels are generally greatest in the kitchen, but levels in the bedroom probably correlate best with allergic sensitization and asthma morbidity [42,46].

The first step in cockroach allergen reduction is cockroach extermination. Initially, this is best delegated to a professional pest control company. An inspection should be performed to identify probable cockroach locations, water sources, and food sources. Storing food in sealed containers, washing dishes daily, removing sources of standing water, and taking the trash outside daily may help reduce cockroach populations [40••]. Pesticides are very effective at reducing cockroach populations. Abamectin 0.05% gel has a relatively low human toxicity and has been used in clinical studies of cockroach allergen abatement. Professional extermination with abamectin significantly reduces cockroach populations, but it only minimally decreases allergen levels in the kitchen [47]. However, if professional extermination is combined with professional cleaning before extermination, then cockroach allergen levels can be reduced about 90% in the kitchen and 75% in the bedroom [48,49]. Whether a 75% reduction in cockroach allergen levels is enough to provide clinical benefit is unclear. Trials that have examined the effects of cockroach extermination on asthma control have failed because they did not achieve significant decreases in cockroach allergen levels [47,50]. This underscores the challenge of reducing cockroach levels, particularly for people who cannot afford professional interventions.

FUNGAL ABATEMENT

At least 80 genera of fungi have been associated with allergic disease. The fungus best linked to asthma is *Alternaria* spp, which have been associated with the presence, severity, and mortality of asthma [51••]. *Alternaria* spp grow on dead and decaying material and are considered outdoor molds, with most indoor exposure attributed to infiltration of spores from outdoors.

Two other fungi, *Penicillium* spp and *Aspergillus* spp, can be recovered at greater rates indoors than outdoors [51••]. Although less often implicated than *Alternaria* spp, these fungi have been associated with allergic disease and some asthma epidemics [52]. Literature reviews [53] have also associated the presence of indoor mold and humidity with wheezing and coughing. Whether the mold has a cause-and-effect relationship to these symptoms is difficult to prove, but it is reasonable to hypothesize that an asthmatic individual sensitized to mold will have worse asthma control with greater exposure.

Indoor fungal exposure can occur from two different sources: infiltration of outdoor spores and growth of fungi indoors [40••]. Both sources of fungal exposure must be considered if attempting an allergen reduction program. Closing windows and doors to air conditioning during warmer months can help reduce the infiltration of outdoor mold spores; however, it may also increase spore levels of indoor fungi. Filtering outdoor air allows indoor fungal metabolites to dissipate but keeps outdoor mold spores from entering [40••].

For the most part, indoor fungal growth occurs in areas of increased moisture, particularly in the presence of condensation. A damp basement or humid bathroom can support fungal growth, producing spores that may travel throughout the house [51••]. Therefore, appropriate humidity-reduction measures are encouraged. Treatment of washable surfaces with commercial fungicides or 5% bleach also helps eradicate fungi, but these chemicals can be quite irritating, and asthmatic patients should wear a respirator while applying them [51••]. Areas of more severe fungal contamination often require the removal of carpet, walls, or even the demolition of a building [40••]. Another reasonable approach to fungal allergen reduction is through HEPA air filters. A study [6] has indicated that these may be as good at reducing fungal exposure as dust mite encasements are at reducing dust mite allergen exposure. Generally, the impact of fungus reduction measures on allergen levels has not been well studied, and the clinical benefit of these measures is still based on deductive reasoning.

REFERENCES AND RECOMMENDED READING

Papers of particular interest, published recently, have been highlighted as:
•   Of importance
••   Of major importance

1.• Eggleston PA, Bush RK: Environmental allergen avoidance: an overview. *J Allergy Clin Immunol* 2001, 107(suppl):403–405.
A quick synopsis of important issues and recommendations.

2.••Arlian LG, Platts-Mills TA: The biology of dust mites and the remediation of mite allergens in allergic disease. *J Allergy Clin Immunol* 2001, 107(suppl):406–413.
A review that relates dust mite biology to specific measures of dust mite allergen reduction.

3. Huss K, Adkinson NF, Jr., Eggleston PA, *et al.*: House dust mite and cockroach exposure are strong risk factors for positive allergy skin test responses in the Childhood Asthma Management Program. *J Allergy Clin Immunol* 2001, 107:48–54.

4.• Shapiro GG, Wighton TG, Chinn T, *et al.*: House dust mite avoidance for children with asthma in homes of low-income families. *J Allergy Clin Immunol* 1999, 103:1069–1074.
A recent study that has found reduced airway responsiveness in children with dust mite avoidance measures.

5. Cloosterman SG, Schermer TR, Bijl-Hofland ID, *et al.*: Effects of house dust mite avoidance measures on Der p 1 concentrations and clinical condition of mild adult house dust mite-allergic asthmatic patients, using no inhaled steroids. *Clin Exp Allergy* 1999, 29:1336–1346.

6. van der Heide HS, Kauffman HF, Dubois AE, *et al.*: Allergen reduction measures in houses of allergic asthmatic patients: effects of air-cleaners and allergen-impermeable mattress covers. *Eur Respir J* 1997, 10:1217–1223.

7. Rains N, Siebers R, Crane J, *et al*: House dust mite allergen (Der p 1) accumulation on new synthetic and feather pillows. *Clin Exp Allergy* 1999, 29:182–185.

8. Walshaw MJ, Evans CC: Allergen avoidance in house dust mite sensitive adult asthma. *Q J Med* 1986, 58:199–215.

9. McDonald LG, Tovey E: The role of water temperature and laundry procedures in reducing house dust mite populations and allergen content of bedding. *J Allergy Clin Immunol* 1992, 90:599–608.

10. Arlian LG, Neal JS, Vyszenski-Moher DL: Reducing relative humidity to control the house dust mite *Dermatophagoides farinae*. *J Allergy Clin Immunol* 1999, 104:852–856.

11. Arlian LG, Neal JS, Morgan MS, *et al.*: Reducing relative humidity is a practical way to control dust mites and their allergens in homes in temperate climates. *J Allergy Clin Immunol* 2001, 107:99–104.

12. Hyndman SJ, Vickers LM, Htut T, *et al.*: A randomized trial of dehumidification in the control of house dust mite. *Clin Exp Allergy* 2000, 30:1172–1180.

13.• Gotzsche PC, Johansen HK, Burr ML, *et al.*: House dust mite control measures for asthma. *Cochrane Database Syst Rev* 2001, CD001187.
A recent meta-analysis addressing the clinical efficacy of dust mite control measures for asthma.

14. Popplewell EJ, Innes VA, Lloyd-Hughes S, *et al.*: The effect of high-efficiency and standard vacuum cleaners on mite, cat and dog allergen levels and clinical progress. *Pediatr Allergy Immunol* 2000, 11:142–148.

15. Htut T, Higenbottam TW, Gill GW, *et al.*: Eradication of house dust mite from homes of atopic asthmatic subjects: a double-blind trial. *J Allergy Clin Immunol* 2001, 107:55–60.

16. Gotzsche PC, Hammarquist C, Burr M: House dust mite control measures in the management of asthma: meta-analysis. *Br Med J* 1998, 317:1105–1110.

17. Hesselmar B, Aberg N, Aberg B, *et al.*: Does early exposure to cat or dog protect against later allergy development? *Clin Exp Allergy* 1999, 29:611–617.

18. Platts-Mills TA, Vaughan JW, Blumenthal K, *et al.*: Decreased prevalence of asthma among children with high exposure to cat allergen: relevance of the modified Th2 response. *Mediators Inflam* 2001, 10:288–291.

19. Sears MR, Herbison GP, Holdaway MD, *et al.*: The relative risks of sensitivity to grass pollen, house dust mite and cat dander in the development of childhood asthma. *Clin Exp Allergy* 1989, 19:419–424.

20.• Chapman MD, Wood RA: The role and remediation of animal allergens in allergic diseases. *J Allergy Clin Immunol* 2001, 107(suppl):414–421.
A review of animal allergen control measures.

21. Custovic A, Simpson A, Chapman MD, *et al.*: Allergen avoidance in the treatment of asthma and atopic disorders. *Thorax* 1998, 53:63–72.

22. Charpin C, Zielonka TM, Charpin D, *et al.*: Effects of castration and testosterone on Fel dI production by sebaceous glands of male cats: II: morphometric assessment. *Clin Exp Allergy* 1994, 24:1174–1178.

23. Custovic A, Simpson A, Pahdi H, *et al.*: Distribution, aerodynamic characteristics, and removal of the major cat allergen Fel d 1 in British homes. *Thorax* 1998, 53:33–38.

24. Wood RA, Chapman MD, Adkinson NF Jr, *et al.*: The effect of cat removal on allergen content in household-dust samples. *J Allergy Clin Immunol* 1989, 83:730–734.

25. van dB, X, Charpin D, Haddi E, *et al.*: Cat removal and Fel d I levels in mattresses. *J Allergy Clin Immunol* 1991, 87:595–596.

26. Vaughan JW, McLaughlin TE, Perzanowski MS, *et al.*: Evaluation of materials used for bedding encasement: effect of pore size in blocking cat and dust mite allergen. *J Allergy Clin Immunol* 1999, 103:227–231.

27. de Blay F, Chapman MD, Platts-Mills TA: Airborne cat allergen (Fel d I). Environmental control with the cat in situ. *Am Rev Respir Dis* 1991, 143:1334–1339.

28. Klucka CV, Ownby DR, Green J, *et al.*: Cat shedding of Fel d I is not reduced by washings, Allerpet-C spray, or acepromazine. *J Allergy Clin Immunol* 1995, 95:1164–1171.

29. Avner DB, Perzanowski MS, Platts-Mills TA, *et al.*: Evaluation of different techniques for washing cats: quantitation of allergen removed from the cat and the effect on airborne Fel d 1. *J Allergy Clin Immunol* 1997, 100:307–312.

30. Perzanowski MS, Wheatley LM, Avner DB, *et al.*: The effectiveness of Allerpet/c in reducing the cat allergen Fel d 1. *J Allergy Clin Immunol* 1997, 100:428–430.

31. Wood RA, Johnson EF, Van Natta ML, *et al.*: A placebo-controlled trial of a HEPA air cleaner in the treatment of cat allergy. *Am J Respir Crit Care Med* 1998, 158:115–120.

32. van der Heide HS, van Aalderen WM, Kauffman HF, *et al.*: Clinical effects of air cleaners in homes of asthmatic children sensitized to pet allergens. *J Allergy Clin Immunol* 1999, 104:447–451.

33. Vaughan JW, Woodfolk JA, Platts-Mills TA: Assessment of vacuum cleaners and vacuum cleaner bags recommended for allergic subjects. *J Allergy Clin Immunol* 1999, 104:1079–1083.

34. Gore, RB, Durrell, B, Bishop, S, *et al.*: Vacuum cleaning in homes with cats increases personal cat allergen exposure [abstract]. *J Allergy Clin Immunol* 2002, 109(suppl):359–359.

35. Ingram JM, Sporik R, Rose G, *et al.*: Quantitative assessment of exposure to dog (Can f 1) and cat (Fel d 1) allergens: relation to sensitization and asthma among children living in Los Alamos, New Mexico. *J Allergy Clin Immunol* 1995, 96:449–456.

36. Hodson T, Custovic A, Simpson A, *et al.*: Washing the dog reduces dog allergen levels, but the dog needs to be washed twice a week. *J Allergy Clin Immunol* 1999, 103:581–585.

37. Green R, Simpson A, Custovic A, *et al.*: Vacuum cleaners and airborne dog allergen. *Allergy* 1999, 54:403–405.

38. Green R, Simpson A, Custovic A, *et al.*: The effect of air filtration on airborne dog allergen. *Allergy* 1999, 54:484–488.

39. Custovic A, Green R, Fletcher A, *et al.*: Aerodynamic properties of the major dog allergen Can f 1: distribution in homes, concentration, and particle size of allergen in the air. *Am J Respir Crit Care Med* 1997, 155:94–98.

40.••Bush RK: Environmental Controls in the Management of Allergic Asthma. *Med Clin North Am* 2002, in press.
A review of allergen reduction measures for dust mite, cockroach, animal, and mold allergens.

41.••Arruda LK, Vailes LD, Ferriani VP, *et al.*: Cockroach allergens and asthma. *J Allergy Clin Immunol* 2001, 107:419–428.
A good review of studies linking cockroach allergen exposure to asthma.

42. Rosenstreich DL, Eggleston P, Kattan M, *et al.*: The role of cockroach allergy and exposure to cockroach allergen in causing morbidity among inner-city children with asthma. *N Engl J Med* 1997, 336:1356–1363.

43. Litonjua AA, Carey VJ, Burge HA, *et al.*: Exposure to cockroach allergen in the home is associated with incident doctor-diagnosed asthma and recurrent wheezing. *J Allergy Clin Immunol* 2001, 107:41–47.

44. Weiss ST, O'Connor GT, DeMolles D, *et al.*: Indoor allergens and longitudinal FEV1 decline in older adults: the Normative Aging Study. *J Allergy Clin Immunol* 1998, 101:720–725.

45.••Eggleston PA, Arruda LK: Ecology and elimination of cockroaches and allergens in the home. *J Allergy Clin Immunol* 2001, 107(suppl):422–429.
A good review of the effects of extermination and cleaning procedures on allergen levels.

46. Eggleston PA, Rosenstreich D, Lynn H, *et al.*: Relationship of indoor allergen exposure to skin test sensitivity in inner-city children with asthma. *J Allergy Clin Immunol* 1998, 102:563–570.

47. Gergen PJ, Mortimer KM, Eggleston PA, *et al.*: Results of the National Cooperative Inner-City Asthma Study (NCICAS) environmental intervention to reduce cockroach allergen exposure in inner-city homes. *J Allergy Clin Immunol* 1999, 103:501–506.

48. Eggleston PA, Wood RA, Rand C, *et al.*: Removal of cockroach allergen from inner-city homes. *J Allergy Clin Immunol* 1999, 104:842–846.

49. Wood RA, Eggleston PA, Rand C, *et al.*: Cockroach allergen abatement with extermination and sodium hypochlorite cleaning in inner-city homes. *Ann Allergy Asthma Immunol* 2001, 87:60–64.

50. Carter MC, Perzanowski MS, Raymond A, *et al.*: Home intervention in the treatment of asthma among inner-city children. *J Allergy Clin Immunol* 2001, 108:732–737.

51.••Bush RK, Portnoy JM: The role and abatement of fungal allergens in allergic diseases. *J Allergy Clin Immunol* 2001, 107(suppl):430–440.
An extensive discussion of the evidence associating fungal allergens with asthma and allergic disease that also includes recommendations on fungal allergen abatement.

52. Codina R, Lockey RF: Possible role of molds as secondary etiologic agents of the asthma epidemics in Barcelona, Spain. *J Allergy Clin Immunol* 1998, 102:318–320.

53. Peat JK, Dickerson J, Li J: Effects of damp and mould in the home on respiratory health: a review of the literature. *Allergy* 1998, 53:120–128.

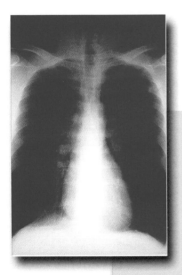

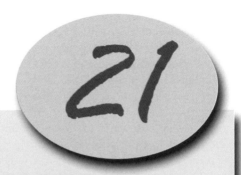

Allergen Immunotherapy in Asthma

Gailen D. Marshall, Jr.

Asthma is now well recognized as an inflammatory condition characterized by reversible airway obstruction, airway hyperresponsiveness, and, at least in some patients, evidence of subepithelial fibrosis and/or smooth muscle hypertrophy and hyperplasia, collectively known as remodeling [1••]. The acute symptomatology is typically related to bronchoconstriction, but the major morbidity (and likely mortality) of the syndrome is linked more to late-phase inflammatory mechanisms. These cause a less reversible airway obstruction (due to inflammation and edema) and hyperactive ("twitchy") airway smooth muscle that constricts to nonspecific stimuli, resulting in worsening acute bronchospasm [2].

The role of allergy as a risk factor for development of asthma has been established [3•]. In children with allergic rhinitis (AR) and a positive family history, the risk of developing allergic asthma (AA) is as high as 40% [4]. When AR is accompanied by atopic dermatitis and food allergy, the risk approaches 80%. This leads to the speculation of a fundamental immunologic relationship between AR and asthma, ie, a systemic immune disease with differing airway phenotypes from patient to patient [5•]. There is evidence of similar inflammatory mechanisms in both AR and AA, including Th1/Th2 cytokine imbalances (excess interleukin [IL]-4, IL-5, IL-13, decreased interferon [IFN]-γ) [6••,7] and excess levels of mast cell (histamine, tryptase) and eosinophil (eotaxin, eosinophil cationic protein) mediators as well as increased numbers of activated T cells, mast cells, and eosinophils in both the upper and lower airways of AR patients with or without accompanying AA (Fig. 21-1) [8].

Therapeutic approaches to asthma management have centered on the use of anti-inflammatory agents to control inflammation and thus chronic symptoms and various bronchodilator agents for relief of acute symptoms [9]. Of note, neither category is considered disease modifying since there is suppression, not elimination, of the underlying immunopathophysiology [10]. With the increasing concern over the significant morbidity of asthma, the small but alarming mortality rate, and improved understanding of mechanisms related to irreversible airway obstruction through remodeling mechanisms, searches for therapeutic approaches that can arrest and reverse or correct the underlying inflammatory mechanisms are at the forefront of developmental asthma pharmacotherapy. With the recognition of the intimate relationships between allergic and asthmatic mechanisms in the majority of afflicted patients [3•,5•], there is a tried and tested therapy that may, at least in part, meet the need for a disease-modifying AA treatment modality.

Allergen immunotherapy (AIT) is the systematic administration (usually parenteral) over an extended period of time of an individualized, defined allergy vaccine composed of specific combinations of allergen extracts that is designed to modify the underlying allergic mechanisms of the afflicted patient [11,12]. There is a certain rationale for using AIT in AA. The most obvious is that AIT has been shown to alter the allergic milieu in patients with AR [13] and *Hymenoptera* sensitivity [14] that correlates with clinical improvement. Although asthma is a complex, multifactorial syndrome, AA patients are worsened clinically when exposed to allergens to which they are sensitive [15]. Further, AIT has been shown to alter the Th1/Th2 cytokine imbalance known to be associated with allergic mechanisms in AR patients [16]. This same imbalance has also been shown to be involved in the immunopathophysiology of asthma [17]. AIT can have a direct effect on eosinophils and mast cells, diminishing their responsiveness and activities in allergic diseases [18]. Additionally, since airway remodeling appears to be a consequence of the chronic airway inflammation characteristic of AA, AIT may well even alter established inflammatory airway changes [19]. Finally, since it is appreciated that AR is a risk factor for the development of asthma in both children and adults, aggressive management with AIT might actually prevent the development of asthma, at least in selected populations [20].

EFFICACY OF ALLERGEN IMMUNOTHERAPY IN ASTHMA

Since the early 1970's, reports have been published that show the positive effects of AIT in treating asthma. Improvements in symptoms, airway function, hospitalization rates, and medication usage have been reported in various combinations depending upon the specific study cited. Recently, several meta-analyses have been published that have examined the efficacy of AIT for AA [21–23]. All of the meta-analyses demonstrated an overall positive effect of AIT for AA. However, what constitutes a positive study needs to be defined. Of course, any asthma therapist wants to see improvements in selected parameters before calling a treatment effective. Varying combinations of symptom scores, nocturnal awakenings, exercise tolerance, and short-acting β-agonist use are used to evaluate efficacy in most therapeutic trials for asthma. Objective measures including changes in forced expiratory volume in 1 second (FEV_1), PC_{20} (dose causing 20% drop in FEV_1) for methacholine, histamine, or even protection against allergen challenges are also used to assess efficacy of specific therapeutic interventions (albeit usually in smaller sample sizes). Several studies also measured AIT effects on concomitant AR symptoms and skin test reactivities in AA patients. Each parameter has studies that show efficacy compared with non–AIT-treated AA patients. Data are often reported as odds ratio with 95% confidence intervals. Various studies have used adults, children, or mixed ages of both genders.

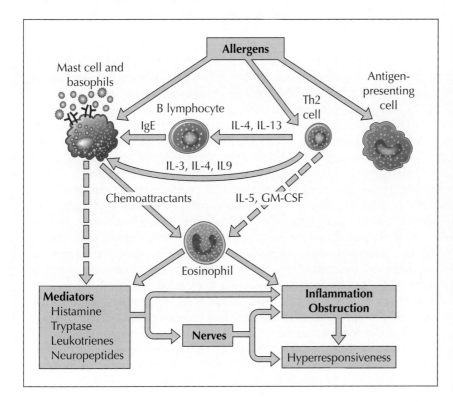

Figure 21-1.
Immunopathophysiology of allergic asthma. The exposure of Th2 cells and B cells to processed antigen causes the production of allergen-specific IgE. This binds to mast cells and awaits subsequent allergen exposure. When exposed, the cross-linked IgE activates mast cells with immediate release of mediators such as histamine and leukotrienes. This causes the immediate symptoms of bronchoconstriction, followed by increased mucus production and recruitment of inflammatory cells (particularly eosinophils), which add to the developing inflammatory milieu. The airway inflammation results in stiff, edematous airways that become hyperresponsive to irritants and otherwise innocuous stimuli such as cold air, exercise, or psychologic stress. GM-CSF—granulocyte-macrophage colony-stimulating factor; IL—interleukin.

Some question how quickly AIT can cause clinical improvement in AA. While treatment protocols of 2 to 5 years are commonly used for AIT in allergic airway disease, several studies show efficacy in terms of reduced airway reactivity to allergen challenge in as few as 3 months [24]. Thus, it is generally not necessary to treat for years to see initial clinical improvement in that fraction of patients who are responsive to AIT. While the duration of treatment varies among practitioners, it is generally acknowledged that clinical responses to AIT should be seen within 1 year of standard treatment and, if patients do not respond, AIT is often interrupted and the patient classified as a nonresponder [25].

Prevention of Asthma with AIT

It is unquestionable that any therapeutic approach that would reduce the incidence of asthma development in at-risk patients would be desirable. It is clear that AR, both seasonal and perennial, is a major risk factor for development of AA in susceptible subpopulations [26••]. This is true for adults as well as children [27]. Particularly susceptible are those AR patients with hyperactive lower airways assessed by methacholine challenge but without any clinical asthma symptoms [28]. Thus it would follow that any disease-modifying therapy for AR could potentially prevent the development of AA. Early studies [29] followed a group of children with AR and positive skin tests to a variety of allergens for 14 years to determine the impact of AIT on the development of AA. Approximately 75% of children who did not receive AIT developed asthma, compared with only 25% of children who received AIT for at least 3 years. Additionally, over half of the children in the control group developed either moderate or severe asthma compared with less than 10% in the AIT group.

Although far from definitive, it is provocative to note that since bronchial hyperresponsiveness (BHR) appears to increase the risk of developing asthma in AR patients [30], any therapy that would lower or prevent BHR might also be expected to lower the asthma risk. Recent studies show that AIT inhibited the development of BHR in a significant proportion of AR patients compared with non–AIT-treated patients [31,32]. This could occur in as little as 3 months [24], and increased by almost threefold the methacholine dose needed to induce significant bronchospasm [33•].

Moller *et al.* [34] reported on the Preventative Allergy Treatment (PAT) study, a prospective, multinational European study that followed 191 children 7 to 15 years of age with documented AR for up to 3 years looking for the development of asthma. More than 90% of the enrolled patients had no asthma symptoms when the study began, and more than 20% of the patients in the control group developed asthma symptoms in the first year compared with 8% in the AIT group. Patients (particularly children) with AR tend to develop additional allergic sensitivities over time [35•].

Studies have demonstrated that AIT with one allergen can diminish or, in some cases, even prevent the development of additional sensitivities to new allergens [36,37]. Up to 10% of subjects developed no new sensitivities to mold, cat, dog, and grass after 3 years of AIT compared with control patients. These data imply that a nonspecific systemic immunomodulatory effect can be attributed to AIT and is the immunologic basis for many new asthma therapies currently in development [38].

Proposed Mechanisms of Efficacy for AIT in Asthma

It is fairly well accepted that asthma can be considered a Th2 disease, *ie*, cytokines such as IL-4, IL-5, IL-9, and IL-13 are responsible for the various inflammatory components involved in AA (Fig. 21-2) [39,40]. IgE is produced as a result of isotype switch from μ to ϵ heavy chain under the direct influence of IL-4 and IL-13 [41]. IL-4, a mast cell growth factor, and IL-5, along with granulocyte-macrophage colony-stimulating factor (GM-CSF), are highly active eosinophil chemotaxins, activators, and anti-apoptotic factors that promote allergic inflammation [42]. Several mechanisms have been proposed to explain the efficacy of AIT in AR (Table 21-1).

It has been well demonstrated in AR that AIT causes an initial increase then a decrease in allergen-specific IgE [43,44] and a blunting of the seasonal increase in pollen-specific IgE [45]. Further, allergen-specific IgG (primarily IgG_1 and IgG_4) increases with AIT [46]. In venom AIT, this has been shown to correlate with efficacy [47]. Regulatory T cells (also known as T_R or Th3 or suppressor T cells) have been noted to increase with AIT [48]. Many or all of these parameters can be attributed to shifts in the Th1/Th2 imbalance noted to occur in AR and AA patients [49]. Indeed, the allergen-specific Th2-predominant cytokine profile is switched to Th0/Th1 (decreased IL-4 and/or increased IFN-γ production in vitro) after successful AIT [50] and correlates with clinical response [51]. Additionally, AIT can directly down-regulate mast cell activity, perhaps through decreased production of histamine-releasing factors [52]. Further, eosinophil numbers and/or activity in nasal secretions [53] and peripheral blood [54] are decreased after AIT. Thus, it appears that AIT can be a disease-modifying therapy for some patients with AR [55].

In AA, the mechanism of AIT efficacy is thought to be similar to that seen in AR. Several studies have shown that AIT decreases IL-4 and IL-13, and increases IFN-γ in treated AA patients [56]. This has correlated with improvements in FEV_1 and decreased symptoms. Additionally, in AA patients with concomitant AR, nasal symptoms improve significantly as well, suggesting that efficacy of AIT for lower airway symptoms may be, at least in part, related to improvements in the upper airway [57]. However, specific lower airway parameters including increased FEV_1 and decreased airway hyperreactivity to methacholine, histamine, and allergen challenges, have all been reported with successful AIT [58]. However, the incomplete response of AA to AIT (*ie*, continued need for controller medications) is disappointing as it is in AR. The exact mechanisms of these incomplete responses are not understood but may involve the known heterogeneity of allergic airway disease to other therapeutic modalities. Major efforts are underway to prospectively identify responders in terms of which and how many allergens cause symptoms, immune changes that are documented, and relative side effects during the AIT treatment protocol.

Risks and Limitations of AIT in Asthma

Because known side effects of AIT include airway compromise (both upper and lower) as well as systemic cardiovascular effects [59], caution is appropriately recommended for treatment in AA patients. Thus, AIT should not be administered to patients with severe persistent AA except under the most extraordinary of circumstances. This is primarily related to safety concerns over surviving a severe idiosyncratic reaction to AIT rather than evidence of lack of efficacy [60]. Indeed, if new pharmaceutical agents (*eg*, anti IgE0) can be demonstrated to increase the safety profile for AIT, studies should be performed to determine whether AIT could be effective in reducing morbidity and decreasing use of controller medications

Several studies have suggested that patients with AA who are optimally treated with pharmacotherapy and environmental control measures may not get as significant a benefit from AIT as those requiring multiple medications for control and may have difficulty minimizing

allergen exposure [61]. Thus, for a patient for whom asthma pharmacotherapy is adequate and AIT impractical (expense of injections, ready access to office of physician with cardiac life support–trained staff, difficulty waiting after injections), current data do not yet support compelling them to undergo AIT in such settings. However, for AA patients for whom a multiplicity of medications and environmental control measures are necessary to control symptoms but who persist in demonstrating clinical exacerbations, decreased airway functions, or multiple allergic triggers, AIT may be considered appropriately as augmentative therapy. This will also depend upon their specific allergen sensitivity, age, and any comorbid conditions that could complicate a systemic reaction to AIT.

RECOMMENDATIONS FOR AIT IN ASTHMA

Based upon National Heart, Lung, and Blood Institute (NHLBI) and World Health Organization (WHO) Allergic Rhinitis and its Impact on Asthma (ARIA) guidelines [26,60], a general scheme for determining the best AA candidates for AIT can developed. First, with current available therapies, AA patients for whom pharmacotherapy is reasonably adequate and whose FEV_1 is consistently less than 70% predicted should not receive AIT. Further, patients receiving β-blockers (including ocular drops) also should not receive AIT due to the reported increased mortality risk should a systemic reaction occur [61]. By extension, AIT should be avoided with any comorbidity (cardiac, metabolic, and neuro-

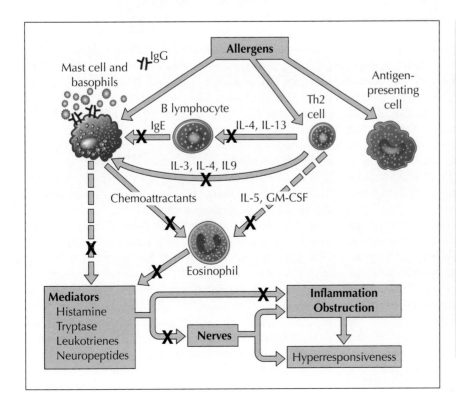

Figure 21-2.
Proposed mechanisms for effects of allergen immunotherapy (AIT) in allergic asthma. Several mechanisms have been proposed to explain the efficacy of AIT in allergic asthma. It may be related to a Th2 to Th1/Th0 shift that has been widely reported. This could account for the observed decrease in allergen-specific IgE, increase in allergen-specific IgG (a Th1-regulated pathway), and decrease in recruitment and activation of eosinophils (interleukin [IL]-5 and granulocyte-macrophage colony-stimulating factor [GM-CSF]–influenced) and mast cells/basophils (IL-4– and IL-9–regulated). The increased number of T regulatory cells are also likely due to the change in cytokine balance induced by AIT.

logic) that would place the patient at increased mortality risk. When contraindications to AIT are listed, immune-based diseases—particularly those with a Th1 compo-nent—are considered contraindications to AIT. While there are little direct data to support this notion, it seems reasonable to assume a conservative approach for those AA patients who are reasonably well-controlled on pharmacotherapy and/or whose asthma is less severe.

In AA patients who have clearly defined allergen triggers that exacerbate their asthma, particularly if they have concomitant AR, AIT is likely to be useful for them. If there are problems with the number of controller med-ications needed, poor clinical control of their asthma, or compliance issues with pharmacotherapy, AIT should be discussed with the patient and family, and a trial of at least 1 year considered. The number of allergens to which a patient should be desensitized varies depending upon the European versus North American perspective [26••,60]. There are data that AIT monotherapy can inhibit new sen-sitizations [37], but whether AIT is safer or more effective in monosensitized versus polysensitized patents remains unclear. The North American experience leans more towards polyallergen therapy, while the European recom-mendations focus more on monotherapy.

FUTURE NEEDS

Disparate opinions on the efficacy of AIT come from world leaders in allergy and asthma research and man-agement. Thus, there are currently few clear answers to the questions of which specific patients should be treated, how many of which specific allergens should be used, and how long AIT should be done. Cooperative studies looking at these parameters should be performed. Standardized allergens and AIT protocols must be developed and followed.

As useful as AIT may be, the responses take time to develop and are often incomplete; pharmacotherapy and other control measures are still required. Given the other anxieties and limitations for AIT described here, predicting who will be most likely to respond to AIT is a high priori-ty for future research. This will be particularly challenging until a standardized AIT protocol with standardized aller-

gens is widely adopted. With the increasing understanding of the genetic basis of allergic and asthmatic susceptibility, genomic studies that accompany efficacy protocols offer promise for practicing allergist-immunologists to someday be able to prospectively identify AA patients who will be high, mid-, or nonresponders.

New agents being developed offer interesting possi-bilities to increase the safety and efficacy of AIT in AA patients. Anti-IgE should decrease the potential for systemic reactions to AIT and may even allow significant increases in allergen doses. Total dose appears to be relat-ed to the efficacy of AIT [11–13,25]. Further, with the development of Th1-stimulating adjuvants such as the oligonucleotide CpG [62], a mixture with allergy vaccines may improve efficacy in terms of both speed and degree of response.

Finally, definitive studies that could show which popu-lation of AR patients at risk for AA will best respond to AIT are still lacking. The data to date are encouraging but do not, for the most part, compare and contrast those patients who do not develop asthma versus those who do. Genetic, immunologic, and clinical profiles before and after treatment must be correlated with environmental factors. In our incredibly mobile and changing societies, this may present the greatest challenge of all. Long-term follow-up studies to determine whether AIT actually prevents or merely delays the onset of are needed as well. Given the worldwide interest in asthma, the future for AIT in AA appears bright provided continued refinement and definition are vigorously pursued.

REFERENCES AND RECOMMENDED READING

Papers of particular interest, published recently, have been highlighted as:
• 　　*Of importance*
•• 　*Of major importance*

1.•• Sears ME: Consequences of long-term inflammation. The natural history of asthma. *Clin Chest Med* 2000, 21:315–329.
A very succinct description of the natural history of asthma.

2. Maddox L, Schwartz DA: The pathophysiology of asthma. *Annu Rev Med* 2002, 53:477–498.

3.• Leynaery B, Neukirch F, Demoly P, Bosquet J: Epidemiologic evidence for asthma and rhinitis comorbidity. *J Allergy Clin Immunol* 2000, 106(5 Suppl):S201–S205.
A comprehensive review of physiologic links between allergic rhinitis and asthma.

4. Braman SS, Barrows AA, DeCotiis BA, *et al.*: Airway hyper-responsiveness in allergic rhinitis. *Chest* 1987, 91:671–674.

5.• Togias AG: Systemic immunologic and inflammatory aspects of allergic rhinitis. *J Allergy Clin Immunol* 2000, 106(5 Suppl):S247–S250.
A description of the rationale for systemic immune derangements in allergic diseases.

6.•• Kay AB: Allergy and allergic diseases. First of two parts. *N Engl J Med* 2001, 344:30–37.
Excellent primer for allergy.

Table 21-1. PROPOSED MECHANISMS FOR EFFICACY OF ALLERGEN IMMUNOTHERAPY

Decrease allergen-specific IgE
Increase allergen-specific IgG (blocking)
Decrease number/activity of inflammatory cells
Increase regulatory T cells
Shift cytokine balance from Th2 to Th0/Th1

7. Barnes PJ: Cytokine modulators for allergic diseases. *Curr Opin Allergy Clin Immunol* 2001, 1:555–560.

8. Spector SL: Allergic inflammation in upper and lower airways. *Ann Allergy Asthma Immunol* 1999, 83:435–444

9. Nicklas RA: National and international guidelines for the diagnosis and treatment of asthma. *Curr Opin Pulm Med* 1997, 3:51–55.

10. Szefler SJ: The changing faces of asthma. *J Allergy Clin Immunol* 2000, 106(3 Suppl):S139–S143.

11. Esch RE, Portnoy J: Allergen immunotherapy. *Curr Allergy Asthma Rep* 2001, 1:491–497.

12. Varga EM, Durham SR: Allergen injection immunotherapy. *Clin Allergy Immunol* 2002, 16:533–549.

13. Theodoropoulos DS, Lockey RF: Allergen immunotherapy: guidelines, update, and recommendations of the World Health Organization. *Allergy Asthma Proc* 2002, 21:159–166.

14. Muller ER: New developments in the diagnosis and treatment of hymenoptera venom allergy. *Int Arch Allergy Immunol* 2001, 124:447–453.

15. Murray CS, Woodcock A, Custovic A: The role of indoor allergen exposure in the development of sensitization and asthma. *Curr Opin Allergy Clin Immunol* 2001, 1:407–412.

16. Nelson HS: Future advances of immunotherapy. *Allergy Asthma Proc* 2001, 22:203–207.

17. Renauld JC: New insights into the role of cytokines in asthma. *J Clin Pathol* 2001, 54:577–589.

18. Weber RW: Immunotherapy with allergens. *JAMA* 1997, 278:1881–1887.

19. Kowalski ML, Jutel M: Mechanisms of specific immunotherapy of allergic diseases. *Allergy* 1998, 53:485–492

20. Yang X: Does allergen immunotherapy alter the natural course of allergic disorders? *Drugs* 2001, 61:365–374.

21. Abramson MJ, Puy RM, Weiner JM: Is allergen immunotherapy effective in asthma? A meta-analysis of randomized controlled trials. *Am J Respir Crit Care Med* 1995, 151:969–974.

22. Abramson MJ, Puy RM, Weiner JM: Immunotherapy in asthma: an updated systematic review. *Allergy* 1999, 54:1022–1041.

23. Ross RN, Nelson HS, Finegold I: Effectiveness of specific immunotherapy in the treatment of asthma: a meta-analysis of prospective, randomized, double-blind, placebo-controlled studies. *Clin Ther* 2000, 22:329–341.

24. Varney VA, Edwards J, Tabbah K, *et al*.: Clinical efficacy of specific immunotherapy to cat dander: a double-blind placebo-controlled trial. *Clin Exp Allergy* 1997, 27:860–867.

25. Portnoy J: Immunotherapy for inhalant allergies. Guidelines for why, when, and how to use this treatment. *Postgrad Med* 2001, 109:89–90, 93–4, 99–100.

26.•• Bousquet J, Van Cauwenberge P, Khaltaev N, *et al*.: Allergic rhinitis and its impact on asthma. *J Allergy Clin Immunol* 2001, 108:S147–S334.
A major summary of evidence linking allergic rhinitis and asthma.

27. Guerra S, Sherrill DL, Martinez FD, Barbee RA: Rhinitis as an independent risk factor for adult-onset asthma. *J Allergy Clin Immunol* 2002, 109:419–425.

28. Polosa R, Ciamarra I, Mangano G, *et al*.: Bronchial hyper-responsiveness and airway inflammation markers in non-asthmatics with allergic rhinitis. *Eur Respir J* 2000, 15:30–35.

29. Johnstone DE, Dutton A: The value of hyposensitization therapy for bronchial asthma in children—a 14-year study. *Pediatrics* 1968, 42:793–802

30. Kusunoki T, Hosoi S, Asai K, *et al*.: Relationships between atopy and lung function: results from a sample of one hundred medical students in Japan. *Ann Allergy Asthma Immunol* 1999, 83:343–347.

31. Lombardi C, Gargioni S, Venturi S, *et al*.: Controlled study of preseasonal immunotherapy with grass pollen extract in tablets: effect on bronchial hyperreactivity. *J Investig Allergol Clin Immunol* 2001, 11(1):41–45.

32. Grembiale RD, Camporota L, Naty S, *et al*.: Effects of specific immunotherapy in allergic rhinitic individuals with bronchial hyperresponsiveness. *Am J Respir Crit Care Med* 2000, 162:2048–2052.

33.• Pichler CE, Helbling A, Pichler WJ: Three years of specific immunotherapy with house-dust-mite extracts in patients with rhinitis and asthma: significant improvement of allergen-specific parameters and of nonspecific bronchial hyperreactivity. *Allergy* 2001, 56:301–306.
Clinical evidence supporting the efficacy of allergen immunotherapy in asthma.

34. Moller C, Dreborg S, Ferdousi HA, *et al*.: Pollen immunotherapy reduces the development of asthma in children with seasonal rhinoconjunctivitis (the PAT- study). *J Allergy Clin Immunol* 2002, 109:251–256.

35.• Nelson HS: The importance of allergens in the development of asthma and the persistence of symptoms. *J Allergy Clin Immunol* 2002, 105:S628–S632.
The rationale linking allergic and asthmatic mechanisms.

36. Des Roches A, Paradis L, Menardo JL, *et al*.: Immunotherapy with a standardized *Dermatophagoides pteronyssinus* extract. VI. Specific immunotherapy prevents the onset of new sensitiza-tions in children. *J Allergy Clin Immunol* 1997, 99:450–453.

37. Pajno GB, Barberio G, De Luca F, *et al*.: Prevention of new sensitizations in asthmatic children monosensitized to house dust mite by specific immunotherapy. A six-year follow-up study. *Clin Exp Allergy* 2001, 31:1392–1397.

38. Babu KS, Holgate ST: Newer therapies for asthma: a focus on anti-IgE. *Indian J Chest Dis Allied Sci* 2002, 44:107–115.

39. Neurath MF, Finotto S, Glimcher LH: The role of Th1/Th2 polarization in mucosal immunity. *Nat Med* 2002, 8:567–573.

40. Barnes PJ: Th2 cytokines and asthma: an introduction. *Respir Res* 2001, 2:64–65.

41. Romagnani S: T-cell subsets (Th1 versus Th2). *Ann Allergy Asthma Immunol* 2000, 85:9–18.

42. Hamelmann E, Gelfand EW: IL-5–induced airway eosinophilia—the key to asthma? *Immunol Rev* 2001, 179:182–191.

43. Peng ZK, Naclerio RM, Norman PS, Adkinson NF Jr: Quantitative IgE- and IgG-subclass responses during and after long-term rag-weed immunotherapy. *J Allergy Clin Immunol* 1992, 89:519–529.

44. Adkinson NF: Immunotherapy for allergic rhinitis. *N Engl J Med* 1999, 341:522–524.

45. Ohashi Y, Tanaka A, Kakinoki Y, *et al*.: Effect of immunotherapy on seasonal changes in serum-specific IgE and IgG4 in patients with pollen allergic rhinitis. *Laryngoscope* 1997, 107:1270–1275.

46. Moverare R, Vesterinen E, Metso T, *et al*.: Pollen-specific rush immunotherapy: clinical efficacy and effects on antibody concen-trations. *Ann Allergy Asthma Immunol* 2001, 86:337–342.

47. Michils A, Baldassarre S, Ledent C, *et al*.: Early effect of ultrarush venom immunotherapy on the IgG antibody response. *Allergy* 2002, 55:455–462.

48. Durham SR, Hamid QA: The effect of immunotherapy on allergen induced late responses. *Arb Paul Ehrlich Inst Bundesamt Sera Impfstoffe Frankf A M* 1997, 91:33–39.

49. Romagnani S: T-cell responses in allergy and asthma. *Curr Opin Allergy Clin Immunol* 2001, 1:73–78.

50. Bellinghausen I, Knop J, Saloga J: The role of interleukin 10 in the regulation of allergic immune responses. *Int Arch Allergy Immunol* 2001, 126:97–101.

51. Ebner C: Immunological changes during specific immunotherapy of grass pollen allergy. *Clin Exp Allergy* 1997, 27:1007–1015.

52. Mosbech H, Malling HJ, Biering I, *et al.*: Immunotherapy with yellow jacket venom. A comparative study including three different extracts, one adsorbed to aluminium hydroxide and two unmodified. *Allergy* 1986, 41:95–103.

53. Wilson DR, Irani AM, Walker SM, *et al.*: Grass pollen immunotherapy inhibits seasonal increases in basophils and eosinophils in the nasal epithelium. *Clin Exp Allergy* 2001, 31(11):1705–1713.

54. Nagata M, Shibasaki M, Sakamoto Y, *et al.*: Specific immunotherapy reduces the antigen-dependent production of eosinophil chemotactic activity from mononuclear cells in patients with atopic asthma. *J Allergy Clin Immunol* 1994, 94:160–166.

55. Jacobsen J: Preventive aspects of immunotherapy: prevention for children at risk of developing asthma. *Ann Allergy Asthma Immunol* 2001, 87(1 Suppl 1):43–46.

56. Majori M, Caminati A, Corradi M, *et al.*: T-cell cytokine pattern at three time points during specific immunotherapy for mite-sensitive asthma. *Clin Exp Allergy* 2000, 30:341–347.

57. Mungan D, Misirligil Z, Gurbuz L: Comparison of the efficacy of subcutaneous and sublingual immunotherapy in mite-sensitive patients with rhinitis and asthma—a placebo controlled study. *Ann Allergy Asthma Immunol* 1999, 82:485–490.

58. Bahceciler NN, Isik U, Barlan IB, Basaran MM: Efficacy of sublingual immunotherapy in children with asthma and rhinitis: a double-blind, placebo-controlled study. *Pediatr Pulmonol* 2001, 32:49–55.

59. Tabar AI, Lizaso MT, Garcia BE, *et al.*: Tolerance of immunotherapy with a standardized extract of *Alternaria tenuis* in patients with rhinitis and bronchial asthma. *J Investig Allergol Clin Immunol* 2000, 10:327–333.

60. National Heart, Lung and Blood Institute. WHO/NHLBI Workshop Report: *Global Strategy for Asthma Management and Prevention*. Bethesda, MD: National Institutes of Health; Pub. No. 95-3659; 1995.

61. Lockey RF, Nicoara-Kasti GL, Theodoropoulos DS, Bukantz SC: Systemic reactions and fatalities associated with allergen immunotherapy. *Ann Allergy Asthma Immunol* 2001, 87(1 Suppl 1):47–55.

62. Kline JN, Kitagaki K, Businga TR, Jain VV: Treatment of established asthma in a murine model using CpG oligodeoxynucleotides. *Am J Physiol Lung Cell Mol Physiol* 2002, 283:L170–L179.

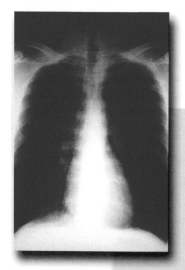

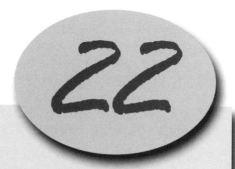

The Role of Anti-IgE in Asthma

Lary Ciesemier and Thomas B. Casale

Allergic disorders, including asthma, allergic rhinoconjunctivitis, and atopic dermatitis, represent a significant health and socioeconomic burden. The prevalence of allergic disorders appears to be increasing around the world. Furthermore, the morbidity from these disorders accounts for significant lost work and school days as well as impairment that leads to decreased productivity at work, home, and school. Atopy is an important factor in the development of asthma. Critical to atopy is the production of allergen-specific IgE [1].

IgE plays a central role in allergic reactions of the respiratory tract. In genetically predisposed individuals, IgE molecules specific for allergens are synthesized and released into the circulation by B cells and plasma cells. The IgE molecule then binds to specific cell-surface receptors located on mast cells, basophils, and other immune effector cells. On subsequent allergen exposure, allergen molecules bind to the Fab portion of the IgE molecule on the surface of mast cells and basophils, forming crosslinks and stimulating degranulation of these cells [2]. The degranulation results in the release of mediators and cytokines that ultimately results in the pathophysiologic consequences and symptoms of allergic diseases such as rhinitis and asthma (Fig. 22-1).

Epidemiologic studies have confirmed the importance of IgE in allergic respiratory disorders [3,4•]. The prevalence of asthma has been shown to be related to the level of serum IgE, and serum IgE levels are also related to persistent wheezing in children. Serum IgE levels have been shown to predict human airway reactivity in vitro. Thus, both epidemiologic and basic research studies have confirmed a clear relationship between IgE and the pathogenesis and development of symptoms associated with allergic respiratory diseases.

Because of the central role that IgE plays in allergic respiratory diseases, therapy to inhibit IgE-mediated responses through the use of anti-IgE antibodies is a logical step. This chapter focuses on the biology of IgE and strategies aimed to counteract its effects via humanized monoclonal antibodies directed against IgE.

IgE SYNTHESIS

The synthesis of IgE occurs after the uptake and processing of allergen and the subsequent presentation of allergen in the context of major histocompatability complex class II (MHC class II) molecules [2]. The switch to the synthesis of IgE by B cells requires two critical signals. The first signal is delivered by interleukin (IL)-4 or -13 when these cytokines bind to receptors on B cells (their receptors both use the same signal transduction pathway, STAT 6). The second signal is delivered when CD40 on B cells binds to its ligand on T cells, the CD40 ligand [2].

REGULATION OF IgE RECEPTOR LEVELS AND PHARMACOKINETICS OF IgE

IgE is capable of modulating the level of expression of its own high- and low-affinity receptors [5]. For example, higher IgE levels are associated with increased numbers of IgE receptors expressed on mast cells and basophils. Thus, IgE affects positive feedback mechanisms that enhance FcεRI receptor density and the excitability of mast cells. IgE-mediated upregulation of FcεRI substantially enhances the ability of mast cells or basophils sensitized with IgE to degranulate in response to allergen. Downregulation of IgE levels and IgE receptor levels on mast cells and basophils decrease the potential of these cells to degranulate [5]. In addition to its effect on FcεRI, IgE is capable of upregulating CD23 in the same manner.

IgE has a very short half-life (< 2 days) and is present in very low concentrations in the circulation—much lower than IgG, IgM, and IgA [6•]. IgE is extremely biologically active despite low concentrations in the circulation. This is because IgE antibodies bind to the high-affinity receptors on mast cells and basophils, so these cells may be primed to respond to allergens even when circulating IgE concentrations are very low.

STRATEGIES TO INHIBIT IgE

Decreasing total serum IgE in atopic patients should decrease the available amounts of antigen-specific IgE to bind to and sensitize tissue mast cells and basophils. This reduction of available IgE should lead to a decrease in IgE-mediated symptoms and improve control of allergic diseases. Indeed, in allergic rhinitis studies, the reduction in serum-free IgE levels caused by an anti-IgE monoclonal antibody was correlated with improvement in symptom scores and rescue medication use [7].

DEVELOPMENT AND CHARACTERISTICS OF OMALIZUMAB

Omalizumab is a recombinant humanized monoclonal anti-IgE antibody that binds to IgE on the same Fc site as FcεRI and contains 5% murine sequences (needed for the IgE-binding portion) and 95% human residues (Fig. 22-2). The antibody was humanized by grafting the mouse amino acid residues responsible for antigen binding onto a human IgG1 framework. Removing murine residues that could trigger an immune response results in the nonanaphylactogenic properties of omalizumab when used in humans [9]. Omalizumab is not able to crosslink IgE molecules that are already bound to the cell surface.

The primary mechanism of action of omalizumab is the binding of free IgE in the circulation [10]. When omalizumab binds to free IgE in the systemic circulation and tissues, it forms small complexes, usually trimers of two omalizumab molecules and one IgE [10]. Some of the characteristics of omalizumab are as follows [11,12]: 1) IgGκ human framework with murine antibody complementary determining regions; 2) humanized monoclonal antibody (mAb) against IgE that binds circulating IgE regardless of specificity; 3) does not activate complement; 4) does not bind cell-bound IgE; and 5) forms small biologically inert omalizumab–IgE complexes.

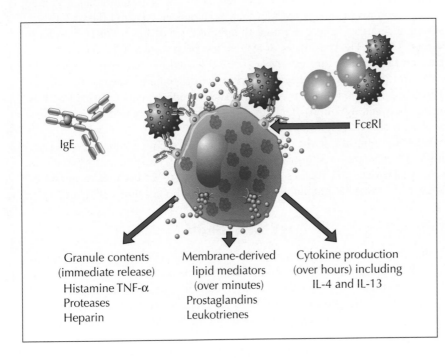

Figure 22-1.
Mast cell and basophil derived mediators. IL—interleukin; TNF—tumor necrosis factor.

IgE

FcεRI

Granule contents (immediate release)
Histamine TNF-α
Proteases
Heparin

Membrane-derived lipid mediators (over minutes)
Prostaglandins
Leukotrienes

Cytokine production (over hours) including IL-4 and IL-13

Omalizumab is thought to have a secondary mechanism of action through the reduction of FcεRI and CD23. Omalizumab resulted in a dramatic reduction in the number of FcεR1 receptors on basophils from about 220,000 receptors per cell to about 8300 receptors per cell [5]. The functional consequence of the FCεR1 downregulation was a 90% decrease in histamine release from basophils in response to ex vivo challenge with dust mites [5]. Only about 2000 IgE molecules are required to elicit a response from a B cell, so reductions in the levels of IgE may still leave enough free IgE to bind to FcεRI and activate effector cells [5]. Nonetheless, the therapeutic efficacy of omalizumab is related to the degree of free IgE reduction in the blood.

To test the therapeutic potential of omalizumab for the therapy of patients with asthma, several proofs of concept studies were done. Omalizumab was found to inhibit both the early and late asthmatic response due to allergen as well as the subsequent development of airway hyperresponsiveness and sputum eosinophilia [13]. Omalizumab was also shown to inhibit allergen-induced skin test responses [14]. Individualized dosing via intravenous bolus administration was used for the pivotal proof of concept phase II study in allergic asthma [15••]. A dosing table based on patient baseline IgE level and body weight has now been developed to assist in the administration of subcutaneous omalizumab.

PHASE III PIVOTAL STUDIES

Clinical protocols designed to study the efficacy of omalizumab in patients with asthma have shown its capacity to be an effective and safe therapy for this disorder. Three large, multicenter, phase III, pivotal trials were designed to assess the efficacy and safety of omalizumab versus placebo in the treatment of patients with moderate to severe allergic asthma. The demographics of study subjects are shown in Table 22-1.

In these three clinical trials, the efficacy and safety of omalizumab versus placebo were examined in symptomatic adults and adolescents (studies 008 and 009) treated with inhaled corticosteroids and asymptomatic children (study 010) treated with inhaled corticosteroids [16,17••,18]. The study design was fundamentally the same for the three studies (Fig. 22-3). The study designs involved a 4- to 6-week run-in phase during which the dose of inhaled beclomethasone was optimized. Subsequently, patients were treated with omalizumab or placebo plus the stable dose of beclomethasone for 16 weeks. Omalizumab dosing was tailored to baseline body weight and serum-free IgE levels. Patients received an approximate dosage of omalizumab of 0.016 mg/kg body weight/IgE (IU/mL) every 4 weeks subcutaneously. The dosing interval was every 2 to 4 weeks. This was followed by a 12-week steroid withdrawal phase in conjunction with continued omalizumab treatment. During this period, an attempt was made to reduce the dose of inhaled beclomethasone by 25% every 2 weeks. Finally, a double-blind (open label in pediatric study) extension phase of 20 weeks was included. The primary outcome measure was the number of asthma exacerbations per patient. Secondary efficacy variables measured throughout the study included daily and nocturnal asthma symptoms, inhaled corticosteroid reduction, quality of life, rescue medication use, and lung functions.

In all three studies, omalizumab was found to decrease the number of asthma exacerbations per patient during the steroid stable dosing period. The reduction in exacerbation rate was significant in the two adult and adolescent studies but did not quite meet statistical significance in the pediatric study. This is likely because the children were asymptomatic and had milder disease at enrollment. During the steroid withdrawal phase, omalizumab resulted in significant reductions over placebo (approximately 50%) in the number of exacerbations per patient in all

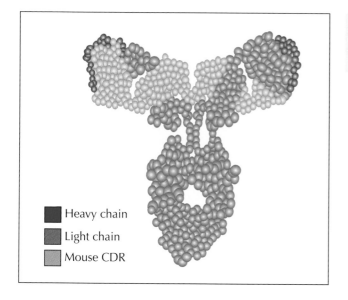

Heavy chain
Light chain
Mouse CDR

Figure 22-2.
Structure of omalizumab. CDR—complementary determining regions. (*Adapted from* Boushey [8].)

three studies (Fig. 22-4). Omalizumab demonstrated greater inhaled corticosteroid dose-reducing capacity than did placebo in all three studies. Furthermore, a greater number of omalizumab patients withdrew completely from inhaled corticosteroids. Approximately twice as many patients were able to withdraw from inhaled corticosteroids in the omalizumab group versus the placebo group.

Omalizumab also demonstrated improvement in typical asthma parameters, both during the steroid stable and steroid reduction phases (Fig. 22-5). Patients treated with omalizumab in all three studies demonstrated improvements in nocturnal symptom scores, daytime symptom scores, and the number of β-agonist puffs per day versus subjects taking placebo. Furthermore, there was a small but statistically significant improvement in FEV_1 (forced expiratory volume in 1 second) percent predicted of approximately 3% to 5% over placebo.

Unscheduled outpatient visits, emergency room treatments, and hospitalizations, which account for a significant amount of the costs attributed to asthma, were significantly reduced in the omalizumab versus placebo groups.

Finally, the ability of omalizumab to improve quality of life was also compared with placebo by the standard questionnaire developed by Juniper *et al.* [19,20]. At the end of the corticosteroid reduction phase, statistically significant improvements versus placebo were observed in all domains in the studies involving adults and adolescents. In the active treatment groups, mean changes from baseline were approximately 1.0 versus 0.6 for the placebo group. Approximately 64% of patients achieved improvements of greater than or equal to 0.5 versus

placebo in the quality of life scores, a measure thought to be clinically significant. In the pediatric study, statistically significant improvements were observed in the activities, symptoms, and overall domains, but not the emotional domain. Approximately 50% more children achieved greater than or equal to 0.5 improvement in the overall quality of life domain versus placebo [18].

The ability of omalizumab to maintain control of asthma symptoms was examined during the extension phase. In the international adult and adolescent study (009), approximately 43% of patients who received omalizumab versus 20% of patients who received placebo were able to withdraw from inhaled corticosteroids during the core treatment phase. After approximately 1 year of treatment, the percentages of patients no longer taking inhaled corticosteroids in the omalizumab and placebo groups were 31% and 11%, respectively. Concomitant with this reduction in the use of corticosteroids was a maintenance in the decrease in the percentage of patients having an exacerbation. During the core treatment phase, 76% of patients treated with omalizumab versus 58% of patients treated with placebo had no asthma exacerbations. After 1 year of treatment, 57% of patients in the omalizumab and 36% of those in the placebo groups had no asthma exacerbations.

In regards to safety, there were no significant adverse events reported in the 767 patients between 6 and 75 years of age who were treated with omalizumab. The adverse event profile was fairly similar in the placebo-treated group. Most adverse events were regarded as mild or moderate in intensity. There were no reported anaphylactic reactions or serum sickness reactions and no drug-related serious adverse events.

Table 22-1. DEMOGRAPHICS OF STUDY SUBJECTS IN OMALIZUMAB VERSUS PLACEBO TRIALS

	Adults and Adolescents (Protocol 008)		Adults and Adolescents (Protocol 009)		Children (Protocol 010)	
	Omalizumab	Placebo	Omalizumab	Placebo	Omalizumab	Placebo
Patients, *n*	268	257	274	272	225	109
Mean age, y *(range)*	39 (12–73)	39 (12–74)	40 (12–76)	39 (12–72)	9 (5–12)	10 (6–12)
Duration of asthma, y *(range)*	21 (1–61)	23 (2–60)	20 (2–68)	19 (1–63)	6 (1–12)	6 (1–12)
Mean serum total IgE, *IU/mL*	172	186	223	206	348	323
Mean FEV_1, *% predicted (range)*	68 (30–112)	68 (32–111)	70 (30–112)	70 (22–109)	84 (49–129)	85 (43–116)
Mean BDP dose, *μg/d (range)*	679 (500–1200)	676 (400–1000)	769 (500–1600)	772 (200–2000)	338 (200–800)	318 (200–600)
Severe asthma, %	22	21	22	22	9	6

Data from *Busse* et al. *[16]; Soler* et al. *[17••]; and Milgrom* et al. *[15].*

Therefore, these three pivotal studies showed that in adults, adolescents, and children with moderate to severe allergic asthma, omalizumab prevented asthma exacerbations while allowing reduction or withdrawal of inhaled corticosteroids to a greater degree than placebo. Concomitant with this reduction in inhaled corticosteroids, patients treated with omalizumab had greater improvements in symptoms, quality of life, and rescue use of β-agonists. Omalizumab appeared to be safe and well tolerated.

OMALIZUMAB AND SEVERE ASTHMA

In study 011, the effects of omalizumab compared with placebo on asthma-related quality of life was investigated in a multicenter, multinational, randomized, double-blind, parallel-group trial involving patients with severe allergic asthma [21]. Subjects began the study with a 6- to 10-week run-in, during which their inhaled corticosteroid dose was switched to fluticasone and optimized. A total of 246 patients with severe allergic asthma requiring regular daily treatment with high-dose inhaled fluticasone (1000 to 2000 µg/d) were randomly assigned to treatment with either omalizumab or placebo, administered subcutaneously every 2 or 4 weeks (at least 0.016 mg/kg body weight/IgE [IU/mL] every 4 weeks) for 16 weeks along with inhaled fluticasone. The inhaled corticosteroid dose was kept constant throughout this corticosteroid-stable phase. Patients then entered a 16-week corticosteroid reduction phase in which attempts were made to gradually reduce the inhaled corticosteroid therapy to the lowest dose required to maintain asthma control. An asthma-related quality of life questionnaire was used to assess patients at baseline and at the completion of the different phases of the study using the asthma-related quality of life questionnaire developed by Juniper *et al.* [18, 19]. The questionnaire looked at four domains: activity limitations, emotions, symptoms, and exposure to environmental stimuli.

Baseline clinical characteristics were as follows: the mean age of the patients was approximately 41 years, the mean FEV_1 values percent predicted were 63% to 66%, the mean fluticasone dose was 1375 µg/d, and the mean duration of asthma was approximately 22.5 years.

At the end of the corticosteroid reduction phase, there was a significant difference in favor of omalizumab for

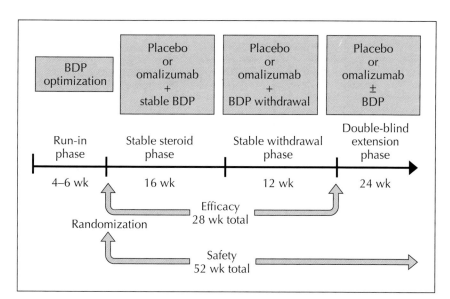

Figure 22-3.
Study design of phase III pivotal omalizumab trials in asthma. BDP—beclomethasone dipropionate.

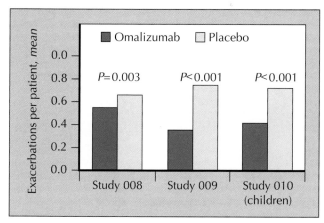

Figure 22-4.
Effects of omalizumab on asthma exacerbations during the steroid withdrawal phase.

the proportion of patients who experienced a clinically meaningful improvement in their asthma-related quality of life. In terms of overall score, 57.5% of patients achieved an increase in score of more than 0.5 U relative to baseline compared with 38.6% of placebo recipients (P < 0.05). The treatment effect was most pronounced for those who experienced a large improvement in quality of life. In terms of overall score, for example, the proportion of patients who achieved an increase in score of more than 1.5 U relative to baseline was nearly threefold higher compared with the effects of placebo (16% and 5.9%, respectively).

The significant improvements in asthma-related quality of life during omalizumab therapy were also accompanied by a meaningful reduction in inhaled corticosteroid use compared with placebo: 1) usage of inhaled fluticasone at end of corticosteroid reduction phase was lower in the omalizumab group compared with placebo (P = 0.01); 2) patients with 50% reduction or more, compared with baseline, in usage of inhaled fluticasone at end of corticosteroid-reduction phase: omalizumab, 74%; placebo, 51%; 3) patients with no usage of inhaled corticosteroid at end

of the corticosteroid-reduction phase: omalizumab, 21%; placebo, 15%; and 4) more patients in the omalizumab group had their fluticasone dose reduced to less than 500 µg/d: omalizumab, 60.3%; placebo, 45.8% (P = 0.026).

The significant improvements in quality of life during omalizumab therapy paralleled the clinically relevant changes in other efficacy measures, such as the use of rescue inhaled β_2-agonist medication and daily asthma symptom scores.

Thus, treatment with omalizumab is associated with a clinically relevant improvement in asthma-related quality of life for patients with severe allergic asthma. Improvement was apparent across all domains of the quality of life questionnaire. The beneficial effect of omalizumab on quality of life increased progressively from completion of the corticosteroid stable phase to the end of the corticosteroid reduction period, despite the clinically relevant reduction in inhaled corticosteroids. Finally, the improvement in asthma-related quality of life during omalizumab therapy was consistent with the significant changes in clinical endpoints, which indicates that such changes are likely to be clinically meaningful from the patient's perspective.

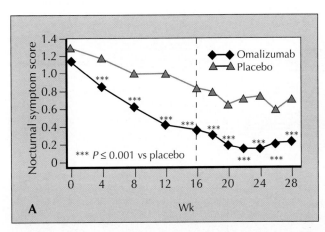

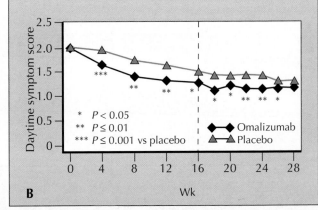

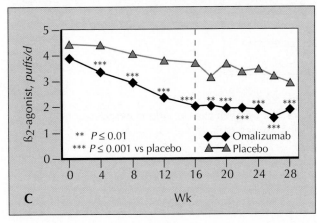

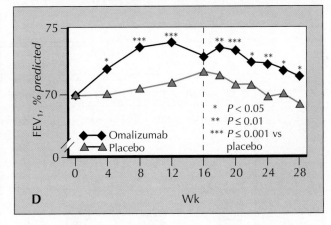

Figure 22-5.
Effects of omalizumab on asthma parameters (**A**, nocturnal symptom score; **B**, daytime symptom score; **C**, use of β_2-agonist; **D**, percent predicted FEV$_1$ [forced expiratory volume in 1 second]) during the steroid stable (*left of dashed line*) and steroid withdrawal (*right of dashed line*) phases of clinical trial 009. (*Adapted from* Soler *et al.* [17••].)

CONCLUSIONS

Omalizumab is a novel agent that should prove useful in the therapy of patients with allergic respiratory disorders. It reduces serum IgE and FcεRI receptors as its mechanism of action. Its been shown to improve asthma in adults, adolescents, and children, allowing reduction in steroid doses. In addition, it also improves symptoms, urgent care visit rates, rescue medication use, and quality of life. In these studies, omalizumab appeared to be safe and well tolerated. It appears that omalizumab will be useful for the therapy of adults and children with moderate to severe allergic asthma who have persistent symptoms despite therapy, intolerable side effects from therapy, or poor compliance. Furthermore, patients with asthma who have concomitant IgE-mediated disorders such as allergic rhinitis and atopic dermatitis are also likely to benefit from this drug.

ACKNOWLEDGMENT

The authors gratefully acknowledge the skilled help of Ms. Barbara Dineen in the preparation of the manuscript.

REFERENCES AND RECOMMENDED READING

Papers of particular interest, published recently, have been highlighted as:
- Of importance
- • Of major importance

1. National Heart, Lung, and Blood Institute, National Asthma Education and Prevention Program: *Expert Panel Report 2: Guidelines for the Diagnosis and Management of Asthma.* Bethesda, MD: National Institutes of Health, Pub. No. 97-4051; 1997.

2. Bacharier LB, Geha RS: Molecular mechanisms of IgE regulation. *J Allergy Clin Immunol* 2000, 105(suppl):547–558.

3. Burrows B, Martinez FD, Halonen M, *et al.*: Association of asthma with serum IgE levels and skin-test reactivity to allergens. *N Engl J Med* 1989, 320:271–277.

4.• Oettgen HC, Geha RS: IgE regulation and roles in asthma pathogenesis *J Allergy Clin Immunol* 2001, 107:429–441.
A review focusing on the mechanisms whereby IgE participates both in immediate hypersensitivity responses in the airways and in the induction of chronic allergic bronchial inflammation.

5. MacGlashen DWJ, Bochner BS, Adelman DC, *et al.*: Down regulation of FcεRI expression on human basophils during in vivo treatment of atopic patients with anti-IgE antibody. *J Immunol* 1997, 158:1438–1445.

6.• Oettgen HC, Geha RS: IgE in asthma and atopy: cellular and molecular connections. *J Clin Invest* 1999, 104:829–835.
A brief overview of the roles of IgE in allergic pathophysiology, and the molecular and cellular factors that ultimately regulate IgE production and Th2 expansion.

7. Casale TB, Condemi J, LaForce F, *et al.*: Effect of omalizumab on symptoms of seasonal allergic rhinitis. *JAMA* 2001, 286:2956–2967.

8. Boushey HA Jr: Experiences with monoclonal antibody therapy for allergic asthma. *J Allergy Clin Immunol* 2001, 108(2 suppl):S77–S83.

9. Breedveld FC: Therapeutic monoclonal antibodies. *Lancet* 2000, 355:735–740.

10. Fox JA, Hotaling TE, Struble C: Tissue distribution and complex formation with IgE on anti-IgE Ab after IV administration in cynomolgus monkeys. *J Pharmacol Exp Ther* 1996, 279:1000–1008.

11. Shields RL, Whether WR, Zioncheck K, *et al.*: Inhibition of allergic reactions with antibodies to IgE. *Int Arch Allergy Immunol* 1995, 107:308–312.

12. Presta LG, Lahr SJ, Shields RL, *et al.*: Humanization of an antibody directed against IgE. *J Immunol* 1993, 151:2623–2632.

13. Fahy JV, Fleming HE, Wong HH, *et al.*: The effect of an anti-IgE monoclonal antibody on the early-and late-phase responses to allergen inhalation in asthmatic subjects. *Am J Respir Crit Care Med* 1997, 155:1828–1834.

14. Togias A, Corren J, Shapiro G, *et al.*: Anti-IgE treatment reduces skin test (ST) reactivity. *J Allergy Clin Immunol* 1998, *101*(suppl):171.

15.•• Milgrom H, Fick RB, Su JQ, *et al.*: Treatment of allergic asthma with monoclonal anti-IgE antibody. *N Engl J Med* 1999, 341:1966–1973.
A study demonstrating that omalizumab has potential as a treatment for subjects with moderate or severe allergic asthma.

16. Busse W, Corren J, Lanier BQ, *et al.*: Omalizumab, anti-IgE recombinant humanized monoclonal antibody, for the treatment of severe allergic asthma. *J Allergy Clin Immunol* 2001, 108:184–190.

17.•• Soler M, Matz J, Townley R, *et al.*: The anti-IgE antibody omalizumab reduces asthma exacerbations and steroid requirement in allergic asthmatics. *Eur Respir J* 2001, 18:254–261.
A study assessing the clinical benefit and steroid-sparing effect of treatment with omalizumab in patients with moderate-to-severe allergic asthma.

18. Milgrom H, Berger W, Nayak A, *et al.*: Treatment of childhood asthma with anti-immunoglobulin E antibody (omalizumab). *Pediatrics* 2001, 108(suppl E):36.

19. Juniper EF, Guyatt GH, Ferrie PJ, *et al.*: Measuring quality of life in asthma. *Am Rev Respir Dis* 1993, 147:832–838.

20. Juniper EF, Guyatt GH, Feeny DH, *et al.*: Measuring quality of life in children with asthma. *Qual Life Res* 1996, 5:35–46.

21. Holgate S, Churchalin A, Herbert J, *et al.*: Omalizumab improves asthma-specific quality of life in patients with severe allergic asthma. *Am J Respir Crit Care Med* 2001, 163(suppl A):858.

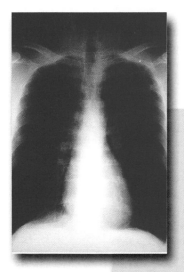

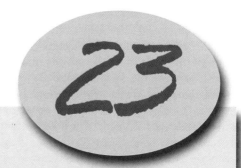

Clinical Pearls

Michael A. Kaliner

I have looked forward to writing this chapter for years. It is intended to share some of the clinical insights in asthma diagnosis and management I have gathered over 30 years of providing care for asthmatic patients. It is not intended to be a scholarly paper; no references will be cited, and no justification for the statements made will be attempted. This chapter is intended to help the clinician who sees asthmatic patients deal with some of the clinical conundrums encountered. Many of the statement reflect my personal opinions, some (perhaps many) of which may be controversial.

DIAGNOSING ASTHMA

When taking an initial history of a patient suspected of having asthma (Table 23-1), I always focus on the evidence of airflow obstruction. Nearly all patients experience wheezing, shortness of breath, and chest tightness. A frequent history is the inability to take a deep breath, as if the lungs are partially full. Some patients have no history of airflow obstruction, but cough instead. These patients belong in a subclass of patients with the "cough variant" of asthma. Others have exercise-induced asthma with symptoms only related to exercise. Most patients report a tight feeling felt below and around the sternum, associated with air hunger and wheezing. For most patients, a wheeze is felt and heard as a prolonged expiration with a whistling sound.

Most asthmatic patients wheeze or get short of breath with exercise; therefore, a detailed history of the patient's exercise program is essential. I always ask about exercise, stairs, or other activities to determine if the patient might have abnormal shortness of breath. Known asthmatic patients may use bronchodilators prior to exercise, and that is an important part of the history. I ask if the patient gets inappropriately short of breath with exercise or if they get out of breath before they should. For children, ask who is the fastest child in their class and how the child compares to this speedster. If they cannot play soccer through a full half, they may be short of breath and have asthma.

Nocturnal awakenings usually indicate that the patient's asthma is relatively severe. Many people wake up once or twice a night for a variety of reasons, and these causes must be distinguished from asthma. If the awakening is due to asthma, patients get up, move around or walk a little, often use their inhaler, and cannot return to sleep for some time. Most asthmatics wake up between 2 and 3 AM, when the plasma cortisol is at its nadir. Congestive heart failure usually occurs 3 to 4 hours after lying down, once the fluid redistributes from the legs to the chest. Thus, determining the time of onset of awakenings can help distinguish between these two causes.

Asthmatic patients whose disease is severe enough to require an emergency room visit or hospitalization are at increased risk for death. Thus, I always ask about these occurrences, as well as how many days of work (or school) the patient misses each year.

COUGH

Cough is frequently encountered in asthmatic patients and is often the presenting symptom. Acute coughing syndromes are usually infectious and often improve, as does the infection. The major causes of chronic cough are listed in Table 23-2.

I ask patients the following questions to determine the most likely cause of their cough. Do you have post-nasal drip? How often do you clear your throat? When you cough, is it in your throat or deep in your chest? (While asking these questions, I indicate my throat and pat myself on the chest to indicate exactly the regions I am asking about). How often do you cough? Every day? Every hour? Every few minutes? Is the cough a single cough or does it occur in spasms? Is the cough wet or dry? If wet, how much sputum do you produce? If I asked you to collect all of the sputum into a coffee cup, how much of the cup would you fill up in 24 hours? Half a cup, a quarter cup, a few teaspoonfuls? What color is the sputum (clear, yellow, or green)? Does the cough interfere with sleep? Do you cough when you lie down or strain at stool? How long have you coughed? Is it getting better, staying the same, or worsening? What helps with your cough?

The answers to these questions and the workup outlined herein nearly always direct the physician in the right direction for the diagnosis and treatment of the cause of cough. I almost never treat cough, focusing instead on the cause of cough.

PATTERNS OF DISEASE

Determining the pattern of disease can assist in uncovering the cause of asthma (Table 23-3). Thus, exposures provoking asthma may suggest an allergic or irritant cause. Cold and exercise are nonspecific causes of asthma, precipitating disease in nearly everyone. Workplace-related disease is often a problem, as there may be secondary gain involved. I usually ask patients to record peak flow readings every 30 to 60 minutes over a weekend, and then during a weekday, including exposure to whatever may be causing the symptoms. This approach can provide valuable insight into what may be causing their symptoms.

Aspirin and other NSAIDs cause asthma in about 3% of asthmatic patients. Such patients often recognize that they cannot take NSAIDs without provoking asthma. These patients usually have concomitant sinusitis, nasal polyposis, and eosinophilia. They should avoid all NSAIDs, but current data suggest COX-2 inhibitors are usually safe.

UNDERLYING CAUSES OF ASTHMA

To treat asthma properly, it is essential to diagnose the underlying causes for the disease (Table 23-4). Allergy is the most common cause and should be pursued in any patient who wheezes more than 2 days a week. A good

---

Table 23-1. DIAGNOSING ASTHMA

Initial history (determine days/week or month for each)
  Do you wheeze?
  Do you experience shortness of breath?
  Do you experience tightness in the chest?
    If so, show where.
  Do you exercise? Is there a need for pretreatment
    with bronchodilator?
  Do you cough (throat vs chest, sputum quality/
    quantity, frequency)?
  Do you use a bronchodilator? How frequently?
  Do you wake up at night?
  Peak flow meter use: average, best, worst reading?
  How many days have you missed from work
    or school each year?
  Have you gone to the emergency room or
    been hospitalized?

Table 23-2. MAJOR CAUSES OF CHRONIC COUGH

Postnasal drip syndromes
  Rhinitis
  Sinusitis
Chest syndromes
  Asthma
  Bronchitis
  Other chest diseases
    Sarcoid
    Tumors
    Others
Gastroesophageal reflux disease
Medication side effects
  ACE inhibitors
Neurogenic cough

historian should be able to ferret out the cause of asthma with a relatively brief history, followed by pulmonary function tests. Allergy skin tests, or radioallergosorbent tests (RAST), are indicated in most patients in order to determine if allergy plays a role.

The role of sinusitis and gastroesophageal reflux disease (GERD) in worsening asthma cannot be stressed enough. For many years, I felt that my real clinical contribution to asthma management was to treat sinusitis and GERD in asthmatic patients who had failed to benefit from standard asthma therapies in other physicians' offices. As many as 75% of severe asthmatic patients have concomitant sinusitis, and more than 60% have GERD. Because either disease worsens asthma, a patient may have to be treated for both before asthma will respond.

PHYSICAL FINDINGS

After the history is completed, a careful physical examination searching for clues to underlying conditions associated with asthma is appropriate. Examination of the eyes for allergic conjunctivitis or steroid-induced cataracts should be performed. Allergic conjunctivitis is indicated by mild swelling of the conjunctiva with some redness but no purulent drainage. Steroid-induced cataracts are seen on the posterior capsule of the lens and are punctate concretions of black pigment, quite distinct from the usual appearance of geriatric cataracts.

The nose in allergic patients is often swollen, with a distinct blue-white color to the mucosa. Secretions are watery and thin. By contrast, sinusitis may be recognized by the presence of green or gray secretions seen posteriorly, usually next to or below the middle turbinate. Allergic disease may also be suggested by the presence of allergic shiners, a long, thin face, and a high, arched palate.

The chest examination of an asthmatic patient may be totally normal, despite abnormal pulmonary function, or terribly abnormal, with less impressive changes in pulmonary function. Wheezing, or a high-pitched expiratory sound, is due to narrowing of small airways with air trapping. Thus, air moves through narrow airways because the lung and the airways widen during inspiration. Expiration is actually associated with narrowing of airways, and therefore, air is trapped in the peripheral lung. As pressure builds up, air can escape through these narrow airways at higher pressure and makes a high-pitched sound, like the sound of air squeezed through the narrow neck of an inflated balloon.

Mucus in larger airways makes a gravelly sound, rhonchi, usually heard in inspiration but also audible during expiration. Airflow obstruction causes a prolongation of expiration. Most breathing is completed in less than 3 seconds, while in asthma and chronic obstructive pulmonary disease (COPD) it may last more than 6 seconds. The chest may appear to be enlarged in the anteroposterior diameter in COPD, while it is normal in asthmatic patients. The breath sounds and cardiac sounds may be quiet or distant in COPD and should be normal in asthma. Be aware, however, that some patients with bronchitis have a pronounced wheeze. By contrast, emphysema is usually not associated with wheezing.

Asthmatic patients do not develop clubbed fingers. With the exception of α_1-antitrypsin deficiency, which may present with wheezing in 15% of patients, few asthmatic patients develop emphysema.

On radiographs, asthmatic patients may have an overinflated chest with a flattened diaphragm. However, infiltrates on chest radiographs are very unusual, except in patients with pulmonary infiltrates with eosinophilia (PIE) syndromes (including acute bronchopulmonary aspergillosis), bronchiectasis (perhaps due to ciliary

---

Table 23-3. PATTERNS OF ASTHMA

Seasonal, perennial

With colds, exercise

Allergen exposure (dust, mold, animals, seasonal with pollen)

Irritant exposure (smoke, odors, pollutants, weather conditions, temperature)

Occupational exposures (irritants, allergens)

Drugs (aspirin or NSAIDs, β-blockers, ACE inhibitors)

Foods and additives (sulfites)

Menses, pregnancy, thyroid disease

Emotional (stress, laughter, crying)

Table 23-4. UNDERLYING CAUSES OF ASTHMA

Allergies
  > 90%, ages 2–16 y
  > 70%, ages 16–30 y
  ≈ 50%, over 30 y
Infections
  Colds, bronchitis, sinusitis
Aspirin (NSAID) sensitivity
  Sinusitis, polyps, eosinophilia, worsened by NSAIDs
Occupational exposures
  Irritants, allergens
Drug and chemical reactions
  β-blockers, sulfites

dyskinesia, which presents as wheezy bronchitis), Löffler's pneumonia, or hypersensitivity pneumonitis.

OFFICE PULMONARY FUNCTIONS

Most asthma specialists have a spirometer in their offices to measure expiratory and inspiratory airflow volumes. In primary care offices where asthma is just one of many diseases encountered every day, a peak flow meter can be substituted for the more expensive spirometer. The most common abnormality observed in asthmatic patients is reduced FEV_1 (forced expiratory volume in 1 second), which is also reflected in a reduced peak flow rate. In addition to measuring FEV and FVC (forced vital capacity), the ratio of FEV_1 to FVC can be calculated. The $FEV_{1\%}$ should be 80% or greater. If the patient has a low FEV_1 or $FEV_{1\%}$, or if the history suggests asthma, a comparison to a post-bronchodilator measurement should be conducted. Traditionally, that study has involved breathing 500 µg of albuterol through a nebulizer. Using 4 to 6 puffs of albuterol by metered-dose inhaler (MDI) with a spacer is as effective, and allows the demonstration of proper use of an MDI at the same time.

Improvement of more than 12% after using a bronchodilator is diagnostic of asthma; however, an improvement of 10% is abnormal and strongly suggests asthma. In such a case, a 4- to 6-week course of inhaled corticosteroid (ICS) is indicated; if the patient improves clinically or by pulmonary function testing, a diagnosis of asthma can be made.

A baseline peak flow can be used to compare with a post-bronchodilator study, although the data may not be as precise as with a spirometer. Thus, the peak flow meter is a reasonable, inexpensive way to screen patients for asthma. The chest radiograph is of limited value in the diagnosis of asthma.

Body plethysmography is helpful to determine if there is a problem with air exchange and to measure residual volumes. In most asthma patients it is not necessary; it is used primarily in individuals where COPD may be combined or differentiated from asthma.

Differential Diagnosis

The history and physical examination need to be capable of differentiating asthma from other diseases (Table 23-5). One disease, which is very confusing to clinicians, is vocal cord dysfunction. This problem is usually found in young female patients often with very difficult to manage disease. Because the disease actually is caused by paradoxical closure of the vocal cords, which causes wheezing, tightness in the throat, and shortness of breath, the usual asthma medications do not work. These patients are often placed on increasing doses of medications, including oral steroids, without much benefit. One hint is that when asked where they feel tightness in the chest, these patients indicate that the tightness is in the throat rather than in

the chest. The diagnosis is confirmed by performing a flow-volume loop, which employs a spirometer recording both inspiration and expiration. Flattening of the loop in both phases of respiration confirms extrathoracic obstruction. Laryngoscopy allows the observer to directly visualize the vocal cords, which may close paradoxically during inspiration. In most cases, a methacholine challenge is negative, where for the overwhelming majority of asthmatic patients it is abnormal. Treatment involves working with an experienced speech pathologist to instruct the patient on vocal cord relaxation techniques. Psychologic treatment may also be necessary.

TREATMENT CONSIDERATIONS

Patients with mild intermittent asthma are treated with inhaled β-agonists on an as-needed basis. Essentially, everyone else is prescribed an ICS at the lowest effective dose. Some children may be treated with montelukast. Principles of asthma treatment are listed in Table 23-6.

Inhaled corticosteroids are the most effective long-term controlling agents available today. I recommend them for all patients with persistent asthma, using lower doses for milder patients and higher doses for more severe patients. If corticosteroids alone are used, the

---

Table 23-5. DIFFERENTIAL DIAGNOSIS OF ASTHMA

Pulmonary embolism
Vocal cord dysfunction
Cardiac failure ("cardiac asthma")
Foreign bodies*
Tumors in the central airways
Aspiration (gastroesophageal reflux)*
Carcinoid syndrome
Laryngo-tracheo-bronchomalacia*
Löffler's syndrome
Bronchiectasis
Tropical eosinophilia
Hyperventilation syndrome
Laryngeal edema
Laryngeal or tracheal obstruction*
Factitious wheezing
α_1-Antitrypsin deficiency
Immotile cilia syndrome, Kartagener's syndrome*
Bronchopulmonary dysplasia*
Bronchiolitis, croup*
Overlapping diseases: chronic bronchitis and emphysema, cystic fibrosis*

Diseases of particular importance in pediatrics.

following list of starting doses, administered twice daily, may prove helpful: for mild persistent asthma, 300 to 600 µg/d; for moderate persistent asthma, 400 to 1000 µg/d; and for severe persistent asthma, 800 to 2000 µg/d.

Inhaled corticosteroids may be toxic at some doses. Chronic exposure above 2000 µg/d is associated with long-term complications.

MDIs should be used with a spacer. Spacers reduce the need for hand-eye coordination and improve the fraction of the dose that gets to the lungs while lowering the amount deposited on the throat. Even after using a spacer, patients should rinse their throats and gargle to get rid of any deposited corticosteroids.

Use the starting dose of ICS for 1 to 3 months, and monitor peak flow rates until they plateau and then assess if the patient is doing well clinically. Use the peak flow as an objective measure of the response to medications. If the patient has not done well and the peak flows remain unimproved, either increase the dose of ICS or add a long-acting β-agonist or a leukotriene antagonist, *eg*, montelukast. Comparative studies have suggested that the combination of a long-acting β-agonist and corticosteroid are better than corticosteroid plus montelukast.

Peak Flow Meters

The peak flow meter is an inexpensive tool used to monitor pulmonary function outside of the office and can provide a "real life" measurement, which often proves invaluable. One way to determine how much medication to use for how long involves monitoring the patient's "personal best" peak flows. Thus, step-up therapy is continued until the patient is well and the personal best peak flow is achieved. After that point, step-down therapy, progressively reducing the strength of the asthma medications, is initiated. During step-down therapy, the patient's symptoms should remain under control, the peak flow should stay at the personal best level, and the need for β-agonist should not increase.

The step-down therapy is continued to the lowest dose where these three criteria can be matched.

Patients are instructed to use their peak flow meters in the morning before dosing with medication and in the evening before bed. If an emergency occurs, the peak flow helps determine the need for treatment.

Emergency Treatment Plans

Each patient should be given a written plan outlining what to do in an asthma emergency. The basic principles are listed in Table 23-7.

Most patients are able to interpret the changes in peak flow and double their ICS without needing support from the physician. With more severe disease, the physician will want to know what is happening and possibly intervene before the need for an emergency interaction. Using this approach, our office of four asthma specialists has not had to hospitalize a patient in years.

Short-acting β-Agonists

Short-acting β-agonists (SABAs) should be used in an emergency and may be used prior to exercise or exposure to a condition known to trigger asthma. β-Agonists should be used only on an "as needed" basis, rather than on a regular schedule. The need for β-agonist use is one of the best ways to gauge how well the patient is doing. Thus, our best-managed patients never use any β-agonist at all. If a patient requires a β-agonist despite adequate therapy, either inadequate control or unnecessary β-agonist use is indicated. If the peak flow rate or office spirometry indicates persistent airflow obstruction, then the selection of medications should be reviewed and changed. On the other hand, many patients use their β-agonist out of habit or for minor symptoms (chest heaviness, slight tightness). These patients should measure their peak flow rates and not resort to the β-agonist unless the peak flows have dropped by 10%.

Table 23-6. PRINCIPLES OF ASTHMA TREATMENT

Daily anti-inflammatory therapy
  (long-term control medications)
Symptomatic use of bronchodilators
  (quick relief medications)
Step therapy
  Aim initial treatment to totally control symptoms
  Step-down to maintain control with lower
    level of treatment
Regular follow-up visits
Written management plan
At-home monitoring with peak flow meters

Table 23-7. PRINCIPLES OF EMERGENCY TREATMENT PLANS

If peak flow falls >10%, double inhaled corticosteroids
If peak flow falls > 20%, use emergency bronchodilator plus corticosteroids; call physician
  (to determine what may have precipitated the
  exacerbation and if antibiotics are necessary)
If peak flow falls 40% to 50%, do everything above
  plus initiate oral corticosteroids; call physician
If peak flow falls > 50%, go to emergency room or
  doctor's office for treatment; call physician

When prescribing beta agonists, write the prescription for 1 to 2 puffs every 4 to 6 hours *as needed*, rather than for regular use. There are now two HFA (hydroflouro-alkane-134a)-propelled β-agonists available: Proventil HFA (Schering, Kenilworth, NJ) and Ventolin HFA (GlaxoSmithKline, Research Triangle Park, NC). Both have softer plumes upon activation than the older chlorofluorocarbon (CFC)-driven products, which make the products more efficient to inhale. Moreover, HFA is not associated with ozone depletion as are the older CFC-propelled MDIs.

Be aware of β-agonist use. A canister of albuterol contains 200 puffs. If the patient is using one canister a month, he is using 7 puffs per day. That much β-agonist use indicates that a patient's asthma is not well-controlled, and the physician should adjust the use of long-acting controller medications to reduce the need for the β-agonist. There have been suggestions that excessive β-agonist use is associated with increased risk of death. Certainly, excessive use indicates inadequate control and puts the patient at some increased risk.

Long-acting β-Agonists

Two long-acting β-agonists (LABAs) are available: salmeterol (Serevent; GlaxoSmithKline, Research Triangle Park, NC) and formoterol (Foradil; Novartis, East Hanover, NJ). Both have prolonged durations of action (12 hours or longer). Formoterol has a rapid onset of action, within a few minutes, while salmeterol requires a few hours to achieve maximal bronchodilation. Foradil is available as a dry powder and employs a cumbersome inhalation device. Salmeterol is available as a dry powder in an extremely convenient device, as an MDI, and is combined with fluticasone in Advair (GlaxoSmithKline, Research Triangle Park, NC).

Not every patient needs an LABA. Certainly, patients with mild intermittent or mild persistent asthma do not need this medication, except under special circumstances. An LABA might be prescribed for a patient with exercise-induced asthma who has mild disease to reduce the need to carry and use an SABA. On the other hand, it has been shown quite convincingly that adding an LABA to an inhaled corticosteroid leads to more effective control with lower doses of corticosteroid. Because controlling asthma with the lowest possible dose of corticosteroid is paramount, those patients requiring substantial doses of inhaled corticosteroid for control are candidates for combined LABA/corticosteroid treatment.

Nocturnal awakenings have always indicated substantial airway hyperreactivity and usually lead to more aggressive management. Lack of sleep has profound effects on function and should push the physician to more intense treatment. An LABA is one means of helping the patient sleep through the night.

Older patients may have cardiac side effects from LABAs, and it is wise to start patients over age 60 on 25

µg of salmeterol if possible (1 puff from the MDI). If no problems occur, increase to 50 µg (2 puffs from the MDI or 1 inhalation from the dry powder inhaler). While formoterol has a rapid onset of action and can be used for patients in acute distress, salmeterol is a prophylactic medication and should NOT be used for emergencies. I advise patients to leave these products at home and to only carry their SABA for emergency use.

Leukotriene Modifiers

Two leukotriene-receptor antagonists are available: montelukast (Singulair; Merck, West Point, PA) and zafirlukast (Accolate; AstraZeneca, Wilmington, DE). Both prevent leukotriene C4/D4 from interacting with its receptor. A leukotriene-synthesis inhibitor, zileuton (Zyflo; Abbott, Abbott Park, IL), is also available. The receptor antagonists are easier to use and are moderately effective, while the synthesis inhibitor is more effective but also more toxic and harder to use. Thus, the first choice among these products would be montelukast, primarily for its ease of use and safety. Because montelukast is a pill, and is not a corticosteroid, it is used extensively by pediatricians who are fearful of any potential systemic effect of inhaled corticosteroids. American patients prefer pills to sprays or inhalers, and tend to be interested in trying montelukast. Comparative studies, however, have shown inhaled corticosteroid and LABAs to be more potent than montelukast for many clinical endpoints. Another issue is the potential effect of these medications on airway inflammation and airway remodeling. Corticosteroids have been shown to reduce inflammation and airway reactivity, while the effects of montelukast are more modest.

Thus, many pediatricians use montelukast as their first-line treatment of patients with mild to moderate persistent asthma. The product is approved for children from 2 years of age, and will soon be available as a sprinkle for infants as young as 1 year of age. I prefer to add montelukast to an ICS, as a means to reduce the corticosteroid dose. However, if patients are afraid of inhaled ICSs, or prefer pills, and respond to montelukast, then it is a fine choice.

General experience has shown that about 50% of patients will respond to montelukast. A trial period of 1 to 2 months, with monitoring of symptoms, β-agonist use, and peak flows, should be employed to determine if this agent will be effective. Pulmonary function changes with montelukast are generally modest, but patients may feel better anyway.

Zileuton is a potent agent, useful in asthma, sinusitis, and polyposis. However, the initial dosage is three or four times a day, and hepatic enzymes need to be monitored periodically. I reserve zileuton for patients with moderate to severe asthma, particularly if they are NSAID-sensitive or if they have nasal polyps. In all cases, after an initial period of 3 to 6 months, I have been able to reduce the dose to twice a day. One out of 33 patients develop liver enzyme elevations, usually asymptomatically, and in all cases, the abnormality reverts to normal within 3 months of stopping the medication.

Oral Corticosteroids

The use of oral corticosteroids is a real art; this brief discussion will leave many points unsaid. I add oral corticosteroids if a patient's peak flows or FEV_1 has fallen sufficiently, usually 40% to 50% from their personal best. In a sick patient with severe asthma or bronchitis who is coughing and short of breath, oral corticosteroids can dramatically shorten the period of illness. Some patients always develop asthma or bronchitis after a cold. These patients benefit from early use of corticosteroids, and in such patients, a supply of prednisone and instructions on its use are provided for early intervention. On occasion, a short course of oral corticosteroids can be employed to determine the maximum reversibility of pulmonary function; ICSs work nearly as well and have fewer side effects.

Prednisone is the drug of choice. Whenever oral corticosteroids are started, the physician should have a therapeutic goal in kind. Generally, patients are kept on a dose of prednisone until peak flow returns to the patient's personal best. In some patients, resolution of coughing may be the endpoint. A dose of prednisone is chosen based upon the patient's sex, weight, and severity of disease. In general, women respond to 20 mg/day, while men need 30 mg/day. Very nervous patients get smaller doses. For very sick patients, an initial plan using 20 mg twice a day is even more effective. Split daily dosing has more side effects but is more potent. As soon as the patient improves, the split doses are consolidated and daily doses reduced as discussed below. Patients should be warned to expect certain short-term side effects from oral corticosteroids, *eg*, increased energy, increased appetite, salt retention, insomnia, euphoria and nervousness. We also inform the patients about potential long-term side effects, should corticosteroids be continued for a prolonged period.

Patients stay on the starting dose until the endpoint is achieved. In this way, the prednisone schedule is individualized. Some patients respond in days while others require weeks. However, once the goal is achieved, most patients can come off prednisone without rebounding. Reducing prednisone is as much an art as is choosing the starting dose. Corticosteroids can be tapered either to an alternate day program or to zero. Tapering to alternate day is appropriate for sicker patients for whom a "soft landing" is desired. A rule of thumb is that if patients have been on corticosteroids for less than a week, the corticosteroid can be stopped abruptly. I never follow this rule, and instead taper everyone off prednisone. For example, an adult male of 200 pounds might require 30 mg/d for 10 days to return to his personal best peak flow after an upper respiratory infection-induced asthma

exacerbation. I would have him take 20, 15, 10, 5, 0 mg/d to taper off. If the same patient was improving but still somewhat symptomatic, the plan might be 30, 20, 30, 15, 30, 10, 30, 5, 30, 0, 20, 0, 15, 0, 10, 0, 5, 0, 0 mg/d. This type of plan must be given to the patient *in writing*.

FOLLOW-UP

The follow-up visit involves a review of the patient's peak flow reading and in-office spirometry, as well as a brief set of questions: Are you wheezing? How many times a week? Are you coughing, experiencing shortness of breath, or chest tightness? How many times per week are you using a bronchodilator? What are your peak flows (review pattern)? Are you exercising? How are you sleeping? Are you having any problems with your medications?

Each visit requires a review of the treatment plan, which should be written. Components of the treatment plan are listed in Table 23-8.

ALLERGEN IMMUNOTHERAPY

If clear-cut allergies are identified and are thought to play a role in the patient's asthma, allergen avoidance techniques need to be reviewed with the patient and instituted. For long-term management, allergen immunotherapy (AIT) might be indicated. There are irrefutable data supporting AIT in allergic asthma, and it remains the only therapeutic choice that has long-term benefit

---

Table 23-8. COMPONENTS OF THE TREATMENT PLAN

Peak flows

LABA (1 or 2 puffs, with or without spacer, dry powder)

Inhaled corticosteroids (number of puffs, frequency; rinse mouth/gargle)

Emergency inhaler (number of puffs, frequency)

Leukotriene modifier (number of pills/day)

Theophylline (dose, frequency, precautions, yearly blood levels)

Oral corticosteroids (provide separate sheet with dose and schedule)

Ipratropium inhaler (number of puffs, frequency)

Nebulizer (when to use and with what)

   Bronchodilator

   Ipratropium

   Combination of beta agonist and ipratropium

   Budesonide

LABA—long-acting β-agonist.

after the treatment is stopped. In fact, I have been extremely impressed that AIT has a powerful, beneficial, long-lasting effect on the majority of allergic asthmatic patients, and AIT is routinely utilized in our office. In fact, it appears that the asthmatic patients may get more benefit from AIT than patients with rhinitis.

There are certain prerequisites when considering AIT. The patient should have unequivocal allergies, exposure to allergens should worsen asthma, skin tests should be significantly positive at the prick skin test level, and the patient should be willing to undergo the process, which is quite time consuming. AIT should be used at concentrations that have been shown to be effective (roughly 10 to 25 µg of allergen per injection), and injections should be given for an adequate period, usually 3 to 5 years. Patients who have undergone effective AIT are far less symptomatic, require less (or sometimes no) medications, and are no longer affected by allergen exposure.

Because allergy is such a frequent underlying cause of asthma, it is appropriate to evaluate every asthmatic patient with persistent wheezing for allergy. If positive, allergen avoidance techniques should be instituted. For patients with persistent disease, AIT might be considered if the criteria listed above are met. AIT is instituted at the same time as standard pharmacotherapy, and its effects become apparent approximately 6 to 12 months later. Once the influence of AIT is observed, step-down therapy can be accelerated.

The risks of AIT are the induction of a systemic allergic reaction, and asthmatic patients are at special risk. From 1 to 3 patients receiving AIT die each year from allergic reactions (out of about 3 million on AIT), and the majority are asthmatic patients experiencing a severe, fatal asthma attack. Thus, the pros and cons of AIT need to be weighed.

GENERAL ADVICE

Here is some general advice about caring for asthmatic patients, each point of which has proven useful to me over many years.

Always assess sinusitis. Sinusitis occurs in more than 50% of asthmatic patients, active sinusitis makes asthma much more difficult to manage, and treating sinusitis has a profound beneficial effect on asthma.

Always assess GERD. GERD also is found in more than 50% of asthmatic patients, and it has a profound effect on the disease. In my opinion, a 24-hour pH monitor is the gold standard for this diagnosis, although endoscopy is also useful. We provide a detailed instruction sheet for patients with GERD to help them initiate the necessary lifestyle changes. In addition to reducing acid secretion, Tums (GlaxoSmithKline, Pittsburgh, PA) can be used as both an antacid and a source of calcium.

Evaluate for allergy. Most younger patients have allergies and many older patients do as well. When present, allergy may play an important role in asthma. Many allergists are

---

Table 23-9. REFERRAL TO THE ASTHMA SPECIALIST

Indications

If the diagnosis of asthma is in doubt (*eg*, persistent coughing)

If the patient is losing time from school or work (8 or more days per year), if their quality of life is seriously affected, or if the patient's activities are limited (including exercise) because of asthma

If the patient requires frequent physician office visits for asthma, is hospitalized for asthma, requires an emergency room visit for asthma, or has moderate to severe asthma

If the patient has highly labile airway function or frequent exacerbations

If the patient requires more than 1 canister of inhaled β-agonist per month, high-dose inhaled corticosteroids (> 1000 µg/day of most corticosteroids or > 660 µg/day of fluticasone), or oral corticosteroids

To determine the extent that allergy plays a role in the disease and to initiate allergy management

To help define the role of occupational exposures

To help manage adverse effects of medications used, to help with complex pharmacotherapy, or to help educate the patient about medications

What the Referring Physician Should Receive from a Consultation on Asthma

Quantitative definition of the severity of asthma

Definition of the underlying cause(s) for the patient's asthma and clarification of the role concomitant diseases which impact on asthma care (such as sinusitis and gastroesophageal reflux) play in the patient

Definition of the role various triggers, including allergy, irritants, and environmental factors, play in the patient's disease

Specific recommendations for therapy, including pharmacotherapy, allergy avoidance, and immunotherapy (if appropriate)

Education of the patient regarding asthma pathophysiology, the mechanisms of action of appropriate medications, and a written treatment plan. Peak flow meters, spacers and emergency treatment plans are important components of an adequate treatment program

firm believers that AIT is useful in long-term management of asthma. At the very least, instituting allergen avoidance techniques warrants the time and expenses of an allergy evaluation. I recommend an allergy evaluation for anyone who experiences symptoms two days a week or more.

Start asthma therapy high, aiming to get the symptoms under complete control, and then step down to the lowest dose of medication that holds the patient stable. Keep the patient at their personal best peak flow reading. Always use β-agonists as "as needed" medications. Patients needing β-agonists on a regular basis are not adequately controlled and might benefit from higher doses of long-term controller medication.

Give good general advice. Patients need calcium (about 1200 mg/d with vitamin D for menstruating women, 1800 mg/d for post-menopausal women, and between 600 to 1000 mg/d for men). Although there is no definite evidence that ICS affects calcium metabolism, I take no chances and always advise patients to exercise and take calcium. For women in particular, I advise upper torso bodybuilding with weight lifting. I encourage all patients to start an aerobic exercise program commensurate with their health, age, and asthma state, so I can judge how their asthma is controlled under the stress of exercise. I may recommend that patients walk, progressing to 30 to 45 minutes at least three times a week. For cardiovascular conditioning, aerobics are better than walking. However, it is better for the patient to walk than not to exercise at all. If feasible, swimming is excellent exercise, but it also builds in a convenient excuse to not exercise because of the need to travel to the pool. Thus, whenever possible, have the patient exercise at or near home or work.

CONCLUSIONS

Asthma is a chronic condition, which can range from an inconvenience to a fatal disease. Excellent management tools are available, but many patients are inadequately treated. Approximately 15 patients die every day in the United States from asthma, and in most cases these deaths could be avoided. The physician who cares for patients with asthma has to be able to visualize the disease, the underlying causes, and the concomitant conditions that affect the disease's course and prognosis and design a comprehensive treatment program with which the patient can comply. Getting advice from a specialist can be very helpful in these respects for many primary care physicians. How to decide when to refer for a consultation and what to expect in return from a consultation is outlined in Table 23-9.

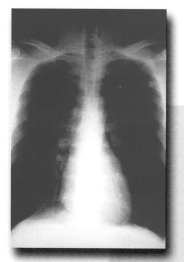

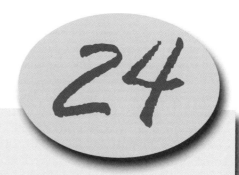

The Internet in Asthma Therapy

Thomas Bell

The revolution in information technology affects medicine in many ways. As doctors, the enhanced speed and ease of medical information exchange via the Internet gives us the ability to be more responsive to rapidly changing therapeutic strategies, research findings, in-home patient monitoring, and physician-patient communication. Networking, made more accessible by the Internet, offers the promise of increased cooperative research, patient and disease-based information databases, patient support groups, and discounted cost of medical supplies. Eventually, therapeutic and diagnostic decision-support engines may be available through the Internet or similar modalities (with wider bandwidth) that may evolve to better serve specialized communities, such as health care networks.

Patients use the Internet for improved communication with the health care community, support from "chat" groups, discounted purchases of medical supplies and prescriptions, advice from "experts," and education on the management of their disease. Asthma-related Internet sites report a steadily increasing volume of traffic, especially from patient users.

WHAT IS THE INTERNET?

The Internet is a vast worldwide network of digitized information that can be rapidly exchanged and shared by telephone, cable, and/or satellite transmission, using computer workstations. Originally conceived to facilitate research and defense communication and networking, it has quickly evolved to serve many other roles, from e-commerce to e-medicine. The hallmark of the Internet has been freedom of information built upon an open architecture to serve the public domain with few constraints. As its role has expanded into areas of privileged information, security measures such as encryption, firewalls, password control, and intranets have appeared on the scene, increasing the complexity of its use but encouraging its increased application in medicine, where security was previously an obstacle.

Although the Internet offers lofty promise, there is a dark side. Users are often unable to assess the veracity and currency of information provided by a system that has not yet fully evolved ethical and legal standards to protect the public from misleading claims and unsubstantiated information. Physicians must be especially wary of outdated "Position Statements" and "Treatment Guidelines" posted to the Internet that may be infrequently reviewed and updated by credible editorial groups. Industry-sponsored sites may present advice to patients and physicians that place their products in more favorable positions, compared with their competitors. Users have recognized the need for site ratings, but have been unable to agree on the agencies that should assume the policing responsibility.

One standard is now evolving called "HONcode" (http://www.hon.ch/Conduct.html), which is sponsored by the Health On the Net Foundation (http://www.hon.ch/home.html), a not-for-profit Swiss organization dedicated to guiding physicians and others to useful and reliable online medical and health information. Their code requires that the information be provided by medically trained and qualified professionals; the information not be aimed at replacing the physician-patient relationship; information provided by users be confidential; the date the information was last revised be provided; data be referenced; claims be supported by balanced evidence; sponsorship and funding be clearly identified; and advertising be clearly identified as such.

HAS THE INTERNET ACTUALLY PROVEN EFFECTIVE IN THE EXECUTION OF ASTHMA THERAPY?

In many ways, the Internet's impact is very difficult to assess with objectivity. In the education arena, for example, how are we to know if a doctor or patient learned of a new asthma therapy or treatment algorithm from the Internet and then successfully applied this knowledge? Polls invariably have considerable bias, but Sharma [1] cites a 2000 Web poll of Internet use among health professionals (http://www.hon.ch/Survey/ResPoll/Total.html) showing that 80% of doctors considered it helpful for patient care, particularly in the area of education. Patients (69%) actually discussed information they derived from the Internet at their health care visit. He further states that there are more than one million health-related Web sites on the Internet, with 1000 new sites being added every month. He added that health is the second most searched topic on the Internet.

The Internet has great potential as a clinical decision support tool, but physicians have been reluctant to embrace similar paper-based guidelines in the past. Would guidelines via the Internet be any more effective? Thomas *et al.* [2] put this question to the test for asthma therapy using an Internet-based decision support system developed from national guidelines. Nurses using the system and physician experts not using the system tested their algorithms. The two groups did not differ significantly in score (89% vs 88%; P = NS). Next, internal medicine residents using the Internet system or a printed version of the National Asthma Education Program guidelines were compared. Those using the computer-assisted guidelines scored significantly higher than those using written guidelines (92% vs 84%; $P < 0.002$). While this study shows Internet guidelines to be more effective than written guidelines, physicians will still have to migrate to this new format before we see an impact on the effectiveness of asthma therapy.

Before using the Internet, you or your patient may need to overcome cyberphobia. Internet users need elementary computer skills. You will need the right equipment: a computer with a modem connected to a phone line or other appropriate data transmission source. The computer will need a browser, such as Netscape or Internet Explorer. Just as with any other new tool, you should spend the time to learn to use it effectively. Both patients and physicians are increasingly more likely to have access to a computer or personal digital assistant with modem capability.

If the Internet connection is next to you as you work, you will be much more likely to venture forth to seek answers to pressing questions at the time information is most needed. In my clinical practice, I enjoyed running computer searches via the Internet with the patient present in response to his or query regarding new therapies or drug interactions, emphasizing that the pace of change in medicine has accelerated, necessitating our use of more advanced technology for up-to-date information retrieval.

INTERNET FOR PATIENT–PHYSICIAN COMMUNICATION: E-MAIL

E-mail is often our first major use of the Internet. It is a rapid, inexpensive means of communication for non-emergency circumstances that is increasing in popularity with physicians and patients. Several of my more secluded patients routinely posted their asthma scores, peak flow records, and medication diaries to me on a weekly or monthly basis via e-mail. I could expeditiously recommend and document minor changes in therapy using e-mail, without costly travel and excessive patient visits. If you choose to use this tool, be certain to keep copies of all communications and request that your patients reply to verify receipt of your e-mail! This can be used as evidence in litigation. Kane and Sands (http://www.amia.org/pubs/fpubl.html) [3] suggest you keep several guidelines in mind (Table 24-1).

INTERNET-BASED TELEMONITORING

Telemonitoring does not necessarily require an Internet connection, but it is facilitated by such an economical network approach. It requires patient acceptance to be effective, but under the right circumstances, this may not be too great an obstacle. In a Canadian study [4], low-income inner-city asthma patients without prior computer experience were enlisted for daily transmission of portable spirometric and symptom diary data using palmtop computers.

Their physicians could read the data via the Internet from nearly any location using a similar device or computer with a Web browser. A constant vigil was also maintained by a computer server programmed to issue alerts if certain data conditions occurred. Only two of the 19 subjects invited declined participation, and after completion of the 3-week study period, 94% "were strongly interested in using home monitoring in the future." Thus it appears Internet-based telemonitoring has a promising future as costs for such devices drop and computer education spreads.

INTERNET RESOURCES FOR THE PHYSICIAN TREATING ASTHMA

The physician who treats asthma has many Internet resources to turn to, including search engines and portals, treatment guidelines and position statements, bibliographic retrieval, e-journals and texts, research trial locators, pharmaceutical and professional association sites, chat groups, news services for asthma, and virtual symposia.

Although I cite as examples only favored Web sites (at the time of this writing), I cannot assume responsibility for the accuracy of their information. Most of my examples will be presented in text or in tables as references to universal resource locators (URLs, *ie*, addresses of Internet sites), the reference format used by the Internet. Just as the information presented on the Internet can change quickly, the addresses can change as well; you may find some of these URLs outdated by the time you try them.

The Internet has two ways to help you around this problem: 1) automatic redirection and 2) search engines. When an address is changed, the prior provider may use a redirection tag to send your browser to the new URL automatically. Search engines are readily available services that will lead you to the more popular sites using key words. Some engines may have commercial or sampling bias, so you must learn which services best suit your needs by trial and error. For example, Medical Matrix might be better than Yahoo as a search engine for *alpha-1-antitrypsin deficiency*, while the reverse may be the case if you are searching for *allergy product retail outlets*. Searches may also harvest too vast a number of URLs to be useful, especially if not restricted by delimiters such as "use the exact phrase." You may find sites that offer

Table 24-1. PROFESSIONAL GUIDELINES FOR E-MAIL

Medicolegal and Administrative Guidelines

Consider obtaining patient's informed consent for use of e-mail. Written forms should
    Itemize terms in Communication Guidelines (below)
    Provide instructions for when and how to escalate to phone calls and office visits
    Describe security mechanisms in place
    Indemnify the health care institution for information loss due to technical failures
    Waive encryption requirement, if any, at patient's insistence
Use password-protected screen savers for all desktop workstations in the office, hospital, and home
Never forward patient-identifiable information to a third party without the patient's express permission
Never use patient's e-mail address in a marketing scheme
Do not share professional e-mail accounts with family members
Use encryption for all messages when encryption technology becomes widely available, user friendly, and practical
Do not use unencrypted wireless communications with patient-identifiable information
Double check all "to:" fields prior to sending messages

Communication Guidelines

Establish turnaround time for messages. Do not use e-mail for urgent matters.
Inform patients about privacy issues. Patients should know who besides addressee processes messages during addressee's usual business hours, and during addressee's vacation or illness. Include this information in the medical record.
Establish types of transactions (*eg*, prescription refill, appointment scheduling) and sensitivity of subject matter (*eg*, HIV, mental health) permitted over e-mail
Instruct patients to put category of transaction in subject line of message for filtering (*eg*, "prescription," "appointment," "medical advice," "billing question")
Request that patients put their name and patient identification number in the body of the message
Configure automatic reply to acknowledge receipt of messages
Print all messages, with replies and confirmation of receipt, and place in patient's paper chart
Send a new message to inform patient of completion of request
Request that patients use autoreply feature to acknowledge reading provider's message

search capabilities as well as other services related to your topic of interest; these are often called "portals." Portals are sites that serve as "traffic cops," pointing you to other sites that share similar information and services. The dividing line between portals and search engines is becoming indistinct as the sites compete to capture consumers on their first pass. Examples of search engines and portals are given in Table 24-2.

The physician most likely to seek help in selecting asthma therapy is often in a broad-based practice at a location distant from a well-stocked medical library and less likely to be an expert in this field. This physician may find Internet sites containing practice guidelines, position statements, or texts covering asthma to be the best early stepping-off points for his or her "asthma quest." The National Guideline Clearinghouse (http://www.guidelines.gov) currently lists 57 guideline documents for asthma and related topics, many of which have been updated as recently as 2001.

The next most likely action for a physician seeking help in treating asthma, in my experience, is bibliographic retrieval using key words or phrases that characterize his or her questions. You may want help in evaluating inhaled corticosteroid therapy in asthma, for example. It would be useful to begin at a site specifically designed for physician use; I currently rely on Medical Matrix (http://www.medmatrix.org), which helps physicians search for titles and/or authors in several different ways. When I tried this search on Medical Matrix, 28 link results appeared for an "all word" search using *inhaled corticosteroid asthma*. Using the same words, an "any word" search yielded 19,703

links; employ "any word" searches with great care, if ever. This service has the advantage of direct full-text retrieval of some of the selected articles without requiring you to subscribe to the linked site. If you wish, you might directly access the National Library of Medicine (NLM) for your searches, or you may use links provided by many of the other sites listed in this article. In most cases, free full-text retrieval is not available, but often it may be obtained for a fee if the abstract does not meet your needs.

If you prefer to use a textbook, you may be disappointed. Even online textbooks are often outdated. One exception is Scientific American Medicine (Table 24-3), which is updated monthly and can be linked to continuing medical education (CME) accreditation via WebMD (http://my.webmd.com/?rdserver=medscapehealth.com). eMedicine is another excellent example of what can be achieved with an electronic text. Its asthma section is authored by experts and provides URL links within the text to help the reader expand the depth of his or her inquiries. Since many of these electronic texts require a subscription fee, you may wish to access them from industry-sponsored, complimentary services for physicians, such as MyHealth.com/mypractice, provided by Schering MyHealth Solutions, Inc. MyHealth provides specific textbook access via Stanford University's SKOLAR, without charge in most cases. Many of these sites also provide CME accreditation.

If you are confronted with a more challenging asthma case and wish to try a therapy only available by a research trial, you could visit an excellent government-sponsored site, ClinicalTrials.gov. Links here will guide you to many of the

Table 24-2. EXAMPLES OF SEARCH ENGINES AND PORTALS

Google www.google.com	A good general search engine with a higher number of returns for specific medical topics than some others
Yahoo! http://www.yahoo.com/	A very popular general public search engine and provider of multiple consumer services, such as e-mail
AltaVista http://www.altavista.com/	Another popular general public search engine
DrugInfo http://www.drugsrnikolov.com/	A portal site oriented toward drug information that also offers search capability
PDR.net http://www.pdr.net/HomePage_template.jsp	Registration required; provides drug information, drug interactions, drug alerts, and other general portal services
The Medical Matrix http://www.medmatrix.org/	A medical portal site with an excellent search engine, bibliographic retrieval, and other services
The MedEngine! http://www.themedengine.com/	Everything you need on one page, including portal service, Toxicology, Audio Medicine, Physicians Online
MedMark http://www.medmark.org/	A specialty-oriented portal with great bibliographic retrieval links; Korean link provided
Medivibe.com http://www.medivibe.com/	MEDLINE and FDA search links and news; multipurpose site

ongoing studies, particularly those that are affiliated with the National Institutes of Health (NIH). Another site, Centerwatch Clinical Trials Listing Service (http://www.centerwatch.com), lists ongoing trials and research centers that subscribe to their proprietary service. There were 351 asthma trials listed on Centerwatch and 22 on ClinicalTrials.gov at the time of this writing. You will find links to these sites on many of the portals listed in Table 24-2.

Many pharmaceutical companies and professional associations provide Internet locations where you can find most of the oft-used services centralized and without charge (Table 24-4). Some are restricted to physicians, and others are open to the public.

What about newsgroups, chat rooms, or "Ask the Expert" forums? These can often be found on professional society or pharmaceutical-sponsored sites, but are rarely useful sources for solutions to immediate problems, since replies may not be prompt. At this point, you may wish to consider using the phone to call your local expert.

Now that you have gained control of your patient's asthma, what's next? An Internet news service customized to your interests is a good way to monitor new developments in asthma therapy (Table 24-5). MDLynx, for example, provides daily abstracts of new medical citations, delivered free to your computer station. Expanded text versions are just a click away! News services are available on many of the professional association sites as well. These locations may also be of interest to your more inquisitive patients.

As time passes, you may wish to attend a symposium on asthma, but may be unable to spare the time to travel from your practice. Check with the professional association sites for virtual symposia that are offered periodically via the Internet. You may wish to consider upgrading to a faster data transmission system to support broadband activities, since the symposia may be multimedia presentations, often including video segments that require huge downloads. Another option is to download a current review on your selected asthma therapy topic. The Cochrane Group (http://www.cochrane.org/cochrane/revabstr/g150index.htm) provides evidence-based reviews and protocols on many key issues in medicine. If you still do not feel you are keeping current, you may subscribe to one of the "Up to Date" services, such as UpToDate in Pulmonary Disease and Critical Care (http://www.uptodate.com/html/spec/pulm/toc.htm), an outstanding clinical information service.

INTERNET RESOURCES FOR THE PATIENT WITH ASTHMA

There are many Internet resources for the patient with asthma, including physician Web sites, general resources,

---

Table 24-3. EXAMPLES OF ONLINE TEXTBOOKS AND JOURNALS

Asthma Disease Management Resource Manual http://allergy.mcg.edu/physicians/manual/manual.html	Links to the American College of Allergy, Asthma & Immunology
Scientific American Medicine http://www.samed.com/cgi-bin/publiccgi.pl?loginOP	Requires annual subscription
Harrison's Online http://www.harrisonsonline.com/	Requires annual subscription
The Journal of Allergy and Clinical Immunology http://www.mosby.com/Mosby/Periodicals/Medical/JACI/ai.html	Abstracts available without subscription. Full text currently free to American Academy of Allergy Asthma & Immunology members
Annals of Allergy, Asthma & Immunology http://www.annallergy.org/standingmatter/howto.html	Requires registration and fee for full services
The American Journal of Respiratory and Critical Care Medicine http://ajrccm.atsjournals.org/	Abstracts available and some full-text articles available without charge. American Thoracic Society members have full privileges
The American Family Physician http://www.aafp.com/afp/	Excellent source of complete review articles
The Internet Journal of Asthma, Allergy, and Immunology http://www.ispub.com/journals/ijaai.htm	A newcomer with potential
eMedicine http://www.emedicine.com/specialties.htm	Advertiser-supported, free access. This popular format for specialty journals has grown rapidly. The site takes 80,000 hits per day
PraxisMD http://praxis.md/praxisgate.asp	Free, subscription-based service. Practical answers for patients and physicians
FindArticles.com http://www.findarticles.com/cf_0/PI/aboutus/index.jhtml	Select the desired journal and search for articles without charge

foundations and user groups, virtual clinics and hospitals, and individual patient's sites.

This area may represent the greatest potential for the treatment of asthma. Many new asthma sufferers are likely to search the Internet for information before or during their physician encounters. If you have a major interest in caring for asthma patients, you should consider establishing an asthma Web site to better serve your community. Medem (http://www.medem.com), a site sponsored by US medical societies, is currently helping physicians develop physician practice communications networks/Web sites.

The proliferation of medical Web sites is phenomenal, but how are consumers responding to this new tool for therapy? To answer this question, let us examine the pub-

lished experience of an independent site, the Asthma Information Center [5], which provided information about asthma to physicians, patients, and other health care professionals. This site (not active at this time) had its own user interactive pages and many links to other information sources. A 5-year analysis of the log files of the Web server showed a progressive increase in the number of page views, which reached 100,000 by the end of the study, when 9000 visitors per month were logged in. Each visitor averaged nearly 2 minutes on the site and appeared to be seeking "fast" information. Certainly, this experience suggests the Internet has already become a powerful tool in asthma therapy.

The majority of URLs on asthma therapy are directed at consumer audiences, but may be very helpful to the

---

Table 24-4. EXAMPLES OF PHARMACEUTICAL AND PROFESSIONAL ASSOCIATION SITES

American Academy of Allergy, Asthma, and Immunology (AAAAI) http://www.aaaai.org/professionals.stm	The AAAAI sites received 1,675,690 visits in 2001. This is one of several portals they offer to physicians
American College of Allergy, Asthma, and Immunology http://allergy.mcg.edu/	Portal for physicians and patients. It includes quizzes, asthma screening, and age-specific sections
Allergy & Asthma Disease Management Center http://www.aaaai.org/aadmc/	An AAAAI site for physicians. Excellent site with CME, quizzes, current literature, and "Ask the Expert" sections
Allergy Learning Lab http://www.asthmalearninglab.com/	Sponsored by the American Academy of Family Physicians and Schering-Plough. Aimed at asthma patients
MerckMedicus http://www.merckmedicus.com/	Primarily for physicians. Provides a broad spectrum of services, including textbooks, engines for diagnosis and antibiotic selection, a special PDA resource, drug information, news, and journal citations. Requires registration
Clearbreathing http://www.clearbreathing.com/	Sponsored by Genentech, Novartis, and National Jewish Hospital. Patient-oriented and age-specific design
Breathingline http://www.breathingline.co.uk/	Sponsored by AstraZeneca, physician and patient services. Try the LinkMedica button, a patient management tool for asthma. Physicians must register

CME—continuing medical education; PDA—personal digital assistant.

Table 24-5. EXAMPLES OF SITES FOR NEWS ON ASTHMA

MDLynx.com http://allergyimmunolinx.com/	Registration required. An excellent, daily service for physicians
Medscape http://www.medscape.com/allergy-immunologyhome	Advertiser supported, free access, good bibliographic retrieval. Registration required
National Institute of Allergy and Infectious Diseases (NIAID) News: Asthma http://www.niaid.nih.gov/cgi-shl/newsroom/default.cfm	NIAID news release archives. Other resources available at this government site. Largely research oriented
American College of Chest Physicians Online Resource Library http://www.chestnet.org/	Service area of a portal site that has an outstanding journal and text surveillance service. Registration required. Try the Online Resource Library link

physician as well (Table 24-6). An outstanding launching point for your patients is provided by the NLM/NIH's Breath of Life, a wonderful multimedia site that contains video and audio resources in addition to rich text covering a broad expanse of asthma background information. Many of the virtual hospital/clinics offer chat groups for patients with specific conditions, such as asthma, that may be useful for patient support.

Once your patient has acquired general information, he or she may wish to interact with others via a user group or a chat room. These can be found at many locations and are sometimes spontaneous or transient. The information may not be monitored by a health professional.

Some patients with asthma may wish to enter a clinic or hospital-like environment provided on the Web. Here we tread on dangerous ground since a patient may perceive that this safely replaces physician consultation. If you provide these URLs, caution your patients to seek your advice if their asthma is changing. I have found the sites listed in Table 24-7 to be of high quality for patient use.

There are numerous sites sponsored by individual patients or patient groups. These present the patient's perspective on asthma and personalize the Web experience for many of your patients. You may not agree with some of the statements on these URLs, but your patients undoubtedly will visit them. One site you can sample is Asthma Online (http://asthmaonline.proboards.com), which is supported by donations.

FUTURE POSSIBILITIES

Future possibilities of Internet use in asthma therapy are limitless and might include registries, collaborative research, prescription transmittal, drug recall services, and patient history repositories. However, this list touches on only a few trends that are already undergoing trials on the Web. Internet registries for less common diseases have been tried, but do not appear to be weathering the current medicolegal seas, where patient confidentiality is a major issue. If adequate security is provided, disease registries could provide information on therapeutic advances with lightning speed to small subgroups of asthma patients. For example, those with aspirin-sensitive asthma (ASA) could be alerted when a safe aspirin sub-

---

Table 24-6. GENERAL PATIENT RESOURCES

Breath of Life http://www.nlm.nih.gov/hmd/breath/breathhome.html	An outstanding, graphic, and interactive site
Asthma Education Network http://www.healthtalk.com/aen/index.html	Contributions from leading physicians in the field, pollen counts, asthma education
PraxisMD http://praxis.md/praxisgate.asp	Free, subscription-based guides. PDA version available. Practical answers for patients and physicians
MEDLINEPlus http://www.nlm.nih.gov/medlineplus/asthma.html	Outstanding portal for asthma news and information. Quick-to-use and well-organized service of the National Library of Medicine
The American Academy of Allergy, Asthma, and Immunology (AAAAI) http://www.aaaai.org/patients.stm	Daily updated news. Patient portal provided by the AAAAI
WebMD http://my.webmd.com/?rdserver=medscapehealth.com	Advertiser-supported patient portal for health information and services. Excellent asthma section that includes a discussion group hosted by Dr. Paul Enright. Select the Newly Diagnosed/Asthma section for starters

---

Table 24-7. VIRTUAL CLINICS AND HOSPITALS

Mayo Clinic: Asthma
http://www.mayoclinic.com/findinformation/diseasesandconditions/invoke.cfm?id=DS00021&

Managing Asthma: Children's Hospital of Iowa with contributions from Dr. Miles Weinberger
http://www.vh.org/Patients/IHB/Peds/Allergy/Asthma/AsthmaHome.html

InteliHealth: A service of Harvard Medical School
http://www.intelihealth.com/IH/ihtIH/WSIHW000/408/408.html

stitute is released. These registries could provide a rich source of information for research as well. For example, the ASA group could be queried for their experience with other anti-inflammatory drugs to help develop better therapeutic guidelines.

Using data reporting forms from a central Internet location, researchers across the globe can pool data instantaneously on research projects requiring large numbers of subjects and broad-based demographics, such as those that compare treatment protocols for severe, corticosteroid-resistant asthma. Restricted intranet groups are currently in use for data transmission in phase III drug trials within the United States. These trials use computer-assisted modem transmission of research data to the internal computer network of the sponsor in a manner that is very similar to Internet data transmission but is more secure.

Networking can provide an economical approach to prescription purchase by centralizing a large volume of orders at a warehouse site, thereby eliminating the middleman. The expense of asthma therapy can be reduced using this technology. Visit Discount Pharmacies Online.com (http://www.discount-pharmacies-online.com) to learn more about this phenomenon. It would appear that patients might easily order drugs from other countries using similar services, although in some cases, this could be hazardous and illegal. The Internet also could provide a means for drug recalls, via e-mail through drug registries, for example. Presently, while the speed might be an advantage, you can never be sure e-mail gets to where it was sent. Perhaps we will have reliable registered e-mail servers soon.

Imagine the time you would save if new patients presented with their prior medical histories available to you by download from the Internet! However, before we can implement large Web repositories for patient histories, we need a universal format, unless the repository is for a restricted health care system. This is a monumental task, and groups have been working during the past several years to develop such a format; more information is available at http://www.uprforum.com/Chapter6.htm. An example of such a system in action can be found at Spacelabs Medical's site (http://www.spacelabs.com/pc/information_systems/). It is doubtful that a universal format for a nationwide Internet-based patient history repository will be put into practice without universal health care/insurance. This is unfortunate because we already have the technology to store this information on a small card, which could be carried by our patients and used, with their permission, when they present to us in emergencies.

The disadvantages posed by a very new, not yet well policed system make the Internet a double-edged sword, but one with great promise. It brings a vast array of information to our doorstep (laptop?) and may eventually provide decision-assisting programs by remote access of more powerful computers. E-mail and physician Web sites can assist our therapy by improving patient-physician communication. Patient home monitoring can also be accomplished inexpensively using this and other new technologies. The greatest impact may result from patient education via the Internet, where we are observing ever-increasing numbers of visitors to asthma education-oriented URLs.

REFERENCES AND RECOMMENDED READING

1. Sharma A: Internet and medicine. http://164.100.9.16/imcwebel01.html. Accessed June 20, 2002.

2. Thomas KW, Dayton CS, Peterson MW: Evaluation of internet-based clinical decision support systems. *J Med Internet Res* 1999, 1(20):E6.

3. Kane B, Sands DZ: Guidelines for the use of electronic mail with patients. *J Am Med Inform Assoc* 1998, 5:104–111.

4. Finkelstein J, Hripcsak G, Cabrera MR: Patients' acceptance of Internet-based home asthma telemonitoring. *Proc AMIA Symp* 1998, 336–340.

5. Wist M: When air is rare: behind the scenes of an asthma web site. *J Asthma* 2001, 38(5):399–404.

Index